From Madness to Mental Health

From
Madness
to
Mental Health

Psychiatric Disorder
and Its Treatment
in Western Civilization

Edited by Greg Eghigian

Rutgers University Press
New Brunswick, New Jersey, and London

Library of Congress Cataloging-in-Publication Data

From madness to mental health : psychiatric disorder and its treatment in Western
  civilization / edited by Greg Eghigian.
        p. ;   cm.
  Includes bibliographical references and index.
  ISBN 978-0-8135-4665-0 (hardcover : alk. paper) — ISBN 978-0-8135-4666-7
    (pbk. : alk. paper)
  1. Psychiatry—History.   I. Eghigian, Greg, 1961–
  [DNLM: 1. Psychiatry—history—Collected Works.   2. Medicine in Literature—
    Collected Works.   3. Mental Disorders—history—Collected Works.
    4. Mental Health Services—history—Collected Works.   5. Mentally Ill
    Persons—history—Collected Works.   6. Western World—history—Collected
    Works.   WM 11.1 F931 2010]
  RC438.F76 2010
  616.89—dc22

                                                              2009008508

A British Cataloging-in-Publication record for this book is available
from the British Library.

This collection copyright © 2010 by Greg Eghigian

For copyrights to individual pieces please see last page of each essay.

Visit our Web site: http://rutgerspress.rutgers.edu

Manufactured in the United States of America

For the countless many

Contents

Part III The Militant Age

War and Neurosis

The New Focus on the Body

Psychiatric Eugenics in Nazi Germany

Illustrations

Acknowledgments

This project was inspired, first and foremost, by students, friends, and colleagues. For some ten years now, I have taught a course on the history of madness and psychiatry in the Western world. Like many of my colleagues who teach their own version of this course, I found myself wishing there were an anthology of primary sources that could provide a glimpse into the long and complex history of mental disorders and their treatment. Over the past decade, historians, social scientists, and former patients have done a remarkable job of rewriting the secondary history of madness and psychiatry. And yet introducing students and other interested readers to the rich fund of primary sources in this history has often been an unwieldy task. After years in which I distributed photocopies and placed books on reserve at the library, the time seemed right to compile a collection of texts from well-known, little-known, and long-since-forgotten sources. I have no doubt that the selections made—and not made—will invariably disappoint. It is my hope, however, that in some small way this collection will kindle insight, provoke discussion, and encourage further reading. The intention is to provide a starting, not an end, point for thought and study.

I am indebted to numerous individuals and institutions for their help and support. Both the College of the Liberal Arts and the Rock Ethics Institute at Penn State University provided needed financial support to see this project through. I am also grateful for the generous assistance given to me by the staff at the National Library of Medicine as well as the Staatsbibliothek in Berlin. I received invaluable suggestions and criticism from numerous colleagues and friends, in particular Jesse Ballenger, Viola Balz, John Burnham, Michael Carhart, Kumkum Chatterjee, Eric Engstrom, Gerald Grob, Baruch Halpern, Volker Hess, Andreas Killen, Ulrike Klöppel, Paul Lerner, Benoit Majerus, Bill Petersen, Hans Pols, Sajay Samuel, Ulf Schmidt, Michael Sokal, and Chloe Silverman. Doreen Valentine has been an ideal editor, shepherding me through the process from idea to artifact. I would be remiss if I did not also single out Gail Hornstein for agreeing to include her unique bibliography of first-person narratives of madness in this volume. Finally, as in most everything in my life, Natascha Hoffmeyer has been a vital source of advice and support.

From Madness to Mental Health

Introduction

More than perhaps any other set of human afflictions, the phenomena that have gone under the names of "madness," "insanity," "lunacy," and "mental illness" have historically provoked a wide variety of often contradictory reactions. Those who have been in the throes of "madness" have described experiences ranging from enjoying an ecstatic sense of holiness to being beset by undeniable impulses to having feelings of unending despair. Observers have sought explanations for the behavior of "touched" and "crazy" individuals by invoking such things as sin, destiny, heredity, moral degeneracy, upbringing, trauma, fatigue, and body chemistry. Those afflicted have been admired, pitied, mocked, hidden from public view, canonized, imprisoned, restrained, operated on, sterilized, hospitalized, killed, counseled, analyzed, and medicated. Why?

This volume is an introductory anthology about the history of madness and its treatment in Western civilization. In part, it is meant to serve as a companion to Rutgers University Press's *Medicine and Western Civilization* (edited by David J. Rothman, Steven Marcus, and Stephanie A. Kiceluk), with the main focus here being scientific and clinical understandings. But attention is also paid to attitudes expressed in theology, art, philosophy, the social sciences, politics, and law, as well as to the perspectives of those directly affected by madness or mental illness.

Rather than provide a broad historical narrative, in this book I present a collection of important and representative historical texts and images that shed light on the development of Western approaches to mental health. Primary sources are an ideal way to both teach and learn about human experiences such as madness that seem to defy simple description and explanation. Rather than reflecting a position on whether insanity is spiritual, social, or biological in origin or whether a given individual was mentally ill, the documents presented here are meant to inspire interpretation, discussion, and debate about how madness has historically been imagined, talked about, and handled. In this sense, madness and mental illness are treated here as what the sociologist Emile Durkheim called "social facts"—that is, as concepts, roles, and experiences that societies have recognized as real and important, even if we today might not.

It is probably safe to say that every society has recognized the existence of something we now generally refer to as "mental illness." That said, the form, substance, and public perception and treatment of that experience have differed greatly over time. To be sure, the history of madness and its treatment in Western society is marked by noteworthy continuities. For instance, the ideas of Hippocrates and Galen influenced medical thinking well into early modern times. But the history of madness also has been punctuated by ruptures and rapid change. One need only look at the late nineteenth century or the late twentieth, when brain science radically altered how people accounted for and treated insanity.

The story of the West's encounter with madness has proved difficult for historians to plot out as one of ever-advancing progress. For centuries, contemporary observers have regularly complained about how ineffective cures have been. And since the late eighteenth century, many have held the view that the prevalence of mental illness actually has increased, rather than decreased, with the passage of time. In addition, it has not escaped the notice of clinicians, scholars, and the lay public that some of what we today might consider among the most ethically questionable forms of treatment—malaria fever therapy, insulin coma therapy, lobotomy, sterilization, euthanasia—were invented and applied only in recent times.

The long history of madness in Western civilization, therefore, cannot be easily characterized as a tale of the gradual triumph of enlightened knowledge. By the same merit, however, it is essential to recognize the good faith and often successful efforts that have been made at comprehending and alleviating the human misery associated with mental illness. Clinicians, caretakers, policymakers, philosophers, theologians, novelists, journalists, and the afflicted themselves—a wide array of professionals and laypeople have wrestled with making sense of madness as a human predicament. In this, they frequently have shown notable insight and compassion.

Of course today, there are prominent individuals and organizations that claim that psychiatry and clinical psychology are pseudosciences, their histories consisting of little more than abuse and torture. Others, on the other hand, proclaim the supremacy of biological psychiatry and disparage any outlook that refuses to accept that madness is anything other than a brain disorder. Such contentiousness appears to be an emblematic feature of our society today. From a historical vantage point, however, it is striking to note that arguments like these actually date back centuries. And beyond the matter of who is right and who is wrong, impassioned debates such as these raise an interesting question: Why does madness seem to compel us to revisit the same issues over and over again?

For its part, *From Madness to Mental Health* has the aim of neither glorifying nor denigrating the contribution of psychiatry, clinical psychology, and psychotherapy (there is ample evidence here to encourage both prospects). Rather, in the volume I approach madness as a historical phenomenon that has sparked a variety of interpretations from sufferers and observers alike. At its heart, madness is an existential matter, meaning that it prompts us to pose fundamental questions about who we are, what makes us human, what constitutes a normal life, and the degree to which we are the authors of that life. Studying the history of madness, then, does not only mean studying deviant ways of perceiving, thinking, and acting. Rather, it is also an exercise in self-exploration, a way of holding up a mirror to ourselves and seeing how we human beings have valued our bodies, minds, and souls.

By and large, the documents in this volume are organized chronologically. The title, *From Madness to Mental Health*, not only refers to the general effort at bringing those deemed insane to a state of relative sanity; it also points to a historical shift from a longtime professional and societal focus on treating severe cases to a more recent focus on promoting the mental well-being of a wide range of individuals. To put it simply, you do not need to be suffering from a mental illness today to call on the know-how of mental health experts.

Over time, certain currents and trends have underscored particular moments in the history of madness. For this reason, the chronology is divided into four major epochs, each characterized by what could be seen as a prevailing attitude or feature of the time. The first and lengthiest period, stretching from the ancient to the early modern, was one in which madness was widely considered to be both material and immaterial, spiritual and somatic in nature. The second period, running from the late eighteenth to the turn of the twentieth century, was a time in which optimistic reformers came to believe in the real possibility of understanding the causes of maladies, discovering cures, and unlocking the full potential of psychiatry. Under the influence of the rise of extreme political ideologies and the two world wars, a third period saw a heightened sense of militancy that helped encourage daring attempts to radically reconceive mental illness and its treatment. Finally, beginning around the middle of the past century, there emerged a period marked by a pronounced expansion and growth in clinical psychology, psychotherapy, and psychopharmacology.

No selection of readings covering such a lengthy period of time could possibly be comprehensive. The emphasis here is on the eighteenth century and after, the period during which "mad-doctors" became professionalized as "psychiatrists" and "clinical psychologists," new asylums and psychiatric clinics were built, and science took on an increasingly important role in shaping how madness was understood and treated. Admittedly, there are glaring absences. Some (such as Ugo Cerletti) result from the fact that copyright permission fees were simply too costly; in other cases (such as William Shakespeare or more recent first-person narratives), versions are readily available elsewhere. In the end, choices have been made that will likely disappoint someone. But the point here is not to attempt to be exhaustive—something that would be impossible anyway—but rather to see a collection such as this as the beginning of an encounter with the history of madness, mental illness, and their treatment.

In the choice of texts and images, emphasis has been placed on exploring three broad dimensions in the history of madness and its treatment:

- *the intellectual history of madness and mental illness*: these are texts that present influential medical, religious, philosophical, scientific, legal, and lay notions about the nature and treatment of mental disorders.
- *the social and institutional history of madness and mental illness*: these are sources that explore the ways in which communities and public institutions have handled the mad and mentally ill.
- *the experiential history of madness and mental illness*: these are personal narratives detailing how individuals have experienced madness and its treatment over time.

Admittedly, direct personal stories make up the smaller share of the sources here. But it should be pointed out that the voices of the afflicted can often be heard within and reconstructed from many of the conventional clinical documents presented here. Case histories, for instance, often provide surprising insight into the tensions and differences between patients and their caretakers. As a reference aid for interested readers, however, a list of first-person narratives about mental illness—put together by Gail A. Hornstein—is provided at the end of this volume.

PART I

The Pneumatic Age

From ancient times until well into the eighteenth century, observers, victims, and healers of madness most often understood and treated it as both a physical and metaphysical malady. This was because it was widely believed that human rationality, passions, and desires had at once somatic and spiritual dimensions. In ancient Greece, for instance, Plato held that different kinds of *psyche*, or "soul," animated organs such as the brain, liver, and heart, while Aristotle equated *psyche* with the very workings of organs. Meanwhile, physicians generally accepted that the human body was composed of the four "humors" of blood, phlegm, yellow bile, and black bile and that health and sickness were the result of some kind of imbalance in their distribution. In turn, the humors were believed to be influenced by the four fundamental elements that composed the universe (fire, air, water, earth). By the second and third centuries C.E., Western medical scholars were arguing that vital *pneuma* (literally "breath" or "wind" in Greek) served as the essential intermediary between the immaterial soul and material organs. These notions continued to inform scholarly and medical thought throughout the Middle Ages (500–1500) and the early modern period (1500–1800).

Madness, however, also carried social and moral meanings. While the mad were first shut up in institutions only in the fourteenth and fifteenth centuries, they were widely feared, ridiculed, and pitied for their apparent foolishness and unpredictable behavior. Relatives or friends were the obvious and primary caretakers for most. But for those who were chronically insane and lacking such support, their care often fell to religious orders and local municipalities, who housed them in a variety of hospices, hospitals, infirmaries, poorhouses, and retreats well into the nineteenth century. Christians, especially, often raised questions about whether, for instance, chronic epilepsy or "idiocy" (an antiquated term for mental retardation) might have been a fate bestowed on a person for a sin committed by the sufferer or his or her family. And right up to modern times, it was not uncommon for charms, amulets, relics, and holy waters to be used to treat and ward off insanity.

Religion thus has played a critical role in the history of madness. Pagan, Jewish, Christian, and Muslim traditions all recognized links, but also boundaries, between expressions of prophecy or devotional ecstasy and madness. And, in fact, religious groups borrowed heavily from one another's worldviews, as in the case of Saint Paul, who adopted the term *pneuma* and applied it to the early Christian concept of the Holy Spirit.

Dating back to ancient times, madness and folly (in Latin, *insania* or *stultitia*) were broad cultural notions. One could apply the terms quite casually to an individual's conduct—"Oh, he must be mad!" or "Look at the old fool!"—without implying the presence of an actual medical disease. The cultural currency of madness allowed poets, essayists, and playwrights to use the figure of the fool to criticize their contemporaries, giving a fool's voice to common deceptions (as in Sebastian Brant's *Ship of Fools*) or having a fool express uncommon wisdom (as in Shakespeare's plays).

These more informal notions clearly inflected and were inflected by legal and medical points of view. Ancient, medieval, and early modern legal systems all considered the chronically insane to be deprived of reason and, therefore, incapable of entering into contracts or assuming criminal responsibility. Distinctions were drawn, however, between those afflicted by temporary bouts of madness and those constantly under its sway. In this regard, idiocy was understood to be a categorically different phenomenon from insanity, in that the former was believed to be a congenital defect.

While there was no universally accepted manual for classifying forms of madness before the twentieth century, ancient, medieval, and early modern physicians did generally agree on there being three classic types of madness: phrenitis, or frenzy (an acute disease associated with delirium); melancholy (a chronic affliction associated with fear, anxiety, and sadness); and mania (another chronic disturbance, characterized by excitement, delusions, and anxiety). A fourth prominent malady, hysteria—thought to chiefly affect women and characterized by dissociation, paralyses, and the loss of various motor skills—was often subsumed under the category of a mania. Medical remedies tended to be whole-body cures (such as throwing a patient into a raging sea), rather than localized treatments, since it was considered essential to restore an equilibrium between the humors. By the end of the eighteenth century, however, humoral medicine was being challenged by scholars who believed that electricity, not fluids, held the key to the human nervous system.

The Ancient World

The Bible, 1 Samuel
(ca. 960 B.C.E.)

Saul was the first king of Israel, reigning between roughly 1020 and 1000 B.C.E. Comparatively little is known about his reign, though he was renowned for leading the Israelites in war against their enemies the Philistines. The Bible devotes a great deal of time to recounting Saul's jealousy of and conflict with his son-in-law and future successor, David. The extent to which the account in Samuel is accurate is, at the very least, difficult to assess. From the standpoint of the history of madness, however, the story of Saul's erratic behavior and his volatile relationship with David provides a glimpse into how the ancient Israelites recognized there to be links and boundaries between religious experience and madness. As the text repeats several times, "Is Saul also among the prophets?"

1 Samuel 10

1 Then Samuel took a vial of oil and poured it on his [Saul's] head, and kissed him and said, "Has not the LORD anointed you to be prince over his people Israel? And you shall reign over the people of the LORD and you will save them from the hand of their enemies round about. And this shall be the sign to you that the LORD has anointed you to be prince over his heritage.

2 When you depart from me today you will meet two men by Rachel's tomb in the territory of Benjamin at Zelzah, and they will say to you, 'The asses which you went to seek are found, and now your father has ceased to care about the asses and is anxious about you, saying, "What shall I do about my son?"'

3 Then you shall go on from there further and come to the oak of Tabor; three men going up to God at Bethel will meet you there, one carrying three kids, another carrying three loaves of bread, and another carrying a skin of wine.

4 And they will greet you and give you two loaves of bread, which you shall accept from their hand.

5 After that you shall come to Gib'e-ath-elo'him, where there is a garrison of the Philistines; and there, as you come to the city, you will meet a band of prophets coming down from the high place with harp, tambourine, flute, and lyre before them, prophesying.

6 Then the spirit of the LORD will come mightily upon you, and you shall prophesy with them and be turned into another man.

7 Now when these signs meet you, do whatever your hand finds to do, for God is with you.

8 And you shall go down before me to Gilgal; and behold, I am coming to you to offer burnt offerings and to sacrifice peace offerings. Seven days you shall wait, until I come to you and show you what you shall do."

9 When he turned his back to leave Samuel, God gave him another heart; and all these signs came to pass that day.

10 When they came to Gib'e-ah, behold, a band of prophets met him; and the spirit of God came mightily upon him, and he prophesied among them.

11 And when all who knew him before saw how he prophesied with the prophets, the people said to one another, "What has come over the son of Kish? Is Saul also among the prophets?"

12 And a man of the place answered, "And who is their father?" Therefore it became a proverb, "Is Saul also among the prophets?"

1 Samuel 15

1 And Samuel said to Saul, "The LORD sent me to anoint you king over his people Israel; now therefore hearken to the words of the LORD.

2 Thus says the LORD of hosts, 'I will punish what Am'alek did to Israel in opposing them on the way, when they came up out of Egypt.

3 Now go and smite Am'alek, and utterly destroy all that they have; do not spare them, but kill both man and woman, infant and suckling, ox and sheep, camel and ass.'"

4 So Saul summoned the people, and numbered them in Tela'im, two hundred thousand men on foot, and ten thousand men of Judah.

5 And Saul came to the city of Am'alek, and lay in wait in the valley.

6 And Saul said to the Ken'ites, "Go, depart, go down from among the Amal'ekites, lest I destroy you with them; for you showed kindness to all the people of Israel when they came up out of Egypt." So the Ken'ites departed from among the Amal'ekites.

7 And Saul defeated the Amal'ekites, from Hav'ilah as far as Shur, which is east of Egypt.

8 And he took Agag the king of the Amal'ekites alive, and utterly destroyed all the people with the edge of the sword.

9 But Saul and the people spared Agag, and the best of the sheep and of the oxen and of the fatlings, and the lambs, and all that was good, and would not utterly destroy them; all that was despised and worthless they utterly destroyed.

10 The word of the LORD came to Samuel:

11 "I repent that I have made Saul king; for he has turned back from following me, and has not performed my commandments." And Samuel was angry; and he cried to the LORD all night.

12 And Samuel rose early to meet Saul in the morning; and it was told Samuel, "Saul came to Carmel, and behold, he set up a monument for himself and turned, and passed on, and went down to Gilgal."

13 And Samuel came to Saul, and Saul said to him, "Blessed be you to the LORD; I have performed the commandment of the LORD."

14 And Samuel said, "What then is this bleating of the sheep in my ears, and the lowing of the oxen which I hear?"

15 Saul said, "They have brought them from the Amal'ekites; for the people spared the best of the sheep and of the oxen, to sacrifice to the LORD your God; and the rest we have utterly destroyed."

16 Then Samuel said to Saul, "Stop! I will tell you what the LORD said to me this night." And he said to him, "Say on."

17 And Samuel said, "Though you are little in your own eyes, are you not

the head of the tribes of Israel? The LORD anointed you king over Israel.

18 And the LORD sent you on a mission, and said, 'Go, utterly destroy the sinners, the Amal'ekites, and fight against them until they are consumed.'

19 Why then did you not obey the voice of the LORD? Why did you swoop on the spoil, and do what was evil in the sight of the LORD?"

20 And Saul said to Samuel, "I have obeyed the voice of the LORD, I have gone on the mission on which the LORD sent me, I have brought Agag the king of Am'alek, and I have utterly destroyed the Amal'ekites.

21 But the people took of the spoil, sheep and oxen, the best of the things devoted to destruction, to sacrifice to the LORD your God in Gilgal."

22 And Samuel said, "Has the LORD as great delight in burnt offerings and sacrifices, as in obeying the voice of the LORD? Behold, to obey is better than sacrifice, and to hearken than the fat of rams.

23 For rebellion is as the sin of divination, and stubbornness is as iniquity and idolatry. Because you have rejected the word of the LORD, he has also rejected you from being king."

24 And Saul said to Samuel, "I have sinned; for I have transgressed the commandment of the LORD and your words, because I feared the people and obeyed their voice.

25 Now therefore, I pray, pardon my sin, and return with me, that I may worship the LORD."

26 And Samuel said to Saul, "I will not return with you; for you have rejected the word of the LORD, and the LORD has rejected you from being king over Israel."

27 As Samuel turned to go away, Saul laid hold upon the skirt of his robe, and it tore.

28 And Samuel said to him, "The LORD has torn the kingdom of Israel from you this day, and has given it to a neighbor of yours, who is better than you.

29 And also the Glory of Israel will not lie or repent; for he is not a man, that he should repent."

30 Then he said, "I have sinned; yet honor me now before the elders of my people and before Israel, and return with me, that I may worship the LORD your God."

31 So Samuel turned back after Saul; and Saul worshiped the LORD.

32 Then Samuel said, "Bring here to me Agag the king of the Amal'ekites." And Agag came to him cheerfully. Agag said, "Surely the bitterness of death is past."

33 And Samuel said, "As your sword has made women childless, so shall your mother be childless among women." And Samuel hewed Agag in pieces before the LORD in Gilgal.

34 Then Samuel went to Ramah; and Saul went up to his house in Gib'e-ah of Saul.

35 And Samuel did not see Saul again until the day of his death, but Samuel grieved over Saul. And the LORD repented that he had made Saul king over Israel.

1 Samuel 16

1 The LORD said to Samuel, "How long will you grieve over Saul, seeing I have rejected him from being king over Israel? Fill your horn with oil, and go; I will send you to Jesse the Bethlehemite, for I have provided for myself a king among his sons."

2 And Samuel said, "How can I go? If Saul hears it, he will kill me." And the LORD said, "Take a heifer with you, and say, 'I have come to sacrifice to the LORD.'

3 And invite Jesse to the sacrifice, and I will show you what you shall do; and you shall anoint for me him whom I name to you."

4 Samuel did what the LORD commanded, and came to Bethlehem. The elders of the city came to meet him trembling, and said, "Do you come peaceably?"

5 And he said, "Peaceably; I have come to sacrifice to the LORD; consecrate yourselves, and come with me to the sacrifice." And he consecrated Jesse and his sons, and invited them to the sacrifice.

6 When they came, he looked on Eli'ab and thought, "Surely the LORD'S anointed is before him."

7 But the LORD said to Samuel, "Do not look on his appearance or on the height of his stature, because I have rejected him; for the LORD sees not as man sees; man looks on the outward appearance, but the LORD looks on the heart."

8 Then Jesse called Abin'adab, and made him pass before Samuel. And he said, "Neither has the LORD chosen this one."

9   Then Jesse made Shammah pass by. And he said, "Neither has the LORD chosen this one."

10   And Jesse made seven of his sons pass before Samuel. And Samuel said to Jesse, "The LORD has not chosen these."

11   And Samuel said to Jesse, "Are all your sons here?" And he said, "There remains yet the youngest, but behold, he is keeping the sheep." And Samuel said to Jesse, "Send and fetch him; for we will not sit down till he comes here."

12   And he sent, and brought him in. Now he was ruddy, and had beautiful eyes, and was handsome. And the LORD said, "Arise, anoint him; for this is he."

13   Then Samuel took the horn of oil, and anointed him in the midst of his brothers; and the Spirit of the LORD came mightily upon David from that day forward. And Samuel rose up, and went to Ramah.

14   Now the Spirit of the LORD departed from Saul, and an evil spirit from the LORD tormented him.

15   And Saul's servants said to him, "Behold now, an evil spirit from God is tormenting you.

16   Let our lord now command your servants, who are before you, to seek out a man who is skilful in playing the lyre; and when the evil spirit from God is upon you, he will play it, and you will be well."

17   So Saul said to his servants, "Provide for me a man who can play well, and bring him to me."

18   One of the young men answered, "Behold, I have seen a son of Jesse the Bethlehemite, who is skilful in playing, a man of valor, a man of war, prudent in speech, and a man of good presence; and the LORD is with him."

19   Therefore Saul sent messengers to Jesse, and said, "Send me David your son, who is with the sheep."

20   And Jesse took an ass laden with bread, and a skin of wine and a kid, and sent them by David his son to Saul.

21   And David came to Saul, and entered his service. And Saul loved him greatly, and he became his armor-bearer.

22   And Saul sent to Jesse, saying, "Let David remain in my service, for he has found favor in my sight."

23   And whenever the evil spirit from God was upon Saul, David took the lyre and played it with his hand; so Saul was refreshed, and was well, and the evil spirit departed from him.

1 Samuel 18

5 And David went out and was successful wherever Saul sent him; so that Saul set him over the men of war. And this was good in the sight of all the people and also in the sight of Saul's servants.

6 As they were coming home, when David returned from slaying the Philistine, the women came out of all the cities of Israel, singing and dancing, to meet King Saul, with timbrels, with songs of joy, and with instruments of music.

7 And the women sang to one another as they made merry, "Saul has slain his thousands, and David his ten thousands."

8 And Saul was very angry, and this saying displeased him; he said, "They have ascribed to David ten thousands, and to me they have ascribed thousands; and what more can he have but the kingdom?"

9 And Saul eyed David from that day on.

10 And on the morrow an evil spirit from God rushed upon Saul, and he raved within his house, while David was playing the lyre, as he did day by day. Saul had his spear in his hand;

11 and Saul cast the spear, for he thought, "I will pin David to the wall." But David evaded him twice.

12 Saul was afraid of David, because the LORD was with him but had departed from Saul.

1 Samuel 19

9 Then an evil spirit from the LORD came upon Saul, as he sat in his house with his spear in his hand; and David was playing the lyre.

10 And Saul sought to pin David to the wall with the spear; but he eluded Saul, so that he struck the spear into the wall. And David fled, and escaped.

11 That night Saul sent messengers to David's house to watch him, that he might kill him in the morning. But Michal, David's wife, told him, "If you do not save your life tonight, tomorrow you will be killed."

12 So Michal let David down through the window; and he fled away and escaped.

13 Michal took an image and laid it on the bed and put a pillow of goats' hair at its head, and covered it with the clothes.

14 And when Saul sent messengers to take David, she said, "He is sick."

15 Then Saul sent the messengers to see David, saying, "Bring him up to me in the bed, that I may kill him."

16 And when the messengers came in, behold, the image was in the bed, with the pillow of goats' hair at its head.

17 Saul said to Michal, "Why have you deceived me thus, and let my enemy go, so that he has escaped?" And Michal answered Saul, "He said to me, 'Let me go; why should I kill you?'"

18 Now David fled and escaped, and he came to Samuel at Ramah, and told him all that Saul had done to him. And he and Samuel went and dwelt at Nai'oth.

19 And it was told Saul, "Behold, David is at Nai'oth in Ramah."

20 Then Saul sent messengers to take David; and when they saw the company of the prophets prophesying, and Samuel standing as head over them, the Spirit of God came upon the messengers of Saul, and they also prophesied.

21 When it was told Saul, he sent other messengers, and they also prophesied. And Saul sent messengers again the third time, and they also prophesied.

22 Then he himself went to Ramah, and came to the great well that is in Secu; and he asked, "Where are Samuel and David?" And one said, "Behold, they are at Nai'oth in Ramah."

23 And he went from there to Nai'oth in Ramah; and the Spirit of God came upon him also, and as he went he prophesied, until he came to Nai'oth in Ramah.

24 And he too stripped off his clothes, and he too prophesied before Samuel, and lay naked all that day and all that night. Hence it is said, "Is Saul also among the prophets?"

Euripides
(484–407/6 B.C.E.)

The Bacchae
(ca. 404 B.C.E.)

Euripides was considered one of the great tragic poets of fifth-century B.C.E. Greece. While little is known about his personal life and intellectual background, we do know that he was prolific (scholars in Alexandria later attributed eighty-eight plays to him) and that he won five different tragic competitions over the course of his life. It is said that upon hearing news of Euripides' death, the famed Sophocles publicly mourned.

As Greek mythology tells it, Dionysus (also known as Bacchus) was the illegitimate offspring of Zeus (king of the gods) and Semele (a Theban princess). According to the myth, Semele's boasting of the pregnancy led Zeus's wife, Hera, and Semele's sisters to become jealous, ultimately leading Hera to kill Semele and her sisters to speak ill about Semele after her death. *The Bacchae* tells the story of the return of the hedonistic Dionysus to Thebes in order to punish Semele's sisters as well as to introduce the city to his new religion. As we join the play, the women of Thebes—including Semele's sister Agave, the daughter of former king Cadmus and mother to the present king, Pentheus—are in the throes of Dionysian ecstasy. In the ancient world, ecstatic states and behavior were associated with both religious devotion and madness, as this excerpt shows.

CHORUS: Speak to me, tell all—
How did death strike him down,
that unrighteous man,
that man who acted so unjustly?

SECOND MESSENGER: Once we'd left the settlements of Thebes,
we went across the river Asopus,
then started the climb up Mount Cithaeron—

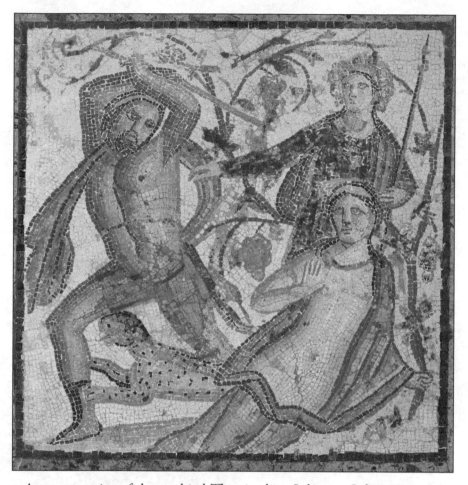

A representation of the mythical Thracian king Lykurgos. Lykurgos, it was said, tried to prevent the spread of the Dionysian cult in his kingdom. In response, Dionysus drove the king mad; the king then killed his own son, believing him to be a vine. From Herculaneum. Museo Archeologico Nazionales, Naples, Italy. © Erich Lessing/Art Resource, NY.

Pentheus and myself, I following the king.
The stranger was our guide, scouting the way.
First, we sat down in a grassy meadow,
keeping our feet and tongues quite silent,
so we could see without being noticed.
There was a valley there shut in by cliffs.
Through it refreshing waters flowed, with pines
providing shade. The Maenads sat there,
their hands all busy with delightful work—

some of them with ivy strands repairing
damaged thyrsoi, while others sang,
chanting Bacchic songs to one another,
carefree as fillies freed from harness.
Then Pentheus, that unhappy man,
not seeing the crowd of women, spoke up,
"Stranger, I can't see from where we're standing.
My eyes can't glimpse those crafty Maenads.
But up there, on that hill, a pine tree stands.
If I climbed that, I might see those women,
and witness the disgraceful things they do."
Then I saw that stranger work a marvel.
He seized that pine tree's topmost branch—
it stretched up to heaven—and brought it down,
pulling it to the dark earth, bending it
as if it were a bow or some curved wheel
forced into a circle while staked out with pegs—
that's how the stranger made that tree bend down,
forcing the mountain pine to earth by hand,
something no mortal man could ever do.
He set Pentheus in that pine tree's branches.
Then his hands released the tree, but slowly,
so it stood up straight, being very careful
not to shake Pentheus loose. So that pine
towered straight up to heaven, with my king
perched on its back. Maenads could see him there
more easily than he could spy on them.
As he was just becoming visible—
the stranger had completely disappeared—
some voice—I guess it was Dionysus—
cried out from the sky, "Young women,
I've brought you the man who laughed at you,
who ridiculed my rites. Now punish him!"
As he shouted this, a dreadful fire arose,
blazing between the earth and heaven.
The air was still. In the wooded valley
no sound came from the leaves, and all the beasts

were silent, too. The women stood up at once.
They'd heard the voice, but not distinctly.
They gazed around them. Then again the voice
shouted his commands. When Cadmus' daughters
clearly heard what Dionysus ordered,
they rushed out, running as fast as doves,
moving their feet at an amazing speed.
His mother Agave with both her sisters
and all the Bacchae charged straight through
the valley, the torrents, the mountain cliffs,
pushed to a god-inspired frenzy.
They saw the king there sitting in that pine.
First, they scaled a cliff face looming up
opposite the tree and started throwing rocks,
trying to hurt him. Others threw branches,
or hurled their thyrsoi through the air at him,
sad, miserable Pentheus, their target.
But they didn't hit him. The poor man
sat high beyond their frenzied cruelty,
trapped up there, no way to save his skin.
Then, like lightning, they struck oak branches down,
trying them as levers to uproot the tree.
When these attempts all failed, Agave said,
"Come now, make a circle round the tree.
Then, Maenads, each of you must seize a branch,
so we can catch the climbing beast up there,
stop him making our god's secret dances known."
Thousands of hands grabbed the tree and pulled.
They yanked it from the ground. Pentheus fell,
crashing to earth down from his lofty perch,
screaming in distress. He knew well enough
something dreadful was about to happen.
His priestess mother first began the slaughter.
She hurled herself at him. Pentheus tore off
his headband, untying it from his head,
so wretched Agave would recognize him,
so she wouldn't kill him. Touching her cheek,

he cried out, "It's me, mother, Pentheus,
your child. You gave birth to me at home,
in Echion's house. Pity me, mother—
don't kill your child because I've made mistakes."
But Agave was foaming at the mouth,
eyes rolling in their sockets, her mind not set
on what she ought to think—she didn't listen—
she was possessed, in a Bacchic frenzy.
She seized his left arm, below the elbow,
pushed her foot against the poor man's ribs,
then tore his shoulder out. The strength she had—
it was not her own. The god put power
into those hands of hers. Meanwhile Ino,
her sister, went at the other side,
ripping off chunks of Pentheus' flesh,
while Autonoe and all the Bacchae,
the whole crowd of them, attacked as well,
all of them howling out together.
As long as Pentheus was still alive,
he kept on screaming. The women cried in triumph—
one brandished an arm, another held a foot—
complete with hunting boot—the women's nails
tore his ribs apart. Their hands grew bloody,
tossing bits of his flesh back and forth, for fun.
His body parts lie scattered everywhere—
some under rough rocks, some in the forest,
deep in the trees. They're difficult to find.
As for the poor victim's head, his mother
stumbled on it. Her hands picked it up,
then stuck it on a thyrsus, at the tip.
Now she carries it around Cithaeron,
as though it were some wild lion's head.
She's left her sisters dancing with the Maenads.
She's coming here, inside these very walls,
showing off with pride her ill-fated prey,
calling out to her fellow hunter, Bacchus,
her companion in the chase, the winner,

the glorious victor. By serving him,
in her great triumph she wins only tears.
As for me, I'm leaving this disaster,
before Agave gets back home again.
The best thing is to keep one's mind controlled,
and worship all that comes down from the gods.
That, in my view, is the wisest custom,
for those who can conduct their lives that way.

[*Exit Messenger*]

CHORUS: Let's dance to honour Bacchus,
Let's shout to celebrate what's happened here,
happened to Pentheus,
child of the serpent,
who put on women's clothes,
who took up the beautiful and blessed thyrsus—
his certain death,
disaster brought on by the bull.
You Bacchic women
descended from old Cadmus,
you've won glorious victory,
one which ends in tears,
which ends in lamentation.
A noble undertaking this,
to drench one's hands in blood,
life blood dripping from one's only son.

CHORUS LEADER: Wait! I see Agave, Pentheus' mother,
on her way home, her eyes transfixed.
Let's now welcome her,
the happy revels of our god of joy!

[*Enter Agave, cradling the head of Pentheus*]

AGAVE: Asian Bacchae . . .

CHORUS: Why do you appeal to me?

AGAVE: [*displaying the head*] From the mountains I've brought home
this ivy tendril freshly cut.

We've had a blessed hunt.

CHORUS: I see it.
As your fellow dancer, I'll accept it.

AGAVE: I caught this young lion without a trap,
as you can see.

CHORUS: What desert was he in?

AGAVE: Cithaeron.

CHORUS: On Cithaeron?

AGAVE: Cithaeron killed him.

CHORUS: Who struck him down?

AGAVE: The honour of the first blow goes to me.
In the dancing I'm called blessed Agave.

CHORUS: Who else?

AGAVE: Well, from Cadmus . . .

CHORUS: From Cadmus what?

AGAVE: His other children laid hands on the beast,
but after me—only after I did first.
We've had good hunting. So come, share our feast.

CHORUS: What? You want me to eat that with you?
Oh you unhappy woman.

AGAVE: This is a young bull. Look at this cheek
It's just growing downy under the crop
of his soft hair.

CHORUS: His hair makes him resemble
some wild beast.

AGAVE: Bacchus is a clever huntsman—
he wisely set his Maenads on this beast.

CHORUS: Yes, our master is indeed a hunter.

AGAVE: Have you any praise for me?

CHORUS: I praise you.

AGAVE: Soon all Cadmus' people . . .

CHORUS: . . . and Pentheus, your son, as well.

AGAVE: . . . will celebrate his mother, who caught the beast,
just like a lion.

CHORUS: It's a strange trophy.

AGAVE: And strangely captured, too.

CHORUS: You're proud of what you've done?

AGAVE: Yes, I'm delighted. Great things I've done—
great things on this hunt, clear for all to see.

CHORUS: Well then, you most unfortunate woman,
show off your hunting prize, your sign of victory,
to all the citizens.

AGAVE: [addressing everyone] All of you here,
all you living in the land of Thebes,
in this city with its splendid walls,
come see this wild beast we hunted down—
daughters of Cadmus—not with thonged spears,
Thessalian javelins, or by using nets,
but with our own white hands, our finger tips.
After this, why should huntsmen boast aloud,
when no one needs the implements they use?
We caught this beast by hand, tore it apart—
with our own hands. But where's my father?
He should come here. And where's Pentheus?
Where is my son? He should take a ladder,
set it against the house, fix this lion's head
way up there, high on the palace front.
I've captured it and brought it home with me.

[Enter Cadmus and attendants, carrying parts of Pentheus' body]

CADMUS: Follow me, all those of you who carry
some part of wretched Pentheus. You slaves,
come here, right by the house.

[They place the bits of Pentheus' body together in a chest front of the palace]

I'm worn out.
So many searches—but I picked up the body.
I came across it in the rocky clefts
on Mount Cithaeron, ripped to pieces,
no parts lying together in one place.
It was in the woods—difficult to search.
Someone told me what my daughter'd done,
those horrific acts, once I'd come back,
returning here with old Tiresias,
inside the city walls, back from the Bacchae.
So I climbed the mountains once again.
Now I bring home this child the Maenads killed.
I saw Autonoe, who once bore
Actaeon to Aristeius—and Ino,
she was with her there, in the forest,
both still possessed, quite mad, poor creatures.
Someone said Agave was coming here,
still doing her Bacchic dance. He spoke the truth,
for I see her there—what a wretched sight!

AGAVE: Father, now you can be truly proud.
Among all living men you've produced
by far the finest daughters. I'm talking
of all of us, but especially of myself.
I've left behind my shuttle and my loom,
and risen to great things, catching wild beasts
with my bare hands. Now I've captured him,
I'm holding in my arms the finest trophy,
as you can see, bringing it back home to you,
so it may hang here.

[offering him Pentheus' head]

Take this, father
let your hands welcome it. Be proud of it,
of what I've caught. Summon all your friends—
have a banquet, for you are blessed indeed,
blessed your daughters have achieved these things.

CADMUS: This grief's beyond measure, beyond endurance.
With these hands of yours you've murdered him.
You strike down this sacrificial victim,
this offering to the gods, then invite me,
and all of Thebes, to share a banquet.
Alas—first for your sorrow, then my own.
Lord god Bromius, born into this family,
has destroyed us, acting out his justice,
but too much so.

AGAVE: Why such scowling eyes?
How sorrowful and solemn old men become.
As for my son, I hope he's a fine hunter,
who copies his mother's hunting style,
when he rides out with young men of Thebes
chasing after creatures in the wild.
The only thing he seems capable of doing
is fighting with the gods. It's up to you,
father, to reprimand him for it.
Who'll call him here into my sight,
so he can see my good luck for himself?

CADMUS: Alas! Alas! What dreadful pain you'll feel
when you recognize what you've just done.
If you stay forever in your present state,
you'll be unfortunate, but you won't feel
as if you're suffering unhappiness.

AGAVE: But what in all this is wrong or painful?

CADMUS: First, raise your eyes. Look up into the sky.

AGAVE: All right. But why tell me to look up there?

CADMUS: Does the sky still seem the same to you,
or has it changed?

AGAVE: It seems, well, brighter . . .
more translucent than it was before.

CADMUS: And your inner spirit—is it still shaking?

AGAVE: I don't understand what it is you're asking.
But my mind is starting to clear somehow.
It's changing . . . it's not what it was before.

CADMUS: Can you hear me? Can you answer clearly?

AGAVE: Yes. But, father, what we discussed before,
I've quite forgotten.

CADMUS: Then tell me this—
to whose house did you come when you got married?

AGAVE: You gave me to Echion, who, men say,
was one of those who grew from seeds you cast.

CADMUS: In that house you bore your husband a child.
What was his name?

AGAVE: His name was Pentheus.
I conceived him with his father.

CADMUS: Well then,
this head your hands are holding—whose is it?

AGAVE: It's a lion's. That's what the hunters said.

CADMUS: Inspect it carefully. You can do that
without much effort.

AGAVE: [inspecting the head] What is this?
What am I looking at? What am I holding?

CADMUS: Look at it. You'll understand more clearly.

AGAVE: What I see fills me with horrific pain . . .
such agony . . .

CADMUS: Does it still seem to you
to be a lion's head?

AGAVE: No. It's appalling—
this head I'm holding belongs to Pentheus.

CADMUS: Yes, that's right. I was lamenting his fate
before you recognized him.

AGAVE: Who killed him?
How did he come into my hands?

CADMUS: Harsh truth—
how you come to light at the wrong moment.

AGAVE: Tell me. My heart is pounding in me
to hear what you're about to say.

CADMUS: You killed him—
you and your sisters.

AGAVE: Where was he killed?
At home? In what sort of place?

CADMUS: He was killed
where dogs once made a common meal of Actaeon.

AGAVE: Why did this poor man go to Cithaeron?

CADMUS: He went there to ridicule the god
and you for celebrating Dionysus.

AGAVE: But how did we happen to be up there?

CADMUS: You were insane—the entire city
was in a Bacchic madness.

AGAVE: Now I see.
Dionysus has destroyed us all.

CADMUS: He took offense at being insulted.
You did not consider him a god.

AGAVE: Father, where's the body of my dearest son?

CADMUS: I had trouble tracking the body down.
I brought back what I found.

AGAVE: Are all his limbs laid out
just as they should be? And Pentheus,
what part did he play in my madness?

CADMUS: Like you, he was irreverent to the god.
That's why the god linked you and him together
in the same disaster—thus destroying
the house and me, for I've no children left,
now I see this offspring of your womb,
you unhappy woman, cruelly butchered
in the most shameful way. He was the one
who brought new vision to our family.

From Euripides, *The Bacchae*, translated by Ian Johnston, http://records.viu.ca/
~johnstoi/euripides/euripides.htm. Courtesy of Ian Johnston.

Hippocrates
(ca. 460–377 B.C.E.)

Writings on Hysteria
(ca. fourth century B.C.E.)

Hippocrates was a physician from the Greek island of Cos. Along
with his ancient counterpart Galen (ca. 129 C.E.–ca. 216 C.E.), his
ideas and practices have shaped medicine in the Western world up
to this very day. The writings attributed to him that have been
passed down over the centuries, Corpus Hippocraticum, cover a
range of topics, from diagnosis and prognosis to professional conduct. It is now accepted, however, that few of these documents
were written by Hippocrates himself, but rather were the work of
his followers.

Hippocrates' followers held that disease was the result of an imbalance within the body of fundamental fluids, referred to as "humors": blood, phlegm, and bile. Hippocratic physicians largely rejected spiritual explanations and treatments, looking instead to environmental factors, diet, and lifestyle. Inspired by Hippocrates and others, doctors for centuries after treated afflictions such as madness in an allopathic manner, that is, applying treatments designed to have the opposite effect of a given symptom. The excerpts below discuss the causes and treatment of one of the most discussed ailments in the history of madness—hysteria, considered to be primarily a female malady.

Displacement of the Womb

As for what are called women's diseases: the womb is responsible for all such diseases. For the womb, when it is displaced from its natural position, whether forward or back, causes diseases. When the neck of the womb has been moved back and does not bring its opening towards or touch the lips of the vagina, the problem is minor. But if the womb falls forward and brings its opening towards the lips, it first of all causes pain when it makes contact, and then because the womb is cut off and obstructed by the contact of its neck with the lips of the vagina, there is no so-called menstrual flow. This flow if retained causes swelling and pain. If the womb descends and is diverted so that it approaches the groin, it causes pain. If it ascends and diverted and cut off, it causes illness through its compression. When a woman is ill because of this problem, she has pains in her thighs and her head. When the womb is distended and swollen, there is no flow, and it becomes filled up. When it is filled, it touches the thighs. When the womb is filled with moisture and distended, there is no flow, and it causes pain in both the thighs and the groin, something like balls roll through the stomach, and cause pain in the head, first in one part, and then in all of it, as the disease develops.

The treatment is as follows: if the womb has only moved forward and it is possible to apply ointment, use any foul-smelling ointment you choose, either cedar or myssoton, or some other heavy and ill-scented substance, and fumigate, but do not use a vapour-bath, and do not give food or a diuretic liquid during this time, or wash her in hot water. If the womb has turned upwards and is not obstructed, use sweet-smelling pessaries that are also inflammatory. These are myrrh, or perfume, or some other aromatic and inflammatory substance. Use these in pessaries, and from below apply fumigations with wine vapour, and wash with hot water, and use diuretics. It is clear that the womb is turned upwards and is not obstructed, because there is a flow.

If the womb is obstructed, then there is no so-called menstrual flow. This disease must be treated first with a vapour-bath; put wild figs into the wine, and heat it and put a gourd around the mouth of the vessel in which the wine is heated. Then do as follows: cut the gourd through the middle and hollow it out, and cut off a bit of its top, as if you were making a nozzle for a bellows, so that the vapour can go through its channel and reach the womb. Wash with hot water, and use pessaries made of inflammatory drugs. The following inflammatory drugs bring on menstruation: cow dung, beef bile, myrrh, alum, galbanum, and anything similar; use as much of these as possible. Evacuate from below by laxative drugs that do not cause vomiting, diluted, so that it does not become a purgative by being too strong. Use pessaries as follows, if you want them to be strong. Use half-cooked honey, and add some of the substances prescribed to bring on menstruation; after you have added them, make the pessaries like pellets used for the anus, but make them long and thin. Make the woman lie down, and elevate the feet of the bed towards her feet, insert the pessary, and apply heat either on a chamber-pot or on some other vessel, so that the pessary melts. If you want to make the pessary less strong, wrap it in linen. And if the womb is filled with fluid, with its mouth swollen, so that amenorrhoea results, heal it by bringing on menstruation with medicinal pessaries, using both inflammatory pessaries as described, as in the case of the preceding amenorrhoea. If there is an excessive flow, do not use hot water or any other kind, nor diuretics or laxative foods. Raise the foot of the bed higher, so that the inclination of the bed does not encourage the flow, and use astringent pessaries. The flow, if her period comes directly, is bloody, if it diminishes, it contains pus. Young women bleed more, and the so-called menstrual periods of older women contain more mucous.

Hysterical Suffocation

When the womb remains in the upper abdomen, the suffocation is similar to that caused by the purgative hellebore, with stiff breathing and sharp pains in the heart. Some women spit up acid saliva, and their mouths are full of fluid, and their legs become cold. In such cases, if the womb does not leave the upper abdomen directly, the women lose their voices, and their head and tongue are overcome by drowsiness. If you find such women unable to speak and with their teeth chattering, insert a pessary of wool, twisting it round the shaft of a feather in order to get it in as far as possible—dip it either in white Egyptian perfume or myrtle or bacchar or marjoram. Use a spatula to apply black medicine (the kind you use for the head) to her nostrils. If this is not available, wipe the inside of her nostrils with silphium, or insert a feather that you have dipped in vinegar, or induce sneezing. If her mouth is closed tight and she is unable to speak, make her drink castoreum in wine. Dip your finger in seal oil and wipe inside her nostrils. Insert a wool pessary, until the womb returns, and remove it when the symptoms disappear. But if, when you take the pessary out, the womb returns to the upper abdomen, insert the pessary as you did before, and apply beneath her nostrils fumigations of ground-up goat or deer horn, to which you have added hot ashes, so that they make as much smoke as possible, and have her inhale the vapour up through her nose as long as she can stand it. It is best to use a fumigation of seal oil: put the coals in a pot and wrap the woman up except for her head. So that as much vapour as possible is emitted, drip a little fat on it, and have her inhale the vapour. She should keep her mouth shut. This is the procedure if the womb has fallen upward out of place. . . .

When the womb moves towards her head and suffocation occurs in that region, the woman's head becomes heavy, though there are different symptoms in some cases. One symptom: the woman says the veins in her nose hurt her and beneath her eyes, and she becomes sleepy, and when this condition is alleviated, she foams at the mouth.

You should wash her thoroughly with hot water, and if she does not respond, with cold, from her head on down, using cool water in which you have previously boiled laurel and myrtle. Rub her head with rose perfume, and use sweet-scented fumigations beneath her vagina, but foul-scented ones at her nose. She should eat cabbage, and drink cabbage juice.

Dislocation of the Womb

If her womb moves towards her hips, her periods stop coming, and pain develops in her lower stomach and abdomen. If you touch her with your finger, you will see the mouth of the womb turned towards her hip.

When this condition occurs, wash the woman with warm water, make her eat as much garlic as she can, and have her drink undiluted sheep's milk after her meals. Then fumigate her and give her a laxative. After the laxative has taken effect, fumigate the womb once again, using a preparation of fennel and absinthe mixed together. Right after the fumigation, pull the mouth of the womb with your finger. Then insert a pessary made with squills; leave it in for a while, and then insert a pessary made with opium poppies. If you think the condition has been corrected, insert a pessary of bitter almond oil, and on the next day, a pessary of rose perfume. She should stop inserting pessaries on the first day of her period, and start again the day after it stops. The blood during the period provides a normal interruption. If there is no flow, she should drink four cantharid beetles with their legs, wings and heads removed, four dark peony seeds, cuttlefish eggs, and a little parsley seed in wine.* If she has a pain and irregular flow, she should sit in warm water, and drink honey mixed with water. If she is not cured by the first procedure, she should drink it again, until her period comes. When it comes, she should abstain from food and have intercourse with her husband. During her period she should eat mercury plant and boiled squid, and keep to soft foods. If she becomes pregnant she will be cured of this disease. . . .

When her womb moves towards her liver, she suddenly loses her voice and her teeth chatter and her colouring turns dark. This condition can occur suddenly, while she is in good health. The problem particularly affects old maids and widows—young women who have been widowed after having had children.

When this condition occurs, push your hand down below her liver, and tie a bandage below her ribs. Open her mouth and pour in very sweet-scented wine; put applications on her nostrils and burn foul-scented vapours below her womb. . . .

---

*Editor's note: Lefkowitz and Fant note that in ancient times ground-up cantharid beetles were used as a diuretic as well as to induce menstruation and abortion.

Hysteria in Virgins

As a result of visions, many people choke to death, more women than men, for the nature of women is less courageous and is weaker. And virgins who do not take a husband at the appropriate time for marriage experience these visions more frequently, especially at the time of their first monthly period, although previously they have had no such bad dreams of this sort. For later the blood collects in the womb in preparation to flow out; but when the mouth of the egress is not opened up, and more blood flows into the womb on account of the body's nourishment of it and its growth, then the blood which has no place to flow out, because of its abundance, rushes up to the heart and to the lungs; and when these are filled with blood, the heart becomes sluggish, and then, because of the sluggishness, numb, and then, because of the numbness, insanity takes hold of the woman. Just as when one has been sitting for a long time the blood that has been forced away from the hips and the thighs collects in one's lower legs and feet, it brings numbness, and as a result of the numbness, one's feet are useless for move-ment, until the blood goes back where it belongs. It returns most quickly when one stands in cold water and wets the tops of one's ankles. This numbness presents no complications, since the blood flows back quickly because the veins in that part of the body are straight, and the legs are not a critical part of the body. But blood flows slowly from the heart and from the phrenes.* There the veins are slanted, and it is a critical place for insan-ity and suited for madness.

When these places are filled with blood, shivering sets in with fevers. They call these "erratic fevers." When this is the state of affairs, the girl goes crazy because of the violent inflammation, and she becomes murder-ous because of the decay and is afraid and fearful because of the darkness. The girls try to choke themselves because of the pressure on their hearts; their will, distraught and anguished because of the bad condition of the blood, forces evil on itself. In some cases the girl says dreadful things: [the visions] order her to jump up and throw herself into wells and drown, as if this were good for her and served some useful purpose. When a girl does not have visions, a desire sets in which compels her to love death as if it

---

*Editor's note: The phrenes, or diaphragm, it was believed, was where the work of mind, thought, and will resided.

were a form of good. When this person returns to her right mind, women give to Artemis various offerings, especially the most valuable of women's robes, following the orders of oracles, but they are deceived. The fact is that the disorder is cured when nothing impedes the downward flow of blood. My prescription is that when virgins experience this trouble, they should cohabit with a man as quickly as possible. If they become pregnant, they will be cured. If they don't do this, either they will succumb at the onset of puberty or a little later, unless they catch another disease. Among married women, those who are sterile are more likely to suffer what I have described.

From Mary R. Lefkowitz and Maureen B. Fant, eds., *Women's Life in Greece and Rome: A Source Book in Translation*, 3rd ed. (Baltimore: Johns Hopkins University Press, 2005), 237–240, 242–243. ©2005 Mary R. Lefkowitz and Maureen B. Fant. Reprinted with permission of the Johns Hopkins University Press and by permission of Gerald Duckworth & Co. Ltd.

The Bible, Mark 5
(ca. 65–75 C.E.)

Of the four Gospels chronicling the life and teachings of Jesus of Nazareth, Mark's is considered to be the oldest. Christianity has historically had a close connection to disease and cure. Like their Jewish, Greek, and Roman predecessors and contemporaries, early and medieval Christians believed that sacred power was something that could be shared by both prophets and madmen alike. Moreover, Jesus' fame spread quickly due, in part, to stories of his alleged ability to cure a host of ailments. The story of Jesus' encounter with the Gerasene demoniac is among the most famous in the gospels. A tenth-century depiction of this scene can be found on the front cover of our volume.*

*Editor's note: Thanks to the late Bill Petersen for his suggestions and advice.

Mark 5

1   They came to the other side of the sea, to the country of the Ger'asenes.

2   And when he had come out of the boat, there met him out of the tombs a man with an unclean spirit,

3   who lived among the tombs; and no one could bind him any more, even with a chain;

4   for he had often been bound with fetters and chains, but the chains he wrenched apart, and the fetters he broke in pieces; and no one had the strength to subdue him.

5   Night and day among the tombs and on the mountains he was always crying out, and bruising himself with stones.

6   And when he saw Jesus from afar, he ran and worshiped him;

7   and crying out with a loud voice, he said, "What have you to do with me, Jesus, Son of the Most High God? I adjure you by God, do not torment me."

8   For he had said to him, "Come out of the man, you unclean spirit!"

9   And Jesus asked him, "What is your name?" He replied, "My name is Legion; for we are many."

10   And he begged him eagerly not to send them out of the country.

11   Now a great herd of swine was feeding there on the hillside;

12   and they begged him, "Send us to the swine, let us enter them."

13   So he gave them leave. And the unclean spirits came out, and entered the swine; and the herd, numbering about two thousand, rushed down the steep bank into the sea, and were drowned in the sea.

14   The herdsmen fled, and told it in the city and in the country. And people came to see what it was that had happened.

15   And they came to Jesus, and saw the demoniac sitting there, clothed and in his right mind, the man who had had the legion; and they were afraid.

16   And those who had seen it told what had happened to the demoniac and to the swine.

17   And they began to beg Jesus to depart from their neighborhood.

18   And as he was getting into the boat, the man who had been possessed with demons begged him that he might be with him.

19   But he refused, and said to him, "Go home to your friends, and tell

them how much the Lord has done for you, and how he has had mercy on you."

20 And he went away and began to proclaim in the Decap'olis how much Jesus had done for him; and all men marveled.

21 And when Jesus had crossed again in the boat to the other side, a great crowd gathered about him; and he was beside the sea.

22 Then came one of the rulers of the synagogue, Ja'irus by name; and seeing him, he fell at his feet,

23 and besought him, saying, "My little daughter is at the point of death. Come and lay your hands on her, so that she may be made well, and live."

24 And he went with him. And a great crowd followed him and thronged about him.

25 And there was a woman who had had a flow of blood for twelve years,

26 and who had suffered much under many physicians, and had spent all that she had, and was no better but rather grew worse.

27 She had heard the reports about Jesus, and came up behind him in the crowd and touched his garment.

28 For she said, "If I touch even his garments, I shall be made well."

29 And immediately the hemorrhage ceased; and she felt in her body that she was healed of her disease.

30 And Jesus, perceiving in himself that power had gone forth from him, immediately turned about in the crowd, and said, "Who touched my garments?"

31 And his disciples said to him, "You see the crowd pressing around you, and yet you say, 'Who touched me?'"

32 And he looked around to see who had done it.

33 But the woman, knowing what had been done to her, came in fear and trembling and fell down before him, and told him the whole truth.

34 And he said to her, "Daughter, your faith has made you well; go in peace, and be healed of your disease."

35 While he was still speaking, there came from the ruler's house some who said, "Your daughter is dead. Why trouble the Teacher any further?"

36 But ignoring what they said, Jesus said to the ruler of the synagogue, "Do not fear, only believe."

37 And he allowed no one to follow him except Peter and James and John the brother of James.

38 When they came to the house of the ruler of the synagogue, he saw a tumult, and people weeping and wailing loudly.

39 And when he had entered, he said to them, "Why do you make a tumult and weep? The child is not dead but sleeping."

40 And they laughed at him. But he put them all outside, and took the child's father and mother and those who were with him, and went in where the child was.

41 Taking her by the hand he said to her, "Tal'itha cu'mi," which means, "Little girl, I say to you, arise."

42 And immediately the girl got up and walked (she was twelve years of age), and they were immediately overcome with amazement.

43 And he strictly charged them that no one should know this, and told them to give her something to eat.

Soranus of Ephesus

(ca. second century C.E.)

"Madness or Insanity (Greek Mania)"

Soranus of Ephesus studied medicine in Alexandria and practiced in Rome during the reigns of the emperors Trajan and Hadrian. Particularly famous for his treatise on gynecology, he was the author of many works, and, along with Hippocrates and Galen, his teachings influenced Western medicine well into the Middle Ages. Soranus was a proponent of a school of medicine known as Methodism, which tended to see the body as composed of moving atoms—as opposed to flowing humors, as the Hippocratic school viewed it—and held that abnormalities in the movements of these atoms caused disease. The excerpt here comes from a treatise titled *On Chronic Diseases*. The original text has been lost, but a reliable Latin translation by the physician Caelius Aurelianus (ca. early fifth century C.E.) provides us with valuable insight into not only the beside manner of the Methodist doctor, but also experiences and understandings of madness in the Roman Empire.

Madness or Insanity (Greek Mania)

In the *Phaedrus*, Plato declares that there are two kinds of mania, one involving a mental strain that arises from a bodily cause of origin, the other divine or inspired, with Apollo as the source of the inspiration. This latter kind, he says, is now called "divination," but in early times was called "madness"; that is, the Greeks now call it "prophetic inspiration" (*mantice*), though in remote antiquity it was called "mania." Plato goes on to say that another kind of divine mania is sent by Father Bacchus, that still another, called "erotic inspiration," is sent by the god of love, and that a fourth kind comes from the Muses and is called "protreptic inspiration" because it seems to inspire men to song. The Stoics also say that madness is of two kinds, but they hold that one kind consists in lack of wisdom, so that they can consider every imprudent person mad; the other kind, they say, involves a loss of reason and a concomitant bodily affection. The school of Empedocles holds that one form of madness consists in a purification of the soul, and the other in an impairment of the reason resulting from a bodily disease or indisposition.

It is this latter form of madness that we shall now consider. The Greeks call it *mania* because it produces great mental anguish (Greek *ania*); or else because there is excessive relaxing of the soul or mind, the Greek word for "relaxed" or "loose" being *manos*; or because the disease defiles the patient, the Greek word "to defile" being *lymaenin*; or because it makes the patient desirous of being alone and in solitude, the Greek word "to be bereft" and "to seek solitude" being *monusthae*; or because the disease holds the body tenaciously and is not easily shaken off, the Greek word for "persistence" being *monia*; or because it makes the patient hard and enduring (Greek *hypomeneticos*).

Mania is an impairment of reason; it is chronic and without fever and in these respects may be distinguished from phrenitis. For mania is not an acute disease, nor is it observed to occur with fever; or, if fever *is* present in case of mania, the case may be distinguished from phrenitis by considerations of time, for in mania the madness precedes any supervening fever and the patient does not have a small pulse. In phrenitis, however, the fever always precedes the madness, and the patient has a small pulse.

Mania occurs more frequently in young and middle-aged men, rarely in old men, and most infrequently in children and women. Sometimes it strikes suddenly, at other times it takes hold gradually. Sometimes it arises from hidden causes, at other times from observable causes, such as exposure to intense heat, the taking of severe cold, indigestion, frequent and uncontrolled drunkenness (Greek *craepale*), continual sleeplessness, excesses of venery, anger, grief, anxiety, or superstitious fear, a shock or blow, intense straining of the sense and the mind in study, business, or other ambitious pursuits, the drinking of drugs, especially of those intended to excite love (Greek *philtropota*), the removal of long-standing hemorrhoids or varices, and, finally, the suppression of the menses in women.

Before the disease emerges, those who are not attacked suddenly by it have the same symptoms as persons on the verge of epilepsy or of apoplexy. These signs may be found, then, in what has already been said. But some seek to distinguish the antecedent signs of these diseases by listing specific signs for each of them in addition to the general signs common to all. Thus deep sleep, they say, is indicative of the coming of epilepsy; light and short sleep, on the other hand, of mania. So, too, they take it as an indication that mania is imminent when a person in a state of anger suffers congestion of the head and believes that he has gone mad or, again, when such a person is overcome by speechlessness resulting from groundless fear. Other such signs, in their opinion, are unhappiness, mental anxiety, tossing in sleep, immoderate appetite, frequent blinking of the eyes, palpitation of the heart, sleep marked by great fear and turmoil, abdominal distention, frequent passing of wind through the anus, and a small, rapid, hard pulse. On the other hand, they say that persons on the verge of epilepsy have a large, rare, and soft pulse. Now these same writers tell us to study the nature of these diseases as they first come to the body, on the theory that they often attack the body by a kind of external contact. But all these methods fail, in our opinion, to provide an accurate and definite means of distinguishing which of the aforesaid diseases is imminent in a given case. . . .

Now when the disease of mania emerges into the open, there is impairment of reason unaccompanied by fever; this impairment of reason in some cases is severe, in others mild; it differs in various cases in its outward form and appearance, though its nature and character are the same. For, when mania lays hold of the mind, it manifests itself now in anger, now in merriment, now in sadness or futility, and now, as some related, in an overpowering fear of things which are quite harmless. Thus the patient will be afraid of caves or will be obsessed by the fear of falling into a ditch or will dread other things which may for some reason inspire fear.

The ancients also associated madness with a kind of prophetic power. And Demetrius calls mania a strain imposed on the mind for a brief period, saying that some persons in a sudden moment of confusion are so terror-stricken that they lose their memory of the past. In fact, Apollonius tells us that when the philologist Artemidorus was lying on the sand he was frightened by the ponderous approach of a crocodile; his mind was so affected by the sudden sight of the reptile's motion that he imagined that his left leg and hand had been eaten by the animal, and he lost his memory even of literature. Apollonius says that melancholy should be considered a form of mania, but we distinguish melancholy from mania. And mania or madness is sometimes continuous and other times relieved by intervals of remission. Thus the patient sometimes does not remember his tasks, sometimes is unaware of his own forgetfulness, sometimes suffers impairment of all the senses, and sometimes is affected by various other types of aberration. Thus one victim of madness fancied himself a sparrow, another a cock, another an earthen vessel, another a brick, another a god, another an orator, another a tragic actor, another a comic actor, another a stalk of grain and asserted that he occupied the center of the universe, and another cried like a baby and begged to be carried in the arms. In most cases of mania, at the time of the actual attack, the eyes become bloodshot and intent. There is also continual wakefulness, the veins are distended, cheeks flushed, and body hard and abnormally strong.

In this disease the whole system of nerves and sinews is affected, as we may gather from the symptoms. But the head is especially affected; and, in fact, most of the discomfort preceding the attack is in the head, the patient being affected by a feeling of pain and heaviness there. Also the senses are individually affected, and these are, as we know, centered in the head. Mania is a major disease; it is chronic and consists of attacks alternating with periods of remission; it involves a state of stricture. . . . Thus, in the interval of remission the patient feels fatigued. Our conclusion is further confirmed by the symptoms that precede the loss of reason, e.g., a feeling of heaviness in the head, pain in the spine and shoulder blades, sluggishness in the movements of the limbs, and abdominal distention. Thus those who imagine that the disease is chiefly an affection of the soul and only secondarily of the body are mistaken. For no philosopher has ever set forth a successful treatment for this disease; moreover, before the mind is affected, the body itself shows visible symptoms. This concludes the Methodist account of the recognition or diagnosis of the disease.

As for the treatment, we hold that measures should be taken similar to those employed in epilepsy. Thus, to begin with, have the patient lie in a moderately light and warm room. The room should be perfectly quiet, unadorned by paintings, not lighted by low windows, and on the ground floor rather than on the upper stories, for victims of mania have often jumped out of windows. And the bed should be firmly fastened down. It should face away from the entrance to the room so that the patient will not see those who enter. In this way the danger of exciting or aggravating his madness by letting him see many different faces will be avoided. And the bedclothes should be soft.

Rub the patient's limbs and hold them gently. If any part of the body is shaken by a throbbing movement, relieve it with warmth, applying soft scoured wool to the head, too, the neck and circularly to the chest. Also employ a fomentation of warm olive oil, sometimes adding, for its soothing properties, fenugreek water (obtained from a decoction of fenugreek; but see that it is not thick), or else an infusion of marsh mallow or flaxseed. Then wash the patient's mouth and have him take a drink of warm water.

Do not permit many people, especially strangers, to enter the room. And instruct servants to correct the patient's aberrations while giving them a sympathetic hearing. That is, have the servants, on the one hand, avoid the mistake of agreeing with everything the patient says, corroborating all his fantasies, and thus increasing his mania; and, on the other hand, have them avoid the mistake of objecting to everything he says and thus aggravating the severity of the attack. . . .

If the patient is excited when he sees people, bind him without doing any injury. First cover his limbs with wool and then fasten with a bandage. Now if there is a person whom the patient has customarily feared or respected, he should not be brought into the sickroom repeatedly. For this frequent repetition gives rise to a lack of regard. But when circumstances require it, as when the patient does not submit to the application of a remedy, this person should then be brought in to overcome the patient's stubbornness, by inspiring fear or respect. And if you observe that the light is upsetting his mind, shade his eyes but let the rest of his body be touched by the light.

Do not give the patient food until the end of the first three-day period; and if his strength permits and the disease requires it, perform venesection before the end of the three-day period. If there is any reason why an adequate withdrawal of blood cannot be made, take the amount required in several operations. But if there is no reason for doing otherwise, perform the venesection at the end of the three-day period.

After venesection anoint the patient, foment his face, and give him a small quantity of light and digestible food, e.g., bread in warm water, spelt groats mixed with honey which has been boiled down moderately, and some other gruel-like or soft food. Thereafter, feed the patient on alternate days, if his strength permits, until the disease declines. And if the case requires it, purge with a simple clyster. Again, relax the precordial region with poultices as an aid to digestion. The purpose is to prevent any state of constriction from causing the pent-up gases to pass to the head. Attention must also be paid to the type of mental aberration involved, for its symptoms will have to be relieved by properly reasonable countermeasures. Thus they [the servants] will soothe a patient with cheerfulness, telling him something to relax his mind.

And when the highest stage of the attack is reached, cut the patient's hair and shave his head; then apply cupping with scarification, beginning with the precordia, and then passing to the region between the shoulder blades (Greek *metaphrenon*). For in these cases the upper parts of the body are apt to be sympathetically affected. Then apply cupping in conjunction with scarification to the occiput, the top of the head, and the temples. And if the face is particularly affected, relax the whole body using leeches, which we call *hirudines*. Then use poultices of bread and other substances with relaxing properties, followed by an application of heat with sponges. And if the disease persists, keep using the same remedies a second or even a third time. If the patient is wakeful, prescribe passive exercise, first in a hammock and then in a sedan chair. The rapid dripping of water may be employed to induce sleep, for under the influence of its sound patients often fall asleep. And heat should then be applied to the eyes with warm sponges, and the stiffness of the lids relaxed; for the beneficial effects of this treatment will pass through the eyes to the membranes of the brain.

When the disease declines and the patient's wakefulness and mental aberration are very much reduced, give him varied food of the middle class. . . . And then prescribe passive exercise, first in a sedan chair and then in a cart drawn by hand. When the patient's body has gained strength, prescribe walking and also vocal exercise, as required by the case. Thus have the patient read aloud even from texts that are marred by false statements. In this way he will exercise his mind more thoroughly. And for the same reason he should also be kept busy answering questions. This will enable us both to detect malingering and to obtain the information we require. Then let him relax, giving him reading that is easy to understand; injury due to overexertion will thus be avoided. For if these mental exercises overtax the patient's strength, they are no less harmful than passive exercise carried to excess.

And so after the reading let him see a stage performance. A mime is suitable if the patient's madness has not manifested itself in dejection; on the other hand, a composition depicting sadness or tragic error is suitable in cases of madness which involve childish playfulness. For the particular characteristic of a case of mental disturbance must be corrected by emphasizing the opposite quality, so that the mental condition, too, may attain the balanced state of health. And as the treatment proceeds, have the patient deliver discourses or speeches, as far as his strength permits. And in this case the speeches should all be arranged in the same way, the introduction to be delivered with a gentle voice, the narrative portions and proof more loudly and intensely, and the conclusion, again, in a subdued and kindly manner. This is in accordance with the precepts of those who have written on vocal exercise (Greek *anaphonesis*). An audience should be present, consisting of persons familiar to the patient; by according the speech favorable attention and praise, they will help relax the speaker's mind. And, in fact, any pleasant bodily exercise promotes the general health. Soon after the discourse or speech, the patient should be taken and gently anointed; he should then take a light walk for exercise.

Now if he is unacquainted with literature, give him problems appropriate to his particular craft, e.g., agricultural problems if he is a farmer, problems in navigation if he is a pilot. And if he is without any skill whatever, give him questions on commonplace matters, or let him play checkers. Such a game can exercise his mind, particularly if he plays with a more experienced opponent. . . .

Serve the patient varied food, as we indicated above in discussing epilepsy. Do not give him wine at first, but add some fruit to his diet to test the body. Afterward give him a small quantity of thin, mild wine at the time of eating. At first, the wine should be given at intervals of five days, and, as times goes on, at intervals of four, three, two, and then on alternate days; finally, it maybe be given every day. But water should be drunk in the intervals, the amount decreasing in proportion as the allotment of wine becomes more liberal.

Then, if the patient shows no new symptoms and has accustomed himself to the various parts of his regimen, change of climate should be prescribed. And if he is willing to hear discussion of philosophers, he should be afforded the opportunity. For by their words philosophers help to banish fear, sorrow, and wrath, and in so doing make no small contribution to the health of the body.

But if the disease persists and becomes chronic, being marked by attacks alternating with intervals of remission, relieve the attacks using the same remedies as those prescribed above for the initial attack of mania. But in the intervals of remission, prescribe, first, the restorative series of treatments including various types of passive exercise, vocal exercise arranged under supervision of a musician, walking, passive exercise, varied food, and the like. Follow this series with the metasyncritic cycle, as we have described it above.

From Soranus of Ephesus, "Madness or Insanity (Greek Mania)" in Caelius Aurelianus, *On Acute Diseases and on Chronic Diseases*, edited and translated by I. E. Drabkin (Chicago: University of Chicago Press, 1950), 535–559. Copyright 1950 by the University of Chicago. All rights reserved. Published 1950. Composed and printed by The University of Chicago Press, Chicago, Illinois, U.S.A.

Medieval and Early Modern Europe

Sarābiyūn Ibn Ibrāhīm, "Three Cases of Melancholia by Rufus of Ephesus"

(ca. 873 C.E.)

Rufus of Ephesus (first century C.E.) was an ancient physician who authored an influential two-volume work on the causes, symptoms, and treatment of melancholia. The work is lost and is now known only from citations in other works. But it was disseminated in Arabic translation throughout the Middle Ages. Rufus's method can be seen in the cases that are reproduced in the ninth-century Arabic textbook of Sarābiyūn Ibn Ibrāhīm. Among those who relied heavily on his understanding of the affliction was the famous Greek physician Galen. There is good evidence to suggest it was Rufus who was responsible for locating the seat of melancholia in the brain.

I knew another man, and he had pain between the ribs every year in the spring, without fever or inflammation but with stinging and pricking. Heat did not appear in the [affected] part. For this condition he used to have his blood let every year and take a purgative. He suffered from the illness between the autumnal equinox and the height of the heat in the spring,

47

when the disease would subside on account of the bleeding and the use of purgatives. When he thought that he did not benefit from the two [treatments], he gave them up. The pain returned for about a month and rose to his chest. Then, he had some blood let and took a purgative. The pain did not subside but extended to the side of his face; he felt it only on one side [of his face], and it affected his jaw for a while. When I feared that it might pass to his eye and brain and that it might kill him, I asked him to have his blood let and to take the purgative three times. Then, I cauterized his ribs where there was pain. The pain subsided completely. He had nothing to complain about for four days. On the fifth day he began to see phantoms before his eyes. I did not risk evacuation because his body was weakened. I prescribed for him a moist diet, so that the evacuation could take place easily if I had to resort to it. The phantoms remained for two more days. On the third day the symptoms of melancholia appeared, and all hope was given up for him, but I was sure that I had stopped the matter. These symptoms did not frighten me. I fed him with barley juice, rock fish, and bean soup for about thirty days. Because everything moistened his body, the symptoms of melancholia receded until he was completely recovered. The symptoms of melancholia were sadness and fear of death. Therefore, I prescribed for him entertainment and pleasure. He was over it in eighty days. The physicians were baffled by his recovery—how the matter was inclined toward the noble part of the body after being evacuated and, then, how the illness left him without any [further] evacuation. I showed them that it was a surplus of black bile that was blocked in some of his arteries. It had changed and had corrupted the blood in the arteries little by little. After we evacuated it, the quality persisted, but we had eliminated its source, so that it decreased gradually. When it reached the brain it had become quite weak. It found in the brain, however, a dry moist humor from the sadness and insomnia that the patient had suffered. Because of this, the rest became like dough; it was changed into black bile and caused melancholia. When we moistened his diet and removed his sadness, the damage ceased.

I know another man with whom melancholia began from the burning of the blood. He was a man of leisure. The anxiety and sorrow that he suffered were not great, for a little joy was mixed with them. The reason [for the melancholia] was his constant preoccupation with mathematical sciences. He was also a courtier. Because of these things, bilious matter collected in him at the age that it is customarily created, that is in the period of decline. Besides, he had a fiery temperament in his youth, so that as he advanced in age, black bile collected in him. He had fits mostly at night because of his insomnia and in the morning. When he slept at daybreak, he saw evil phantoms in his sleep because of lethargy (*subāt*) caused by the insomnia. He was treated by an inexperienced physician who evacuated him many times with strong emetics. He neglected the balance of his [patient's] temperament. The restoration of the temperament in diseases like these is the best treatment because the badness of the temperament produces such a humour as this one. The creation of the humour is not stopped except by the restitution of the temperament. When his temperament was agitated by these treatments, the burning in his body increased. His condition led to madness (*junūn*); he continued not to eat or drink until he died.

Another man who was 21 years old was rescued from drowning. He suffered from melancholia on account of the fear caused by it. A physician treated him with methods like the ones that have been described, i.e. repeated evacuation by means of emetics. In the end, [the doctor] evacuated him with black hellebore, but he didn't know any better. Then, another physician treated him by moistening, nourishment, and amusement. The man was rightly guided and recovered. His recovery was really due to both the doctors because the first physician evacuated the matter and the second corrected the temperament.

From Michael W. Dols, *Majnun: The Madman in Medieval Islamic Society*, edited by Diana E. Immisch (Oxford: Clarendon, 1992), 479–480. By permission of Oxford University Press.

Ibn Sīnā [Avicenna]

(ca. 980–1037)

"Lovesickness"

(first Latin translation, twelfth century)

The Persian philosopher and physician Ibn Sīnā—known in the Latin-speaking world as Avicenna—was one of the most esteemed thinkers of the medieval period. His renowned medical text, *Al-Qānuñ* (*The Canon*), was an attempt to harmonize Aristotelian philosophy with Galenic medicine, and it remained an essential medical text throughout the Middle East and Europe for centuries.

Among the topics Ibn Sīnā discussed was the ailment known as "lovesickness." A malady that can be traced back to ancient times, lovesickness was viewed as a potentially lethal affliction (Thomas, Archbishop of York, is purported to have died of it in 1114). The existence and disappearance of the diagnosis of lovesickness raises some interesting questions. As one historian has put it: "Was lovesickness real, simply to evolve into the erotomania of the Victorians? Is it the cause of stalking in our times? Or maybe even the source of fidelity and genuine sacrifice?"*

This is a delusionary (*waswāsī*) illness, which is similar to melancholia. The individual brought it about in his own psyche (*nafs*) by his obsession that overwhelmed his discretion about appearances and character. It helped him to attain his desire, or it did not. The characteristics of the illness are hollowness of the eyes and their dryness, the lack of moisture except when weeping, continuous movement of the eyelids, and laughing as if he sees something pleasant or hears happy news or jokes. His psyche is full of alienation and withdrawal, so that there is much deep sighing. His condition changes from exhilaration and laughter to sadness and weeping when he hears love poetry (*ghazal*), especially when he remembers the separation

---

*W. F. Bynum, "Lovesickness," *Lancet* 357 (2001): 403.

and distance from his beloved. All of his bodily parts are moist except the eyes; besides their hollowness, the eyelids are heavy because of insomnia and sighing. His behavior is disordered, and his pulse is irregular, like those who are anxious. His pulse and his condition change at the mention of the beloved (ma'shūq) especially and when he meets his beloved suddenly. It is possible, therefore, to learn the identity of the beloved person if the patient will not reveal it, and the knowledge of the beloved is the best way of treating the patient. The way of doing this is to mention many names repeatedly while the finger is kept on his pulse, and when it becomes very irregular and almost stops, you should then repeat the procedure. I have tried this method several times, and I have learned the name of the beloved. Then, in a similar manner, the lanes, houses, professions, crafts, families, and countries are mentioned, combining each of them with the name of the beloved, while you keep your hand on the pulse. When it changes at the mention of one thing several times, you will know from this method all the particulars of the beloved—the name, appearance, and occupation. We have tried this procedure and have discovered the useful information.

If you cannot find any cure except to unite the two in a manner that is permitted by religion and the law (sharī'a), do it. We have seen cases where health and strength were fully regained and the flesh restored. [In one instance] wasting had progressed and overcome a man; he had suffered severe chronic illness and prolonged fevers as the result of his bodily weakness that was caused by the strength of 'ishq. When he experienced union with his beloved, recovery occurred in a very short time. We were astonished at it and realized the subordination of the constitution (tabī'a) to mental delusions (awhām).

Treatment: You should consider whether his condition is attributable to the burning of the humor by the signs that you know; if so, you should evacuate. Then, concern yourself with moisturizing their bodies, lulling them to sleep, and nourishing them with good foods, and help them to preserve their equanimity in disputes, activities, and quarrels—matters that generally preoccupy men's minds. If that were done, it sometimes makes them forget what caused them to be seriously ill. Or you can deceive them by joining the lover with someone other than the beloved, whom the law permits; then, their thinking about the second person should be cut off before it grows stronger and after they have forgotten about the first. When the lover is a reasonable person, he can be given sincere advice and warning, as well as being ridiculed and rebuked. The image that he has within himself is nothing but a delusion and a kind of madness. Medical advice about it, as in this chapter, is useful, as well as the power of old women over it. For the women make the beloved hateful to him; they report the beloved's unclean conditions, and they tell him repulsive things about the one he loves, and they convey the beloved's considerable loathing for him. All of this is something that is very calming [for the lovesick]. If it were so, it may bring about other [benefits]. Among the useful things in this situation is for these old women to mimic the appearance of the beloved with ugly imitations and to present parts of the body in a shameful parody. They continue to do that and to speak about the beloved in great detail because it is their job. They are more proficient at it than men, except for the effeminate men whose skill is not inferior to that of the old women. They are also able to transfer gradually the lust (hawā) of the lover to someone other than the beloved. Then, they stop their actions before the second lust gains ground. Among the recommended activities are also the buying of slave-girls and the increase of sexual intercourse, acquiring new partners and taking pleasure in them. Some people are consoled with entertainment and recitation, while for others it only increases their infatuation; it is possible to discover which is which. Or hunting, different kinds of games, renewed patronage, and the company of important people—all of these ways bring consolation. Sometimes it is necessary that you arrange these things for those who suffer from melancholia, mania, and lycanthropy (qutrub) and that they are evacuated with strong laxatives (ayārjāt) and moistened with what has been said [in this section] on moisturizers. Therefore, if men are changed in their character and in the appearance of their bodies to resemble this [condition], you must concern yourself with moisturizing their bodies.

From Michael W. Dols, *Majnun: The Madman in Medieval Islamic Society*, edited by Diana E. Immisch (Oxford: Clarendon, 1992), 484–485. By permission of Oxford University Press.

Julian of Norwich
(1342–ca. 1416)
Revelations of Divine Love
(ca. 1390s)

Julian was a Christian mystic and anchoress in the English town of Norwich. As she later recounted in *Revelations of Divine Love*, while gravely ill in 1373, she began to have a series of visions of Jesus. These "shewings," as she referred to them, convinced her to dedicate herself to living a life aimed at spiritual perfection. To do this, she subsequently shut herself up in an isolated cell attached to what is now known as St. Julian's Church.

Experiences like Julian's and those of her contemporary Margery Kempe raise challenging questions about how societies and individuals differentiate between legitimate and illegitimate spiritual experiences. Does this constitute a case of "lovesickness" or does it, rather, simply represent an example of profound devotion? Like their ancient counterparts, observers during the second millennium C.E. frequently considered unusual or unconventional expressions of religious faith to be signs of insanity. This is not meant to say that Julian was, in fact, mad. Rather, it is important to consider Julian's case in relation to those of, for instance, Saul and Jesus in the ancient world or Daniel Paul Schreber or Thea H. (discussed later in this volume) in the modern period, in order to understand what makes a community consider an experience a case of religious transcendence or evidence of madness.

Chapter II

A simple creature unlettered.—
Which creature afore desired
three gifts of God

THESE Revelations were shewed to a simple creature unlettered, the year of our Lord 1373, the Thirteenth day of May. Which creature [had] afore desired three gifts of God. The First was mind of His Passion; the Second was bodily sickness in youth, at thirty years of age; the Third was to have of God's gift three wounds.

As to the First, methought I had some feeling in the Passion of Christ, but yet I desired more by the grace of God. Methought I would have been that time with Mary Magdalene, and with other that were Christ's lovers, and therefore I desired a bodily sight wherein I might have more knowledge of the bodily pains of our Saviour and of the compassion of our Lady and of all His true lovers that saw, that time, His pains. For I would be one of them and suffer with Him. Other sight nor shewing of God desired I never none, till the soul were disparted from the body. The cause of this petition was that after the shewing I should have the more true mind in the Passion of Christ.

The Second came to my mind with contrition; [I] freely desiring that sickness [to be] so hard as to death, that I might in that sickness receive all my rites of Holy Church, myself thinking that I should die, and that all creatures might suppose the same that saw me: for I would have no manner of comfort of earthly life. In this sickness I desired to have all manner of pains bodily and ghostly that I should have if I should die, (with all the dreads and tempests of the fiends) except the outpassing of the soul. And this I meant for [that] I would be purged, by the mercy of God, and afterward live more to the worship of God because of that sickness. And that for the more furthering in my death: for I desired to be soon with my God.

These two desires of the Passion and the sickness I desired with a condition, saying thus: *Lord, Thou knowest what I would,—if it be Thy will that I have it—; and if it be not Thy will, good Lord, be not displeased: for I will nought but as Thou wilt.*

For the Third [petition], by the grace of God and teaching of Holy Church I conceived a mighty desire to receive three wounds in my life: that is to say, the wound of very contrition, the wound of kind compassion, and the wound of steadfast longing toward God. And all this last petition I asked without any condition.

These two desires aforesaid passed from my mind, but the third dwelled with me continually.

Chapter III

I desired to suffer with Him

AND when I was thirty years old and a half, God sent me a bodily sickness, in which I lay three days and three nights; and on the fourth night I took all my rites of Holy Church, and weened not thought of, designed to have lived till day. And after this I languored forth two days and two nights, and on the third night I weened oftentimes to have passed; and so weened they that were with me.

And being in youth as yet, I thought it great sorrow to die;—but for nothing that was in earth that meliked to live for, nor for no pain that I had fear of: for I trusted in God of His mercy. But it was to have lived that I might have loved God better, and longer time, that I might have the more knowing and loving of God in bliss of Heaven. For methought all the time that I had lived here so little and so short in regard of that endless bliss,— I thought [it was as] nothing. Wherefore I thought: *Good Lord, may my living no longer be to Thy worship!* And I understood by my reason and by my feeling of my pains that I should die; and I assented fully with all the will of my heart to be at God's will.

Thus I dured till day, and by then my body was dead from the middle downwards, as to my feeling. Then was I minded to be set upright, backward leaning, with help,—for to have more freedom of my heart to be at God's will, and thinking on God while my life would last.

My Curate was sent for to be at my ending, and by that time when he came I had set my eyes, and might not speak. He set the Cross before my face and said: *I have brought thee the Image of thy Master and Saviour: look thereupon and comfort thee therewith.*

Methought I was well [as it was], for my eyes were set uprightward unto Heaven, where I trusted to come by the mercy of God; but nevertheless I assented to set my eyes on the face of the Crucifix, if I might; and so I did. For methought I might longer dure to look evenforth than right up.

After this my sight began to fail, and it was all dark about me in the chamber, as if it had been night, save in the Image of the Cross whereon I beheld a common light; and I wist not how. All that was away from the Cross was of horror to me, as if it had been greatly occupied by the fiends.

After this the upper part of my body began to die, so far forth that scarcely I had any feeling;—with shortness of breath.

And then I weened in sooth to have passed. And in this [moment] suddenly all my pain was taken from me, and I was as whole (and specially in the upper part of my body) as ever I was afore.

I marvelled at this sudden change; for methought it was a privy working of God, and not of nature. And yet by the feeling of this ease I trusted never the more to live; nor was the feeling of this ease any full ease unto me: for methought I had liefer have been delivered from this world.

Then came suddenly to my mind that I should desire the second wound of our Lord's gracious gift: that my body might be fulfilled with mind and feeling of His blessed Passion. For I would that His pains were my pains, with compassion and afterward longing to God. But in this I desired never bodily sight nor shewing of God, but compassion such as a kind soul might have with our Lord Jesus, that for love would be a mortal man: and therefore I desired to suffer with Him.

The First Revelation

Chapter IV

I saw . . . as it were in the time of His
Passion . . . And in the same Shewing
suddenly the Trinity filled my heart
with utmost joy

IN this [moment] suddenly I saw the red blood trickle down from under the Garland hot and freshly and right plenteously, as it were in the time of His Passion when the Garland of thorns was pressed on His blessed head who was both God and Man, the same that suffered thus for me. I conceived truly and mightily that it was Himself shewed it me, without any mean.

And in the same Shewing suddenly the Trinity fulfilled my heart most of joy. And so I understood it shall be in heaven without end to all that shall come there. For the Trinity is God: God is the Trinity; the Trinity is our Maker and Keeper, the Trinity is our everlasting love and everlasting joy and bliss, by our Lord Jesus Christ. And this was shewed in the First [Shewing] and in all: for where Jesus appeareth, the blessed Trinity is understood, as to my sight.

And I said: *Benedicite Domine!* This I said for reverence in my meaning, with mighty voice; and full greatly was astonied for wonder and marvel that

I had, that He that is so reverend and dreadful will be so homely with a sinful creature living in wretched flesh.

This [Shewing] I took for the time of my temptation,—for methought by the sufferance of God I should be tempted of fiends ere I died. Through this sight of the blessed Passion, with the Godhead that I saw in mine understanding, I knew well that *It* was strength enough for me, yea, and for all creatures living, against all the fiends of hell and ghostly temptation.

In this [Shewing] He brought our blessed Lady to my understanding. I saw her ghostly, in bodily likeness: a simple maid and a meek, young of age and little waxen above a child, in the stature that she was when she conceived. Also God shewed in part the wisdom and the truth of her soul: wherein I understood the reverent beholding in which she beheld her God and Maker, marvelling with great reverence that He would be born of her that was a simple creature of His making. And this wisdom and truth: knowing the greatness of her Maker and the littleness of herself that was made,—caused her to say full meekly to Gabriel: *Lo me, God's handmaid!* In this sight I understood soothly that she is more than all that God made beneath her in worthiness and grace; for above her is nothing that is made but the blessed Manhood Of Christ, as to my sight.

Chapter V

God, of Thy Goodness, give me
Thyself;—only in Thee I have all

IN this same time our Lord shewed me a spiritual sight of His homely loving. I saw that He is to us everything that is good and comfortable for us: He is our clothing that for love wrappeth us, claspeth us, and all encloseth us for tender love, that He may never leave us; being to us all-thing that is good, as to mine understanding.

Also in this He shewed me a little thing, the quantity of an hazel-nut, in the palm of my hand; and it was as round as a ball. I looked thereupon with eye of my understanding, and thought: What may this be? And it was answered generally thus: It is all that is made. I marvelled how it might last, for methought it might suddenly have fallen to naught for little[ness]. And I was answered in my understanding: It lasteth, and ever shall [last] for that God loveth it. And so All-thing hath the Being by the love of God.

In this Little Thing I saw three properties. The first is that God made it, the second is that God loveth it, the third, that God keepeth it. But what is to me verily the Maker, the Keeper, and the Lover,—I cannot tell; for till I am Substantially oned to Him, I may never have full rest nor very bliss: that is to say, till I be so fastened to Him, that there is right nought that is made betwixt my God and me.

It needeth us to have knowing of the littleness of creatures and to hold as nought all-thing that is made, for to love and have God that is unmade. For this is the cause why we be not all in ease of heart and soul: that we seek here rest in those things that are so little, wherein is no rest, and know not our God that is All-mighty, All-wise, All-good. For He is the Very Rest. God willeth to be known, and it pleaseth Him that we rest in Him; for all that is beneath Him sufficeth not us. And this is the cause why that no soul is rested till it is made nought as to all things that are made. When it is willingly made nought, for love, to have Him that is all, then is it able to receive spiritual rest.

Also our Lord God shewed that it is full great pleasance to Him that a helpless soul come to Him simply and plainly and homely. For this is the natural yearnings of the soul, by the touching of the Holy Ghost (as by the understanding that I have in this Shewing): *God, of Thy Goodness, give me Thyself: for Thou art enough to me, and I may nothing ask that is less that may be full worship to Thee; and if I ask anything that is less, ever me wanteth,—but only in Thee I have all.*

And these words are full lovely to the soul, and full near touch they the will of God and His Goodness. For His Goodness comprehendeth all His creatures and all His blessed works, and overpasseth without end. For He is the endlessness, and He hath made us only to Himself, and restored us by His blessed Passion, and keepeth us in His blessed love; and all this of His Goodness.

Chapter IX

If I look singularly to myself,
I am right nought

BECAUSE of the Shewing I am not good but if I love God the better: and in as much as ye love God the better, it is more to you than to me. I say not this to them that be wise, for they wot it well; but I say it to you that be simple, for ease and comfort: for we are all one in comfort. For truly it was not shewed me that God loved me better than the least soul that is in grace; for I am certain that there be many that never had Shewing nor sight but of the common teaching of Holy Church, that love God better than I. For if I look singularly to myself, I am right nought; but in [the] general [Body] I am, I hope, in oneness of charity with all mine even-Christians.

For in this oneness standeth the life of all mankind that shall be saved. For God is all that is good, as to my sight, and God hath made all that is made, and God loveth all that He hath made: and he that loveth generally all his even-Christians for God, he loveth all that is. For in mankind that shall be saved is comprehended all: that is to say, all that is made and the Maker of all. For in man is God, and God is in all. And I hope by the grace of God he that beholdeth it thus shall be truly taught and mightily comforted, if he needeth comfort.

I speak of them that shall be saved, for in this time God shewed me none other. But in all things I believe as Holy Church believeth, preacheth, and teacheth. For the Faith of Holy Church, the which I had aforehand understood and, as I hope, by the grace of God earnestly kept in use and custom, stood continually in my sight: [I] willing and meaning never to receive anything that might be contrary thereunto. And with this intent I beheld the Shewing with all my diligence: for in all this blessed Shewing I beheld it as one in God's meaning.

All this was shewed by three [ways]: that is to say, by bodily sight, and by word formed in mine understanding, and by spiritual sight. But the spiritual sight I cannot nor may not shew it as openly nor as fully as I would. But I trust in our Lord God Almighty that He shall of His goodness, and for your love, make you to take it more spiritually and more sweetly than I can or may tell it.

From Julian of Norwich, *Revelations of Divine Love* (Grand Rapids: Christian Classics Ethereal Library, 1901), 2–13.

Desiderius Erasmus
(ca. 1466–1536)

The Praise of Folly
(1511)

Erasmus was a Catholic theologian and writer and a key figure in the sixteenth-century scholarly movement known as humanism. His insistence that classical Greek and Roman teachings were vital in the quest for wisdom led him at times to be critical of the Church. Still, when Martin Luther (1483–1546) began contesting official doctrine, Erasmus remained steadfastly loyal to the Catholic faith.

Soon after arriving in England in 1509, Erasmus began writing *Moriae Encomium* (*The Praise of Folly*) while staying at the house of his good friend Thomas More (1478–1535). The text begins satirically, as Folly—in female voice—explains her origins and accomplishments. Later on, Erasmus turns his attention to what he considered to be some of the Church's failings. In the context of the history of madness, *The Praise of Folly* offers a chance to appreciate the broader cultural connotations of the terms folly and foolishness (in Latin, *stultitia* or *insania*), beyond the medical setting.

Of my name I have informed you, Sirs; what additional epithet to give you I know not, except you will be content with that of most foolish; for under what more proper appellation can the goddess Folly greet her devotees? But since there are few acquainted with my family and original, I will now give you some account of my extraction.

First then, my father was neither the chaos, nor hell, nor Saturn, nor Jupiter, nor any of those old, worn out, grandsire gods, but Plutus, the very same that, maugre Homer, Hesiod, nay, in spite of Jove himself, was the primary father of the universe; at whose alone beck, for all ages, religion and civil policy, have been successively undermined and re-established; by whose powerful influence war, peace, empire, debates, justice, magistracy, marriage, leagues, compacts, laws, arts, (I have almost run myself out of breath, but) in a word, all affairs of church and state, and business of private concern, are severally ordered and administered; without whose assistance all the Poets' gang of deities, nay, I may be so bold as to say the very majordomos of heaven, would either dwindle into nothing, or at least be confined to their respective homes without any ceremonies of devotional address: whoever he combats with as an enemy, nothing can be armour-proof against his assaults; and whosoever he sides with as a friend, may grapple at even hand with Jove, and all his bolts. Of such a father I may well brag; and he begot me, not of his brain, as Jupiter did the hag Pallas, but of a pretty young nymph, famed for wit no less than beauty: and this feat was not done amidst the embraces of dull nauseous wedlock, but what gave a greater gust to the pleasure, it was done at a stolen bout, as we may modestly phrase it. But to prevent your mistaking me, I would have you understand that my father was not that Plutus in Aristophanes, old, dry, withered, sapless and blind; but the same in his younger and brisker days, and when his veins were more impregnated, and the heat of his youth somewhat higher inflamed by a chirping cup of nectar, which for a whet to his lust he had just before drank very freely of at a merry-meeting of the gods. And now presuming you may be inquisitive after my birth-place (the quality of the place we are born in, being now looked upon as a main ingredient of gentility), I was born neither in the floating Delo's, nor on the frothy sea, nor in any of these privacies, where too forward mothers are wont to retire for an undiscovered delivery; but in the fortune islands, where all things grow without the toil of husbandry, wherein there is no drudgery, no distempers, no old age, where in the fields grow no daffodils, mallows, onions, pease, beans, or such kind of trash, but there give equal divertisement to our sight and smelling, rue, all-heal, bugloss, marjoram, herb of life, roses, violets, hyacinth, and such like fragrances as perfume the gardens of Adonis. And being born amongst these delights, I did not, like other infants, come crying into the world, but perked up, and laughed immediately in my mother's face. And there is no reason I should envy Jove for having a she-goat to his nurse, since I was more creditably suckled by two jolly nymphs; the name of the first drunkenness, one of Bacchus's offspring, the other ignorance, the daughter of Pan; both which you may here behold among several others of my train and attendants, whose particular names, if you would fain know, I will give you in short. This, who goes with a mincing gait, and holds up her head so high, is Self-Love. She that looks so spruce, and makes such a noise and bustle, is Flattery. That other, which sits hum-drum, as if she were half asleep, is called Forgetfulness. She that leans on her elbow, and sometimes yawningly stretches out her arms, is Laziness. This, that wears a plighted garland of flowers, and smells so perfumed, is Pleasure. The other, which appears in so smooth a skin, and pampered-up flesh, is Sensuality. She that stares so wildly, and rolls about her eyes, is Madness. As to those two gods whom you see playing among the lasses the name of the one is Intemperance, the other Sound Sleep. By the help and service of this retinue I bring all things under the verge of my power, lording it over the greatest kings and potentates.

You have now heard of my descent, my education, and my attendance; that I may not be taxed as presumptuous in borrowing the title of a goddess, I come now in the next place to acquaint you what obliging favours I everywhere bestow, and how largely my jurisdiction extends: for if, as one has ingenuously noted, to be a god is no other than to be a benefactor to mankind; and if they have been thought deservedly deified who have invented the use of wine, corn, or any other convenience for the well-being of mortals, why may not I justly bear the van among the whole troop of gods, who in all, and toward all, exert an unparalleled bounty and beneficence?

For instance, in the first place, what can be more dear and precious than life itself? And yet for this are none beholden, save to me alone. For it is neither the spear of throughly-begotten Pallas, nor the buckler of cloud-gathering Jove, that multiplies and propagates mankind: but that prime father of the universe, who at a displeasing nod makes heaven itself to tremble, he (I say) must lay aside his frightful ensigns of majesty, and put away that grim aspect wherewith he makes the other gods to quake, and, stage player-like, must lay aside his usual character, if he would do that, the doing whereof he cannot refrain from, i.e., getting of children. The next place to the gods is challenged by the Stoicks; but give me one as stoical as ill-nature can make him, and if I do not prevail on him to part with his beard, that bush of wisdom, (though no other ornament than what nature in more ample manner has given to goats,) yet at least he shall lay by his gravity, smooth up his brow, relinquish his rigid tenets, and in despite of prejudice become sensible of some passion in wanton sport and dallying. In a word, this dictator of wisdom shall be glad to take Folly for his diversion, if ever he would arrive to the honour of a father. And why should I not tell my story out? To proceed then: is it the head, the face, the breasts, the hands,

the ears, or other more comely parts, that serve for instruments of generation? I trow not, but it is that member of our body which is so odd and
uncouth as can scarce be mentioned without a smile. This part, I say, is that
fountain of life, from which originally spring all things in a truer sense than
from the elemental seminary. Add to this, what man would be so silly as to
run his head into the collar of a matrimonial noose, if (as wise men are wont
to do) he had before-hand duly considered the inconveniences of a wedded
life? Or indeed what woman would open her arms to receive the embraces
of a husband, if she did but forecast the pangs of child-birth, and the plague
of being a nurse? Since then you owe your birth to the bride-bed, and (what
was preparatory to that) the solemnizing of marriage to my waiting-woman
Madness, you cannot but acknowledge how much you are indebted to me.
Beside, those who had once dearly bought the experience of their folly,
would never re-engage themselves in the same entanglement by a second
match, if it were not occasioned by the forgetfulness of past dangers. And
Venus herself (whatever Lucretius pretends to the contrary), cannot deny,
but that without my assistance, her procreative power would prove weak
and ineffectual. It was from my sportive and tickling recreation that proceeded the old crabbed philosophers, and those who now supply their
stead, the mortified monks and friars; as also kings, priests, and popes, nay,
the whole tribe of poetic gods, who are at last grown so numerous, as in the
camp of heaven (though ne'er so spacious), to jostle for elbow room. But it
is not sufficient to have made it appear that I am the source and original of
all life, except I likewise shew that all the benefits of life are equally at my
disposal. And what are such? Why, can any one be said properly to live to
whom pleasure is denied? You will give me your assent; for there is none I
know among you so wise shall I say, or so silly, as to be of a contrary opinion. The Stoics indeed contemn, and pretend to banish pleasure; but this is
only a dissembling trick, and a putting the vulgar out of conceit with it, that
they may more quietly engross it to themselves: but I dare them now to
confess what one stage of life is not melancholy, dull, tiresome, tedious, and
uneasy, unless we spice it with pleasure, that hautgoust of Folly. Of the
truth whereof the never enough to be commended Sophocles is sufficient
authority, who gives me the highest character in that sentence of his,

To know nothing is the sweetest life.

Yet abating from this, let us examine the case more narrowly. Who
knows not that the first scene of infancy is far the most pleasant and

delightsome? What then is it in children that makes us so kiss, hug, and play with them, and that the bloodiest enemy can scarce have the heart to hurt them; but their ingredients of innocence and Folly, of which nature out of providence did purposely compound and blend their tender infancy, that by a frank return of pleasure they might make some sort of amends for their parents' trouble, and give in caution as it were for the discharge of a future education; the next advance from childhood is youth, and how favourably is this dealt with; how kind, courteous, and respectful are all to it? and how ready to become serviceable upon all occasions? And whence reaps it this happiness? Whence indeed, but from me only, by whose procurement it is furnished with little of wisdom, and so with the less of disquiet? And when once lads begin to grow up, and attempt to write man, their prettiness does then soon decay, their briskness flags, their humours stagnate, their jollity ceases, and their blood grows cold; and the farther they proceed in years, the more they grow backward in the enjoyment of themselves, till waspish old age comes on, a burden to itself as well as others, and that so heavy and oppressive, as none would bear the weight of, unless out of pity to their sufferings. I again intervene, and lend a helping-hand, assisting them at a dead lift, in the same method the poets feign their gods to succour dying men, by transforming them into new creatures, which I do by bringing them back, after they have one foot in the grave, to their infancy again; so as there is a great deal of truth couched in that old proverb, *Once an old man, and twice a child.* Now if any one be curious to understand what course I take to effect this alteration, my method is this: I bring them to my well of forgetfulness, (the fountain whereof is in the Fortunate Islands, and the river Lethe in hell but a small stream of it), and when they have there filled their bellies full, and washed down care, by the virtue and operation whereof they become young again. Ay, but (say you) they merely dote, and play the fool: why yes, this is what I mean by growing young again: for what else is it to be a child than to be a fool and an idiot? It is the being such that makes that age so acceptable: for who does not esteem it somewhat ominous to see a boy endowed with the discretion of a man, and therefore for the curbing of too forward parts we have a disparaging proverb, *Soon ripe, soon rotten?* And farther, who would keep company or have any thing to do with such an old blade, as, after the wear and harrowing of so many years should yet continue of as clear a head and sound a judgment as he had at any time been in his middle-age; and therefore it is great kindness of me that old men grow fools, since it is hereby only that they are freed from such vexations as would torment them if they were more wise; they can drink briskly, bear up stoutly, and lightly pass over such infirmities, as a far stronger constitution could scarce master. Sometime, with the old fellow in Plautus, they are brought back to their horn-book again, to learn to spell their fortune in love. Most wretched would they needs be if they had but wit enough to be sensible of their hard condition; but by my assistance, they carry off all well, and to their respec-tive friends approve themselves good, sociable, jolly companions. Thus Homer makes aged Nestor famed for a smooth oily-tongued orator, while the delivery of Achilles was but rough, harsh, and hesitant; and the same poet elsewhere tells us of old men that sate on the walls, and spake with a great deal of flourish and elegance. And in this point indeed they surpass and outgo children, who are pretty forward in a softly, innocent prattle, but otherwise are too much tongue-tied, and want the other's most acceptable embellishment of a perpetual talkativeness. Add to this, that old men love to be playing with children, and children delight as much in them, to ver-ify the proverb, that *Birds of a feather flock together*. And indeed what differ-ence can be discerned between them, but that the one is more furrowed with wrinkles, and has seen a little more of the world than the other? For otherwise their whitish hair, their want of teeth, their smallness of stature, their milk diet, their bald crowns, their prattling, their playing, their short memory, their heedlessness, and all their other endowments, exactly agree; and the more they advance in years, the nearer they come back to their cra-dle, till like children indeed, at last they depart the world, without any remorse at the loss of life, or sense of the pangs of death.

And now let any one compare the excellency of my metamorphosing power to that which Ovid attributes to the gods; their strange feats in some drunken passions we will omit for their credit sake, and instance only in such persons as they pretend great kindness for; these they transformed into trees, birds, insects, and sometimes serpents; but alas, their very change into somewhat else argues the destruction of what they were before; whereas I can restore the same numerical man to his pristine state of youth, health and strength; yea, what is more, if men would but so far consult their own interest, as to discard all thoughts of wisdom, and entirely resign themselves to my guidance and conduct, old age should be a paradox, and each man's years a perpetual spring. For look how your hard plodding students, by a close sedentary confinement to their books, grow mopish, pale, and meagre, as if, by a continual wrack of brains, and torture of invention, their veins were pumped dry, and their whole body squeezed sapless; whereas my followers are smooth, plump, and bucksome, and altogether as lusty as so many bacon-hogs, or sucking calves; never in their career of pleasure be arrested with old age, if they could but keep themselves untainted from the contagiousness of wisdom, with the leprosy whereof, if at any time they are infected, it is only for prevention, lest they should otherwise have been too happy.

For a more ample confirmation of the truth of what foregoes, it is on all sides confessed, that Folly is the best preservative of youth, and the most effectual antidote against age. And it is a never-failing observation made of the people of Brabant, that, contrary to the proverb of *Older and wiser*, the more ancient they grow, the more fools they are; and there is not any one country, whose inhabitants enjoy themselves better, and rub through the world with more ease and quiet. To these are nearly related, as well by affinity of customs, as of neighbourhood, my friends the Hollanders: mine I may well call them, for they stick so close and lovingly to me, that they are styled fools to a proverb, and yet scorn to be ashamed of their name. Well, let fond mortals go now in a needless quest of some Medea, Circe, Venus, or some enchanted fountain, for a restorative of age, whereas the accurate performance of this feat lies only within the ability of my art and skill.

It is I only who have the receipt of making that liquor wherewith Memnon's daughter lengthened out her grandfather's declining days: it is I that am that Venus, who so far restored the languishing Phaon, as to make Sappho fall deeply in love with his beauty. Mine are those herbs, mine those charms, that not only lure back swift time, when past and gone, but what is more to be admired, clip its wings, and prevent all farther flight. So then, if you will all agree to my verdict, that nothing is more desirable than the being young, nor any thing more loathed than contemptible old age, you must needs acknowledge it as an unrequitable obligation from me, for fencing off the one, and perpetuating the other.

From Desiderius Erasmus, *Erasmus in Praise of Folly, Illustrated with Many Curious Cuts, Designed, Drawn, and Etched by Hans Holbein, with Portrait, Life of Erasmus, and His Epistle Addressed to Sir Thomas More*, 8–22 (London: Reeves & Turner, 1876).

Robert Burton
(1577–1640)

The Anatomy of Melancholy
(1621)

The writer and Anglican clergyman Robert Burton led, by his own account, an inconspicuous, solitary life. His work *The Anatomy of Melancholy*, first published in 1621, went through four editions in his own lifetime and became one of the most cited discussions of the subject for centuries to come. Rather than being a clinical examination of melancholy, *The Anatomy* is really a collection of thoughts and reflections on the topic that had been passed down until the early seventeenth century. In this regard, Burton gives us a sense of the varied ways in which he and his contemporaries perceived melancholy as well as how melancholic experiences had been discussed over time.

Melancholy, What It Is

Melancholy, the subject of our present discourse, is either in disposition or habit. In disposition, is that transitory melancholy which goes and comes upon every small occasion of sorrow, need, sickness, trouble, fear, grief, passion, or perturbation of the mind, any manner of care, discontent, or thought, which causeth anguish, dulness, heaviness, and vexation of spirit, causing frowardness in us, or a dislike. In which equivocal and improper sense, we call him melancholy that is dull, sad, sour, lumpish, ill-disposed, solitary, any way moved, or displeased. And from these melancholy dispositions, no man living is free, no stoic, none so wise, none so happy, none so patient, so generous, so godly, so divine, that can vindicate himself; so well composed, but more or less, some time or other he feels the smart of it. Melancholy in this sense is the character of mortality. "Man that is born of a woman, is of short continuance, and full of trouble." Zeno, Cato, Socrates himself, whom Aelian so highly commends for a moderate temper, that "nothing could disturb him, but going out, and coming in, still Socrates kept the same serenity of countenance, what misery soever befel him," (if we may believe Plato his disciple) was much tormented with it. . . . No man can cure himself; the very gods had bitter pangs, and frequent passions, as their own poets put upon them. In general, "as the heaven, so is our life, sometimes fair, sometimes overcast, tempestuous, and serene; as in a rose, flowers and prickles; in the year itself, a temperate summer sometimes, a hard winter, a drought, and then again pleasant showers: so is our life intermixed with joys, hopes, fears, sorrows, calumnies": there is a succession of pleasure and pain. "Even in the midst of laughing there is sorrow" (as Solomon holds). . . . And it is most absurd and ridiculous for any mortal man to look for a perpetual tenure of happiness in this life. Nothing so prosperous and pleasant, but it hath some bitterness in it, some complaining, some grudging; it is all a mixed passion, and like a chequer table, black and white men, families, cities, have their falls and wanes; now trines, sextiles, then quartiles, and oppositions. We are not here as those angels, celestial powers and bodies, sun and moon, to finish our course without all offense, with such constancy to continue for so many ages: but subject to infirmities, miseries, interrupted, tossed and tumbled up and down, carried about with every small blast, often molested and disquieted upon each slender occasion, uncertain brittle, and so is all that we trust unto. "And he that knows not this is not armed to endure it, is not fit to live in this world (as one condoles our times), he knows not the condition of it, where with a reciprocality, pleasure and pain are still united, and succeed one another in a ring." Get thee gone hence if thou canst not brook it; there is no way to avoid it, but to arm thyself with patience, with magnanimity, to oppose thyself unto it, to suffer affliction as a good soldier of Christ; as Paul adviseth constantly to bear it. . . .

Symptoms, or Signs of Melancholy in the Body

Fear. Arculanus will have these symptoms to be definite, as indeed they are, varying according to the parties, "for scarce is there one of a thousand that dotes alike." Some few of greater note I will point at; and amongst the rest, fear and sorrow, which as they are frequent causes, so if they persevere long, according to Hippocrates and Galen's aphorisms, they are most assured signs, inseparable companions and characters of melancholy. Many fear death, and yet in a contrary humor, make away themselves. Some are afraid that heaven will fall on their heads: some they are damned, or shall be. They are troubled with scruples of consciences, disturbing God's mercies, think they shall go certainly to hell, the devil will have them, and make great lamentation. Fear of devils, death, that they shall be so sick of some such or such disease, ready to tremble at every object they shall die themselves forthwith, or that some of their dear friends or near allies are certainly dead; imminent danger, loss, disgrace, still torment others, etc.; that they are all glass, and therefore will suffer no man to come near them: that they are all cork, as light as feathers; others as heavy as lead; some are afraid their heads will fall off their shoulders, that they have frogs in their bellies, etc. Montanus speaks of one "that durst not walk alone from home, for fear he should swoon or die." A second "fears every man he meets will rob him, quarrel with him, or kill him." A third dares not venture to walk alone, for fear he should meet the devil, a thief, be sick; fears of all old women as witches, and every black dog or cat he sees suspecteth to be a devil, every person comes near him is malificiated, every creature, all intend to hurt him, to seek his ruin; another dares not go over a bridge, come near a pool, rock, steep hill, lie in a chamber where cross beams are, for fear he be tempted to hang, drown, or precipitate himself. If he be in a silent auditory, as at a sermon, he is afraid he shall speak aloud at unawares, something indecent, unfit to be said. If he be locked in a close room, he is afraid of being stifled for want of air. . . .

Suspicion, jealousy. Suspicion and jealousy are general symptoms: they are commonly distrustful, apt to mistake, and amplify, testy, pettish, peevish, and ready to snarl upon every small occasion. If they speak in jest, he takes it in good earnest. If they be not saluted, invited, consulted with, called to council, etc., or that any respect, small compliment, or ceremony be omitted, they think themselves neglected, and contemned; for a time that tortures them. If two walk together, discourse, whisper, jest, or tell a tale in general, he thinks presently they mean him, applies all to himself. Or if they talk with him, he is ready to misconstrue every word they speak, and interpret it to the worst; he cannot endure any man to look steadily on him, speak to him, laugh, jest, or be familiar, or hem, or point, cough, or spit, or make a noise sometimes, etc. He thinks they laugh or point at him, or do it in disgrace of him, circumvent him, contemn him; every man looks at him, he is pale, red, sweats for fear and anger, lest somebody should observe him. He works upon it, and long after this conceit of an abuse troubles him.

Inconstancy. Inconstant they are in all their actions, vertiginous, restless, unapt to resolve of any business, they will and will not, persuades to and fro upon every small occasion, or word spoke: and yet if once they be resolved, obstinate, hard to be reconciled. If they abhor, dislike, or distaste, once settled, though to be removed by odds, by no counsel, or persuasion to be removed. Yet in most things wavering, irresolute, unable to deliberate. Now prodigal, and then covetous, they do, and by and by repent them of that which they have done, so that both ways they are troubled, whether they do or do not, want or have, hit or miss, disquieted of all hands, soon weary, and still seeking changes, restless, I say, fickle, fugitive, they may not abide to tarry in one place long. . . .

Humorous. Humorous they are beyond all measure, sometimes profusely laughing, extraordinarily merry, and then again weeping without a cause (which is familiar with many gentlewomen), groaning, sighing, pensive, sad, almost distracted, they feign many absurdities, vain, void of reason: one supposeth himself to be a dog, cock, bear, horse, glass, butter, etc. He is a giant, a dwarf, as strong as an hundred men, a lord, duke, prince, etc. And if he be told he hath a stinking breath, a great nose, that he is sick, or inclined to such or such a disease, he believes it eftsoons, and peradventure by force of imagination will work it out. Many of them are immovable, and fixed in their conceits, others vary upon every object, heard or seen. If they see a stage-play, they run upon that a week after; if they hear music, or see dancing, they have nought but bagpipes in their brain; if they see a combat, they are all for arms. . . . This progress of melancholy you shall easily observe in them that have been so affected, they go smiling to themselves at first, at length they laugh out; at first solitary, at last they can endure no company: or if they do they are now dizzards, past sense and shame, quite moped, they care not what they say or do, all their actions, words, gestures, are furious or ridiculous. At first his mind is troubled, he doth not attend to what is said, if you tell him a tale, he cries at last, what said you? but in the end he mutters to himself as old women do many times, or old men when they sit alone, upon a sudden they laugh, whoop, halloo, or run away, and swear they see or hear players, devils, hobgoblins, ghosts, strike, or strut, etc, grow humorous in the end; he will dress himself and undress, careless at last, grows insensible, stupid, or mad. He howls like a wolf, barks

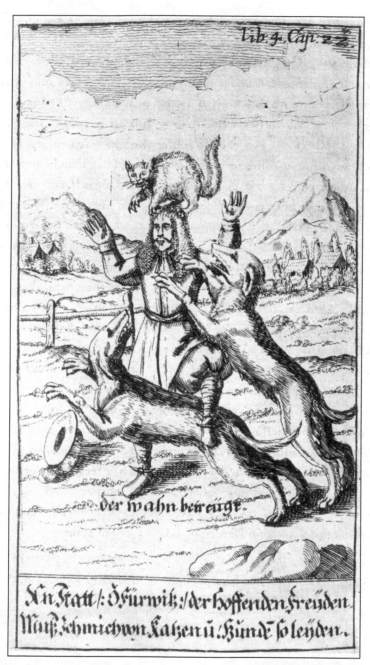

Madness Is Deceptive (1669). This is an illustration from *Der Abentheuerliche Simplicissimus, Teutsch* (*The Adventurous Simplicissimus*), written by Hans Jakob Christoffel von Grimmelshausen (1621–1676). The novel, based on Grimmelshausen's own life, chronicles the development of a child against the backdrop of the brutal Thirty Years' War (1618–1648). Nuremberg. Bibliothèque Nationale, Paris, France. © Snark/Art Resource, NY.

like a dog, and raves like Ajax and Orestes, hears music and outcries, which no man else hears. . . .

Solitariness. Most part they will scarce be compelled to do that which concerns them, though it be for their good, so diffident, so dull, of small or no compliment, unsociable, hard to be acquainted with, especially of strangers; they had rather write their minds than speak, and above all things love solitariness. Are they so solitary for pleasure (one asks) or pain? for both; yet I rather think for fear and sorrow. They delight in floods and waters, desert places, to walk alone in orchards, gardens, private walks, back lanes, averse from company, as Diogenes in his tub, or Timon Misanthropus, they abhor all companions at last, even their nearest acquaintances, and most familiar friends, for they have a conceit (I say) every man observes them, will deride, laugh to scorn, or misuse them, confining themselves therefore wholly to their private houses or chambers, they will diet themselves, feed and live alone. . . . But this and all precedent symptoms, are more or less apparent, as the humor is intended or remitted, hardly perceived in some, or not at all, most manifest in others. Childish in some, terrible in others; to be derided in one, pitied or admired in another; to him by fits, to a second continuate: and howsoever these symptoms be common and incident to all person, yet they are most remarkable, frequent, furious, and violent in melancholy men. To speak in a word, there is nothing so vain, absurd, ridiculous, extravagant, impossible, incredible, so monstrous a chimaera, so prodigious and strange, such as painters and poets durst not attempt, which they will not really fear, feign, suspect, and imagine unto themselves. . . . The tower of Babel never yielded such confusion of tongues, as the chaos of melancholy doth variety of symptoms.

From Robert Burton, *The Essential Anatomy of Melancholy* (Mineola, NY: Dover, 2002), 15–17, 97–108. With the generous permission of Dover Press.

John Brydall

(ca. 1635–ca. after 1705)

The Law Relating to Natural Fools, Mad-Folks, and Lunatick Persons

(1700)

John Brydall was a conservative Oxford-trained lawyer who wrote on a wide range of legal topics. In this commentary on English law, Brydall set about to summarize the contemporary legal status of those deemed to be mentally incompetent, that is, "idiots," "mad persons," "lunatics," and "drunken persons." Since English law was a form of customary law—meaning, it was based on historical practices rather than written statutes—Brydall relied on the writings and statements of jurists, medical observers, and the lay public to provide a kind of snapshot of how mental incompetence was seen at the time.

The Author to the Reader

Seeing there have been exposed to Publick View, a couple of Tracts, the one entituled, *The Woman's Lawyer*; and the other stiled, *The Infant's Lawyer*; I have been induced to [ ] a Publication of this perexiguous [ ]iece, and have named it, *The Law of Non Compos Mentis*:* It being no other than a Collection (methodically digested) of such Laws, with Cases, Opinions, and Resolutions, of our common Law Sages, as do properly concern the Rights of all such, as are wholly destitute of Reason: Some whereof are become so by a perpetual Infirmity, as *Idiots*, or *Fools Natural*: Some, who were once of good and sound Memory, but by the Visitation of God, are deprived of it, as Persons, in a high Degree, Distracted: Some, that have their lucid intervals, (sometimes in their Wits, sometimes Out) as Lunatick Persons: And some, who are made so by their own Default; as Persons overcome with

---

*Editor's note: *Non compos mentis* translates as "not having mastery of one's mind."

Drink, who during the time of their Drunkenness, are compared to Mad-Folks. All which Sorts of *Non Compos Mentis*, are the Subject Matter of the ensuing Sheets.

. . . Take no Pleasure in the Folly of an Idiot, nor in the Fancy of a Lunatick, nor in the Frenzy of a Drunkard; make them the Object of thy Pity, not of thy Pastime. When thou beholdest them, behold, how thou art beholding to Him, that suffered thee not to be like them. This wholsome Counsel of his, to embrace, will be look'd on as an Act of Prudence: But to reject it, will be such a piece of Folly, as will undoubtedly bring him, that shall be guilty of it, under the hard Sentence, of our old *English* Proverb, *Let him be begg'd for a Fool.*

Part the First. Of him that is an Idiot Born

SEC. I. AN IDIOT OR NATURAL FOOL, WHO.

Before a Description be given of an Idiot, that from his Nativity, by a perpetual Infirmity; is *Non Compos Mentis*, it will not be much amiss to give some Account of the first Original of the Word [*Idiot*]; *Idiota* or *Idiotes*, is a Greek Word, and properly signifies a private Man, who is not employed in any Publick Office. Amongst the Latines it is taken for illiterate or foolish; and hence in *Cicero*, and other good Authors, *Idiota* signifies commonly an unlearned and illiterate Person; In *Herodian*, he is said to be [ ] *qui rei alicujus est imperitus, ut* [ ]. But among the English Jurists, Idiot is a Term of Law, and taken for one that is wholly deprived of his Reason and Understanding from his Birth; and with us in our common Speech is called a *Fool Natural*; of whom there has been given a Description by several of our Law-Authors.

Master *Fitzherbert* describes an Idiot thus: *He who shall be said to be an Idiot from his Birth, is such a Person, who cannot account or number twenty pence, or cannot tell who is his Father or Mother, or how old he is, etc. So that it may appear that he hath no understanding of Reason, what shall be for his Profit, or what shall be his Loss.*

. . . An Idiot by Civilian *Swinbourn*, is thus described. *An Idiot, or a natural Fool is he, who notwithstanding he be of lawful Age, yet he is so witless that he cannot number to Twenty, nor can tell what Age he is of, nor knoweth who is his Father or Mother, nor is able to answer to any such easie Question; whereby it may plainly appear that he hath not reason to discern what is to his profit or* damage, though it be notorious, nor is apt to be informed or instructed by any other. . . .

SEC. II. OF THE REMARKS CONCERNING IDIOTS

I. If a person hath so much knowledge that he can read, or learn to read by Instruction and Information of others, or can measure an Ell of Cloth, or name the days of the Week, or beget a Child, Son or Daughter, or such like, whereby it may appear that he hath some light of Reason, then such a one is no Idiot naturally. . . .

II. An Idiot or Fool Natural, is uncapable of making a Testament; nor can he dispose of his Lands or Goods. . . .

IV. If a person be so very foolish, so very simple and sottish that he may be made believe things incredible or impossible, as that an Ass can fly, or that in old-times Trees did walk, Beasts and Birds could speak, as it is in *Aesop's Fables*; for he that is so foolish, cannot make a Testament because he hath not so much wit, as a Child of ten or eleven years old, who is therefore intestable, namely, for want of Judgment. . . .

VI. Notwithstanding all which, if it may appear by sufficient conjectures and circumstances, that such Idiots had the use of Reason and Understanding at such time as they did make their Testament, then are such Testaments good and valid in law [according to Godolphin]. . . . And yet (says the same *Godolphin*) if he be an Idiot indeed, albeit he may make a wise reasonable, and sensible Testament as to the matter of it, yet it will be void.

XIII. There is required in them who do contract Matrimony, a sound and whole Mind to consent; for he that is either an Ideot or Madman, without intermission of Fury cannot Marry. . . . This consent (saith *Amesius*) must be voluntary and free, else it's not esteemed a humane consent; and hence the consent of such as have not the use of Reason is no force to such a Contract. . . .

XVI. It appears in the old Books of Law, that it was expedient that Ideots should have a Curator or Tutor, or one that should take the charge of their Persons, Lands and Good, which Office since is devolved to the King, and made parcel of his Prerogative. . . . As *Fitzherbert* very well saith, in his *Natura Brevium*. The King is the Protector of all his Subjects, their Goods, Lands and Tenements, and therefore of such as cannot govern themselves. . . .

Part the Second. Of him who is by
Accident wholly deprived of his Wits.

SEC . I. THIS SORT OF <u>NON COMPOS MENTIS</u> HOW DESCRIBED.

He is said to be one, that was of good and sound Memory, and by the visitation of God, through some Sickness, Grief, or other Accident, utterly loseth his Memory and Understanding; and so falls into some high, or low degree of Fury or Madness. . . .

SEC . II. THE REMARKS CONCERNING MAD,
OR DISTRACTED PERSONS.

I. The true account of the Cause of Distraction is this: When the Animal Spirits, by some Accident or other, are so over-heated, that they become unserviceable to cold and sedate Reasoning; and then Reason being thus laid aside, Fancy gets the Ascendent, and *Phaeton*-like, drives on furiously, and inconsistently. This Combustion of the Spirits happens, sometimes by over-great Intention of the Mind, in long and constant Study; sometimes by a Fever, which inflaming the Blood, that communicates the *Incendium* to the Spirits, which take the Original from it; But most usually by the Rage and Violence of some of the Passions (whether Irascible, or Concupiscible, as they are wont to be distinguished) a Man setting his Heart vehemently upon some Object or other, the Spirits are set on fire, by the Violence of their own Motion; and in that Rage are not to be governed by Reason. This we have sad Examples of, in Love, in Grief, in Jealousie, in Wrath, and Vexation; and indeed, (saith my Author) *Bethlehem* is filled with the Instances.

II. By the Statute of *Praerogativa Regis*, the King of England is to provide, that the Lands of the Furor Men be safely kept, without waste; and that they, and their Families (if they have any) shall be maintained with the Profits thereof; and that the Residue be kept for their use, and delivered unto them, when they come to be of right Mind: So as their Land shall not be aliened, neither shall the King have any profit thereof to his own use: But if they die in such Estate, the Residue shall be distributed for their Souls, by the Advice of the Ordinary. . . .

VI. Tho' Furor, or Madness, hinders the contracting of Matrimony, yet it shall not take away that Marriage that is already contracted, as appears by the Civil and Canon Laws. . . .

Part the Third. Of the Lunatick having
sometime his Reason, and sometimes not.

SEC. I. THE DESCRIPTION OF A LUNATICK, AND THE WORD, WHENCE DERIVED

As for the Origination of the word *Lunaticus, Lunatick,* we are told, it comes
from *Luna,* the *Moon;* and so the Party is said to be Moon-sick. . . .

This Lunatick, according to the Law of *England,* is one, that hath sometime his Understanding, and sometime not. . . .

SEC. II. THE REMARKS CONCERNING LUNATICKS

I. . . . Those that are born during the Interlune, or Conjunction of the
Sun and Moon, are liable to the Disease of lunacy: For, according to the
Opinion of Star-Gazers, if the Moon be ill set, or placed, it causeth Men
to be subject, either to Convulsions, to Lunacy, or the Falling-sickness:
And concerning the last of these, Physicians have a Rule, viz. *They who
are troubled with the Fallingsickness, upon their good Days are not accounted
whole.* . . .

III. The King of *England,* by his Prerogative is *Summus Regni Custos,* and
hath the Custody of the Person, and Estates of such, as for want of Reason
and Understanding, cannot govern themselves, or manage their Estates; so
that the Persons and Estates of Lunaticks, are as well in the Custody of the
King, as of Idiots; but with this difference: That of Idiots to his own use,
and that of Lunaticks to the use of the next Heir. . . .

XX. A Mad-man or a Lunatick, may be imprisoned by another, to pre-
vent killing of him, or burning of his House, and justifiable. The Lord
Hobart says, That the necessity of avoiding greater Inconvenience, is a good
Plea in Law; as where one kills a Thief, or a Burglar, in defence of his Per-
son, or House; so also is the binding and beating of a Person Mad or
Lunatick. . . .

SEC. III. THE QUERIES WITH THEIR SOLUTIONS, RELATING TO LUNATICKS

I. Whether the Testament made by a Lunatick, during his mad Fits, be
valid in Law, when he is come to himself?

Solution: Such as are Lunaticks, can make no Testament, during the
time of their Furor, or Mad Fits; no, not so much as *adpios usus:* Nay, the

Testament made at such a time, shall not stand good, when the Madness is past. . . .

VI. Whether a Lunatick be punishable for hurting a Man?

Solution: If a Lunatick kill a Man, this is no felony; because Felony must be done, *Animo Felonico*; yet in Trespass, which tends only to give Damages; according to Hurt or Loss, it is not so: And therefore if a Lunatick hurt a Man, he shall be answerable in Trespass, and therefore no Man shall be excused in Trespass. . . .

Part the Fourth. Of Him that is Drunken.

SEC. I. A DRUNKEN MAN, HOW DESCRIBED.

The Fourth Sort of *Non sane Memories*, according to the Law of *England*, is he that is Drunk; one, that (not by the visitation of God, but) by his own vicious Act and Folly, is so overcome with Drink, that he is deprived, for a time, of the free Use and Exercise of his Reason and Understanding. . . .

SEC. II. REMARKS CONCERNING DRUNKENNESS, AND HIM THAT IS DRUNKEN.

III. That which we do, being Evil, is notwithstanding by so much the more pardonable, by how much the Exigence of so doing, or the Difficulty of doing otherwise is greater; unless the Necessity, or Difficulty, have originally risen from our selves; it is no Excuse therefore unto him, who being Drunk, committeth Incest, and alledgeth, that his Wits were not his own; inasmuch as himself might have chosen, whether his Wits should by that means have been taken from him. . . .

V. The Moralists in resolving the Quest, *Whether Ebriety can excuse, or extenuate a Fault*? do make a Distinction betwixt Actual, and Habitual Drunkenness: The former is, when any Man beside Intention, being ignorant as well of the Weakness of his Brain, as of the Strength of the Liquor, is overcome with it. The latter is, when a Man is delighted with it, and knowingly, and willingly, makes himself Drunk. That of Actual Drunkenness does, they say, somewhat excuse and extenuate the Fault; and consequently, there is allowed some mitigation of the Punishment: But that which is termed *Habitual Drunkenness*, does not at all excuse the Fault committed, nor mitigate the Punishment. . . .

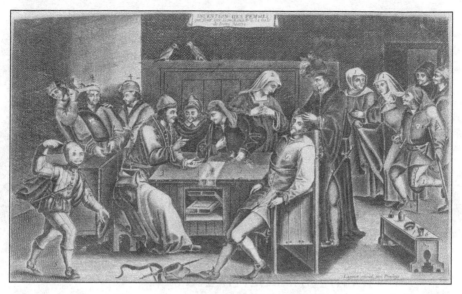

Laginet, *Allegory: Women Have the Stones of Folly Removed from Their Husbands' Heads.* The extraction of a stone from the head to cure folly was a common artistic motif dating back to at least the fifteenth century. There is no evidence to suggest that this operation was actually ever performed (although trepanation, or drilling into the skull, dates back to ancient times). Some medical and art historians contend that sham extractions like this were performed by charlatans, though there is no agreement on this point. Engraving, France, eighteenth century. © Snark/Art Resource, NY.

SEC. III. THE QUERIES WITH THEIR SOLUTIONS, RELATING TO HIM THAT IS DRUNKEN.

I. Whether a Man's Drunkenness can by any good Plea in the Courts at *Westminster,* either in Criminal, or Civil Acts?

Solution: The Judges, in *Beverley's Case,* tho' they have admitted a drunken Man to be, for the time, a *Non compos mentis*; yet have pronounced, that his Drunkenness shall not extenuate his Act, or Offence, not turn to his Avail, but it is a great Offence in it self, and therefore doth aggravate Offence, and doth not derogate from the thing he doth in that time, and that in Case as well touching his Life, as his Goods, Chattels, or Lands, or any other thing, concerning him. . . .

II. A Drunken Person, whether he may make a Testament?

He (saith *Swinburn*) that is overcome with Drink during the time of his Drunkenness, is compared to a Mad-man; and therefore, if he make his Testament at that time, it is void in Law: Which is to be understood, when he is so excessively drunk, that he is utterly deprived of the use of Reason and Understanding. Otherwise, if he be not clean spent, albeit his Understanding be obscured, and his Memory troubled, yet may he make his Testament being in that Case.

From John Brydall, *Non Compos Mentis; or, the Law Relating to Natural Fools, Mad-Folks, and Lunatick Persons Inquisited and Explained for Common Benefit* (London: Richard & Edward Aktins, 1700), A2–A3, 6–14, 52–56, 93–107, 119–124.

Hermann Boerhaave
(1668–1738)
"Aphorisms"
(1765)

Educated in both philosophy and medicine, Hermann Boerhaave was one of the most influential physicians of the eighteenth century. The son of a Dutch clergyman, he spent most of his life as a professor at the University of Leyden, teaching botany, chemistry, and medicine. In part, his influence resulted from his teaching students from across Europe, who, in turn, imported his ideas into their homelands. But his reputation was sealed by a number of textbooks he wrote in which he attempted to systematize the wealth of medical knowledge he had gained over the years. The following excerpts come from lengthy commentaries made by the physician Gerhard Freiherr van Swieten on Boerhaave's 1709 *Aphorisms on the Recognition and Treatment of Diseases.* (Note that Boerhaave's aphorisms are followed by Swieten's comments, which are indented below the former). The combination of aphorisms and commentaries provides an opportunity to see how Boerhaave's ideas were interpreted and expanded upon over the years.

Of the Melancholy-Madness

This distemper therefore arises from that malignant indisposition of the blood, which the ancients have termed atrabilis; and on the other hand, when the same distemper springs primarily from the mind affected, although the body be in health, it soon introduces a like atrabilis throughout the habit.*

We are taught by physiology, that man is compounded of two distinct beings, united one to the other; namely, the mind, and the body, which however different in their nature, do yet appear from undoubted observation to be so linked one to the other, that certain thoughts of the mind are ever united with determinate changes, or conditions of the body; and on the contrary the same, or the like thoughts, which spring up in the mind, without previous change of the body, are even able to produce, especially if they stay long in the intellect, the same, or a like change, and condition, as was excited in the will by those ideas which first impressed their force upon the body. And although any knowledge we have either of the body, or the mind, is insufficient to explain why these two, so very different beings, should thus mutually actuate and influence each other, and suffer from the other, yet we are no less certain, by experience, that this is truly matter of fact. . . . When a woman is seized with an hysterical fit, the stomach is often inflated, and intolerable uneasiness and anguish is thereby produced; and that again often renders the mind so sorrowful, that sometimes life itself is judged burdensome; but when the cramp of this convulsive malady is relaxed, the flatulences are expelled, the anguish goes off, and the mind recovers its former calm and serene state. But if the same woman shall be affected with some remarkable scandal or affront, she shall presently fall again into all like bodily complaints, although the thoughts of the mind only were first changed as the instrumental cause. So an inflammation only in the common membrane of the brain, turns the modest and beneficent person into a raving madness, from whence is urged to make fierce attacks upon every one that comes in his way. . . .

These particulars being first considered, it now remains for us to enquire how the atrabilis can be formed in the blood, and from what causes it may principally proceed.

---

*Editor's note: *Atrabilis* was another term used for black bile, thought to be a cause of melancholy.

If the more fluxile, or movable parts, are any way exhausted from the entire mass of blood, the more sluggish, or immoveable parts will be left in cohesion one with the other; whereupon the blood will become thick, black, oily, and gross, or earthy. But to the blood thus conditioned we shall give the name of an atrabiliary humour, or a melancholic juice.

The cause of which atrabiliary tenacity, may be every thing that expels the more moveable parts of our juices, and fixes the rest; such as a violent application of the mind, taken up both day and night almost upon one and the same object; too long continued wakefulness; violent passions, or commotions of the mind, whether cheerful or sorrowful; violent or laborious exercises of body, too long continued, especially in an air that is very hot and dry; to which add immoderate venery; foods that are austere, hard, dry, and earthy, taken for a long time under an idle or studious course of life, with drinks of the like sort; and hitherto also belong foods of the animal kind hardened by salting and drying in the air of smoak, and especially from old or tough animals, with crude or unripe fruits, mealy substances not fermented; medicines too astringent, coagulating, fixing, or cooling, slow poisons, and the like; ardent fevers, long continued, or often returning, or departing, without coming to a good crisis, and without the use of the proper diluents, &c. . . .

Now whenever this vice, or tenacity, springing from its respective causes, does as yet equally infest all the whole mass of the circulating juices, it becomes the author of certain complaints that immediately shew themselves to the observation; and among these principally are the following; the external and internal colour of the body appears first pale, then yellowish, brown, livid, or black, with spots on the same appearance; the pulse becomes slow, the chill, or coldness of the body is great, the breathing slow; the circulation through the red blood vessels continues laudable; but that through the pellucid or lateral vessels is not so free; from thence there follows a diminution of all the secretions and excretions of the humours, which make thus a more slow thick discharge; the fluids are less wasted, the appetite weakens, and the persons turn lean, sorrowful, and desirous of retirement, or solitude; the passions of the mind of every sort become very obstinate and intense; but in other matters the mind is indifferent, or unconcerned, while the body is sluggish, or lazy towards exercise; but yet they have an indefatigable constancy in their chosen labours and studies of every kind. . . .

As soon as the said melancholy shews itself by the leading signs, whether they be causes or effects, the mind is to be continually entertained with a variation of objects, while the patient is not made acquainted with your design; but for this such objects are to be chosen, as are commonly known to excite passions, or affections, in the patient, perfectly contrary to those that are at present known to prevail over him; sleep is to be reconciled to him by use of medicine that are diluent, sweetening, mitigative, and even stupifactive, or narcotic, together with silence; the air is to be rendered warm and moist. . . .

Of the Maniacal, or Raving-Madness

If the melancholy foregoing grows up to such a heighth, as to disturb or agitate the juices of the brain enough to throw the patient into violent ragings, the distemper is then called a *Mania*, or the raving-madness.

The raving madness therefore differs only in degree from the more sorrowful melancholy, of which it is the offspring; owing its birth to the same causes, and its cure generally to remedies almost of the like nature. . . .

But it is to be observed that by anatomical dissections the brain of such person has appeared hard, dry, and friable, with a yellowness in its cortext; but the vessels have been turgid, best with varices, and distended with a tough blood.

Moreover in this distemper almost all the excretions of the body are likewise put to a stand.

Here then, the throwing of the patient into the sea, and there keeping him under water as long as he can bear, makes the principal remedy.

In the cure of a melancholy at §1123, and the following, such remedies were recommended as by resolving or attentuating, inciting, and stimulating the atrabiliary matter into fusion, might remove its lodgments within the abdominal viscera, and cause it to be afterwards expelled from the body. But besides these remedies, such things were also recommended as might gradually change, and at length wholly efface, or at least so far weaken the common idea about which the mind is delirious, that it may not affect the common sensory more powerfully than other ideas that are received by the senses. . . . And therefore we see such numerous methods have been used by prudent physicians to change the present state or condition of the sensory, by disturbing the whole body with violent remedies and commotions. For this purpose hellebore, antimonial vomits, mercurials, and the like have been put in practice, not so much to operate by evacuations, as rather by disturbing the whole body to shake all the viscera and vessels, and by resolving all the humours, to change their present diseased state, than which nothing can be more miserable; since raving mad persons must, like wild beasts, be confined with chains, and imprisoned from the conversation of mankind. . . . But when all these methods have been found fruitless, the unhappy patient must be either left to his deplorable condition, or else plunging in the sea must be tried as the last remedy, that the patient being almost half-dead under-water, may have all ideas extinguished. The success observed from this practice by physicians in the cure of an *hydrophobia*, as we shall hereafter declare, seems to have been the occasion of their putting it in force upon persons desperately maniacal; and promiscuous experiences have taught the happy issue of it. . . .

The like remedy therefore seems applicable to the cure of a desperate mania or raving madness, since the patient's life is in no absolute danger; namely, that by effacing all the ideas for a short time, while there are no apparent signs of life, the latent indisposition of the common sensory, that is productive of the madness, may also be removed. For thus sometimes, rash, or "daring experiments recover those who are not within the compass of reasonable methods." . . . At the same time too it seems to appear from hence, that submersion in the sea is of no more importance towards this end, than the submersion that is made in any other water.

From Gerard Freiherr van Swieten, *The commentaries upon the aphorisms of Dr. Herman Boerhaave, . . . concerning the knowledge and cure of the several diseases incident to human bodies*, Vol. 11 (London: Printed for Robert Horsfield and Thomas Longman, 1765), 4–6, 12–13, 27–28, 41–42, 132–134, 138–145.

William Cullen

(1710–1790)

Lectures on the Materia Medica

(1773)

William Cullen was a Scottish chemist and physician. While serving as a professor of chemistry at Edinburgh University beginning in 1755, he also continued to have a private medical practice. In 1760–1761, he gave a series of lectures on the subject of *materia medica*, a Latin term referring to those substances with therapeutic properties in medicine (later known as *pharmacology*). Much to his exasperation, an unauthorized published version of his lectures began appearing in 1772. He was eventually convinced to authorize a reissue of the volume with corrections.

Cullen was part of an eighteenth-century scholarly movement that placed the human nervous system at the center of medicine. While Boerhaave and others continued to follow the humoral tradition of understanding the workings of the body in hydraulic terms, others such as Cullen, Friedrich Hoffmann (1660–1742), and John Brown (1735–1788) began the process of thinking about nerves as analogous to wires. Cullen is perhaps most famous for introducing the term *neurosis* to medicine.

Of all the plans of a Materia Medica, that of Boerhaave, in his posthumous book *De viribus Medicamentorum*, to me seems the best. There are, indeed, several mistakes in the introductory chapters of that performance, not to be attributed to him, as that book was printed from erroneous notes of his scholars. In imitation of Boerhaave, I shall begin with some physiological observations. I am more willing to do this, as I have some peculiar notions on this subject; and although this be no reason for thinking others in the wrong, yet it is a very good one for explaining them here, in order that, afterwards, I may be better understood.

First, we adopt this maxim, viz. *Medicamentum non agit in Cadaver*: because the operation of medicine does not depend on laws of matter and motion, but on the vital principle.* We must therefore enquire into these principles, but they run so much in a circle, that we do not know where to begin. The circulation, however, seems to be the vital principle on which the others depend. This leads me to examine into the cause of its motion, namely, the heart. Some have stopped here, and considered the body *entirely* as a hydraulic machine, without enquiring upon what *power* the contraction of the heart *depends*. But this is manifestly owing to some power, inherent in its muscular fibres, which disappear entirely soon after death. This then may be called a vital principle, which is independent of the fluids, as the contractile power continues after the fluids are taken away. This is not peculiar to the *heart*, but common to all the muscles and contractile membranes. This contractile power again is manifestly connected with nerves; for by tying or dividing a nerve, distributed to particular muscles, it entirely ceases in those muscles. All these nerves have a *common origin* from the medullary substance, and by this we see a manifest connection between the brain, medulla, spinalis, nerves, and moving fibres. To what extent this connection goes has been much disputed. There are some experiments where part of the brain is said to have been cut out, and the cranium stuffed with tow, part of the brain has been wasted, by wounds and abscesses, and the whole observed to be ossified, and, in all these cases, without great injury to the vital functions. None of these experiments are conclusive, as we are not sure but that some part of the medullary substance remained, sufficient to form a common origin to all the nerves. This common origin, which may be called *sensorium commune*, is connected with the soul. Here a dispute has arisen, concerning the nature of the soul, as to its materiality, or immateriality. The latter opinion is evident, from observing laws in the animal oeconomy absolutely incompatible with mere matter and motion. . . .

The communication between the common origin of the nerves, and sensible and moving fibres, seems to be kept up by something passing along the nerves, in the case of the *sensation* from the extremity to the *sensorium commune*, and in case of *motion*, from the latter to the former. This nervous power seems different from everything else in our body, and seems not

---

*Editor's note: *Medicamentum non agit in Cadaver* translates as "Medication does not work on cadavers."

peculiar to it, but a general principle in nature, particularly *modified* in our system. This may be easily understood from the nature of magnetism or electricity, which in this respect seem analogous to it.

For my part, I am not able to conceive, that a watery fluid, secreted by the nerves, is capable of performing the actions of the body; though I do not at all doubt, but that the brain secretes a fluid of considerable use. Our opinion, of a general principle operating upon our system by means of the nerves, is strengthened by what we observe in the vegetable kingdom; all plants being, in some degree, sensible and irritable. These principles in the vegetable oeconomy are equally difficult of solution with those in the animal, and seem to depend on the same principle.

We have now shewn, that in the fibres of animal bodies there is *sensibility* and *irritability*, on which the motion of their fluids depends. This vital power is intimately connected with the *sensorium commune*, and this with the soul, which certain is of use in the medical system, though by no means a rational conductor. The soul influences the body, not as a *prime mover*, but as a *modifier* of external sense. . . .

In the common system great stress is laid on the *laxity* and *rigidity* of the *simple* solid fibres. Although these properties are not altogether to be disregarded, yet there are few instances of any sudden changes in the simple fibres, but they seem to increase uniformly in *firmness*, as the person is advanced in age; and I have no idea of any disease in old people depending on their laxity. I believe, in general, that it is little in our power to change *their* laxity or rigidity; and that such changes ought to be imputed to an alteration in the *vital moving fibre*. Application of medicines, therefore, ought to be direct to this nervous power, and diseases, for the most part, deduced from it. . . .

Operation of medicines depends somewhat on their own nature, but as much on the particular modification of the system to which they are applied. Instead, therefore, of spending time in examining the different *figure* of the particles of medicine, their sharpness, oilyness, etc., it will be more useful to say somewhat on temperaments. Temperament is the general state of the system; idiosyncrasy the *peculiar* state of a *particular* part. The variety of temperaments is prodigious. The ancients have confined them to four, and we, through a blind attachment to antiquity, have made few farther advancements in this distinction. It would be difficult to enumerate all the different temperaments; I shall therefore consider, rather, the several particulars in the system that are apt to be varied in different constitutions, and whose varieties constitute diversity of temperaments. These particulars may be reduced to five: 1. The state of the simple solids. 2. The proportion of the fluids to the solids. 3. The state of the fluids. 4. The distribution of the fluids, i.e. of particular determination to this or that part of the system. 5. The state of the nervous power. . . .

Different state of the nervous power, with regard to sensibility, irritability, celerity, mobility, and strength. By sensibility we mean the different forces of impression necessary to move different persons: By irritability the extent of the sensation, e.g. two persons, on taking the same dose of an emetic, will be very differently affected. . . . Of the difference of sensibility we are able to judge but grossly, as it does not depend entirely on the degree of force impressed, but is greatly improveable by custom and practice, e.g. there may be two persons equally sensible to the smallest impressions of any sapid body on the tongue, and yet the one may be able only to distinguish green tea from bohea in infusion, while the other can not only tell a number of *different species* of the same kind of tea are employed in infusion, but also the different proportion in which the teas are employed. . . . Irritability must absolutely be connected with sensibility, as being both excited from the same cause; the one making us sensible of the *simple* impression, the other *propagating* the sensation over the body. Irritability is often connected with weakness of the nervous power; sensibility, more remarkably with its strength: Independent of the nervous power, irritability is also varied in proportion to greater or less tension of the moving fibres: The more accurately, therefore, the vessels are *filled*, the fibres will be more stretched, and the irritability greater.

Another particular, in which there may be a difference of nervous power, is in *mobility* or *celerity*, with which actions are excited. This may be different, even when the sensibility and irritability are the same, though it is generally connected with them, as mobility is greater in more sensible and irritable systems. Another variation of the nervous power is the *duration of impressions*. In some the effects of impression are transitory, and therefore the body is left open to new. This is called levity. In others these effects are longer of *duration*, and the motions excited are more steady. Lastly, the nervous power differs in strength. Some have supposed this to depend entirely on the state of the simple fibres, and, indeed, I allow, that it is often connected with it. But most of the changes of debility and strength are owing to a change in the nervous power. Thus, at the invasion of fevers, where we cannot suppose any change in the state of the simple fibres, we see often remarkable debility in performing the functions, connected also with an increased irritability. Again, in maniac persons there is often an incredible degree of strength exerted, which cannot possibly conceive to proceed from rigidity of simple fibres so suddenly produced. This strength of the nervous power is opposed to sensibility, as appears from a much stronger dose of any medicine required, to produce the same effect on the above-mentioned maniac than other persons.

From William Cullen, *Lectures on the Materia Medica* (New York: Classics of Medicine Library, Gryphon Editions, 1993), 2–8, 11–12.

PART II

The Age of Optimism

While ancient, medieval, and early modern healers were far from passive in their treatment of the mad, during this time there was a degree of acceptance that incurable madnesses were a fact of human existence, that the world would never rid itself of the affliction. This viewpoint began to be challenged, however, in the eighteenth century. The intellectual movement known as the Enlightenment (1730–1800)—stressing a faith in the inherent equality of men (while typically excluding women), the end of deference to traditional authorities, confidence in the power of reason, and trust in scientific and social progress—inspired generations of researchers, physicians, and policymakers to reconsider what they dismissed as their ancestors' ignorant fatalism. Over the course of the late eighteenth and into the nineteenth centuries, many expressed the buoyantly optimistic sentiment that not only could insanity be definitively understood, it could be cured. Not everyone shared this opinion, but it spurred scientific, medical, and institutional experimentation.

In the years 1770–1850, the catalysts of change were reform-minded asylum directors, who believed that the trade of "mad-doctoring" constituted its own worthy specialization. One of the earliest and most famous of the mad-doctors was the Englishman Francis Willis (1718–1807). Willis established a private lunatic retreat in Lincolnshire for an elite clientele, offering a regimen that stressed patient tranquility, subordination to authority, and self-control. Reports of his success led advisors to King George III (1760–1820)—who fell ill with a raving madness in 1788—to call on Willis to treat the monarch. Willis's direct appeal to the intellect and emotions of his charges encouraged others, such as William Tuke (1732–1822) and Philippe Pinel (1745–1826), to articulate what came to be known as the "moral treatment" of madness. In subsequent years, reformers on both sides of the Atlantic drew on the example of the moral treatment to demand what they considered to be a more holistic and humane approach to insanity.

Although the first institutions of confinement for the insane were constructed between 1400 and 1800, it was only over the course of the nineteenth century that large, public asylums were built throughout Europe and the United States. The years 1820–1870 in particular witnessed a surge in asylum building. Whereas in 1800 only a small number of individuals were housed in asylums, by the end of the century, France had more than one hundred separate facilities, Germany could boast of having two hundred state asylums along with another two hundred private institutions, and the city of London alone had sixteen asylums to call on. Historians have not agreed on the reasons for this spurt. Was it because societies were responding to an actual increase in mental disorders caused by modernization? Or was it a function of the fact that states were becoming more intolerant of disruptive behavior? Or might it have more to do with the growing professional power of physicians and alienists (as mad-doctors were often referred to by this time)?

Whatever the reasons for the growth, the nineteenth century created a new image for both patient and physician, associating the madman and the alienist with the specter of the asylum or madhouse. The fact that asylums were often imposing structures and deliberately placed outside residential areas only fed the popular imagination. Lurid tales were told of horrible abuses there, and curious sightseers found opportunities to visit facility buildings and grounds in hopes of catching a glimpse of raving residents.

At the same time that asylums were being built, other developments were under way that quickly changed how insanity and its treatment were viewed. The proliferation of specialized scientific disciplines around 1800 and the increasing reliance of scholars on material explanations encouraged the growth of laboratory research. Nowhere was this trend more apparent than in Germany, where university-based institutes and clinics became hubs for experimental research and student instruction by the last quarter of the century. The rise there of university psychiatric clinics—set in urban environments and intended for the study of a large variety of short-term patients with acute symptoms—encouraged a shift in professional power within psychiatry away from alienists and toward researcher practitioners.

The impact of experimental methods on the study of human physiology, and especially the central nervous system, was profound. What began with phrenology during the first half of the nineteenth century became the professionalized discipline of neurology. By the 1880s, neurology's claims about the integrated nature of the central nervous system, the key role played by nerve cells, and the importance of the reflex provided a new model for understanding insanity. Seen from this perspective, madness was not a form of mental alienation, but rather represented a nervous or brain pathology.

The scientific emphasis on nerves contributed to the popular nineteenth-century belief that nervousness and nervous disorders were rampant. Talk was of having "strong" or "weak" nerves, of buckling under the pressures of modern life and suffering "shattered nerves," a "nervous collapse," or "nervous exhaustion" or having a "nervous breakdown." The symptoms of the nervous breakdown—typically, a sense of emptiness and hopelessness, obsessive thoughts and anxieties, sluggishness, and a generalized indifference—reveal the extent to which both professionals and the lay public had come to think of the human body electrically, as a kind of machine propelled by a fund of nervous energy that, if one were not careful, could be dangerously depleted. The fact that so many of those who complained of having nervous ailments showed no signs of an organic lesion did not dissuade belief in their existence. Instead, physicians simply categorized them as "functional illnesses," requiring alternative or future explanation.

Enlightenment, Romanticism, and Reform

Philippe Pinel
(1745–1826)

A Treatise on Insanity
(1801)

In overturning the old, feudal order, the French Revolution (1789–1799) opened up leadership positions to a new class and generation of eager men and women schooled in Enlightenment thought. One such individual was the physician Philippe Pinel. Born into a family of doctors, Pinel had long criticized the traditional Paris Faculty of Medicine for being insular and elitist, and he had been unafraid of expressing his reformist ideas and leanings. After the revolution, as the new government began reorganizing hospitals, poorhouses, prisons, and schools, Pinel was recruited, in 1792, to serve as chief physician at the Bicêtre Hospital in Paris, then asked a few years later to become director of the Salpêtrière asylum. In both facilities, he set about establishing what contemporaries were calling "the moral treatment." As the famous painting by Charles Muller shows, the changes Pinel instituted at Bicêtre were heralded as an emblem of enlightened Reason's triumph over a backward Old Regime.

Nothing has more contributed to the rapid improvement of modern natural history, than the spirit of minute and accurate observation which has

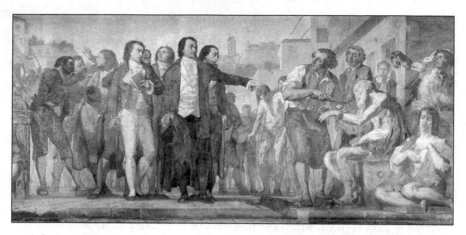

Philippe Pinel has the irons removed from the insane at Bicêtre. Mural by
Charles Louis Muller (1815–1892). Académie de Médecine, Paris, France.
© Bridgeman-Giraudon/Art Resource, NY.

distinguished its votaries. The habit of analytical investigation, thus
adopted, has induced an accuracy of expression and a propriety of classification, which have themselves, in no small degree, contributed to the
advancement of natural knowledge. Convinced of the essential of the
same means in the illustration of a subject so new and so difficult as that
of the present work, it will be seen that I have availed myself of their application, in all or most of the instances of this most calamitous disease,
which occurred in my practice at the Asylum de Bicêtre. On my entrance
upon the duties of that hospital, every thing presented to me the appearance of chaos and confusion. Some of my unfortunate patients laboured
under the horrors of a most gloomy and desponding melancholy. Others
were furious, and subject to the influence of a perpetual delirium. Some
appeared to possess a correct judgment upon most subjects, but were
occasionally agitated by violent sallies of maniacal fury; while those of
another class were sunk into a state of stupid ideotism and imbecility.
Symptoms so different, and all comprehended under the general title of
insanity, required, on my part, much study and discrimination; and to
secure order in the establishment and success to the practice, I determined upon adopting such a variety of measures, both as to discipline and
treatment, as my patients required, and my limited opportunity permitted. From systems of nosology, I had little assistance to expect; since the
arbitrary distributions of Sauvages and Cullen were better calculated to

impress the conviction of their insufficiency than to simplify my labour. I, therefore, resolved to adopt that method of investigation which has invariably succeeded in all the departments of natural history, viz. to notice successively every fact, without any other object than that of collecting materials for future use; and to endeavour, as far as possible, to divest myself of the influence, both of my own prepossessions and the authority of others. With this view, I first of all took a general statement of the symptoms of my patients. To ascertain their characteristic peculiarities, the above survey was followed by cautious and repeated examinations into the condition of the individuals. All our new cases were entered at great length upon the journals of the house. Due attention was paid to the changes of the seasons and the weather, and their respective influences upon the patients were minutely noticed. Having a peculiar attachment for the more general method of descriptive history, I did not confine myself to any exclusive mode of arranging my observations, nor to any one system of nosography. The facts which I have thus collected are now submitted to the consideration of the public, in the form of a regular treatise.

Few subjects in medicine are so intimately connected with the history and philosophy of the human mind as insanity. There are still fewer, where there are so many errors to rectify, and so many prejudices to remove. Derangement of the understanding is generally considered as an effect of an organic lesion of the brain, consequently as incurable; a supposition that is, in a great number of instances, contrary to anatomical fact. Public asylums for maniacs have been regarded as places of confinement for such of its members as are become dangerous to the peace of society. The managers of those institutions, who are frequently men of little knowledge and less humanity, have been permitted to exercise towards their innocent prisoners a most arbitrary system of cruelty and violence; while experience affords ample and daily proofs of the happier effect of a mild, conciliating treatment, rendered effective by steady and dispassionate firmness. Availing themselves of this consideration, many empirics have erected establishments for the reception of lunatics, and have practiced this very delicate branch of the healing heart with singular reputation. A great number of cures have undoubtedly been effected by those base born children of the profession; but, as might be expected, they have not in any degree contributed to the advancement of science by any valuable writings. It is on the other hand to be lamented, that regular physicians have indulged in a blind routine of inefficient treatment, and have allowed themselves to be confined within the fairy circle of antiphlogisticism, and by that means to be diverted from the more important management of the mind. Thus, too generally, has the philosophy of this disease, by which I mean the history of its symptoms, of its progress, of its varieties, and of its treatment in and out of hospitals, been most strangely neglected.

. . . The successful application of moral regimen exclusively, gives weight to the supposition, that, in a majority of instances, there is no organic lesion of the brain nor of the cranium. In order however to ascertain the species, and to establish a nosology of insanity, so far as it depends upon physical derangement, I have omitted no opportunities of examination after death. . . . By these and other means, which will be developed in the sequel, I have been enabled to introduce a degree of method into the service of the hospital, and to class my patients in a great measure according to the varieties and inveteracy of their complaints. . . .

Periodical Insanity Independent of the Influence of the Seasons

. . . From a general examination of the patients, at the Asylum of Bicêtre, in the second year of the republic, which was undertaken for the purpose of ascertaining the relative number of each variety of the disease; it appeared, that, out of two hundred maniacs, there were fifty-two of the class subject to paroxysms of insanity at irregular periods; and only six, whose periods of accession observed a regular intermission. . . . I shall be excused, if I mention three more cases, whose paroxysms invariably returned after an interval of eighteen months, and lasted precisely six months. The peculiar character of those unfortunate cases consisted in a few but well marked circumstances. Their ideas were clear and connected;—as they indulged in no extravagances of fancy;—they answered with great pertinence and precision to the questions that were proposed to them: but they were under the dominion of a most ungovernable fury, and of a thirst equally ungovernable for deeds of blood. In the mean time, they were fully aware of their horrid propensity, but absolutely incapable, without coercive assistance, of suppressing the atrocious impulse. How are we to reconcile these facts to the opinion which Locke and Condillac entertained with regard to the nature of insanity, which they made to consist exclusively in a disposition to associate ideas naturally incompatible, and to mistake ideas thus associated for real truths?

The Character of Maniacal Paroxysms Not Depending upon the Nature of the Exciting Causes, but upon the Constitution

. . . I cannot here avoid giving my most decided suffrage in favour of the moral qualities of maniacs. I have no where met, excepting in romances, with fonder husbands, more affectionate parents, more impassioned lovers, more pure and exalted patriots, than in the lunatic asylum, during their intervals of calmness and reason. A man of sensibility may go there every day of his life, and witness scenes of indescribable tenderness associated to a most estimable virtue.

Maniacal Paroxysms Characterised by a High Degree of Physical and Mental Energy

It is to be hoped, that the science of medicine will one day proscribe the very vague and inaccurate expression of "images traced in the brain, the unequal determination of blood into different parts of this viscus, the irregular movements of the animal spirits," &c. expressions which are to be met with in the best writings that have appeared on the human understanding, but which do not accord with the origin, the causes, and the history of insanity. The nervous excitement, which characterises the greatest number of cases, affects not the system physically by increasing muscular power and action only, but likewise the mind, by exciting a consciousness of supreme importance and irresistible strength. Entertaining a high opinion of his capacity of resistance, a maniac often indulges in the most extravagant flights of fancy and caprice; and, upon attempts being made to repress or coerce him, aims furious blows at his keeper, and wages war against as many of the servants or attendants as he supposes he can well master. If met, however, by a force evidently and convincingly superior, he submits without opposition or violence. This is a great and invaluable secret in the management of well regulated hospitals. I have known it prevent many fatal accidents, and contribute greatly toward the cure of insanity. I have, however, seen the nervous excitement in question, in some few instances, become extremely obstinate and incoercible.

The Variety and Profundity of Knowledge Requisite on the Part of
the Physician, in Order to Secure Success in the Treatment of Insanity

The time, perhaps, is at length arrived when medicine in France, now lib-
erated from the fetters imposed upon it, by the prejudices of custom, by
interested ambition, by its association with religious institutions, and by
the discredit in which it has been held in the public estimation, will be able
to assume its proper dignity, to establish its theories on facts alone, to gen-
eralise those facts, and to maintain its level with the other departments of
natural history. The principles of free enquiry, which the revolution has
incorporated with our national politics, have opened a wide field to the
energies of medical philosophy. But, it is chiefly in great hospitals and asylums, that those advantages will be immediately felt, from the opportunities
which are there afforded of making a great number of observations, experiments, and comparisons. . . .

The Author's Inducements to Study the Principles of Moral Treatment

About that time I was engaged to attend, in a professional capacity, at an
asylum, where I made observations upon this disease [insanity] for five successive years. My opportunities for the application of moral remedies, were,
however, not numerous. Having no part of the management of the interior
police of that institution, I had little or no influence over its servants. The
person who was at the head of the establishment, had no interest in the
cure of his wealthy patients, and he often, unequivocally, betrayed a desire,
that every remedy should fail. At other times, he placed exclusive confidence in the utility of bathing or in the efficacy of petty and frivolous
recipes. The administration of the civil hospitals, in Paris, opened to me in
the second year of the republic a wide field of research, by my nomination
to the office of chief physician to the national Asylum de Bicêtre, which I
continued to fill for two years. In order, in some degree, to make up for the
local disadvantages of the hospital, and the numerous inconveniences
which arose from the instability and successive changes of administration,
I determined to turn my attention, almost exclusively, to the subject of
moral treatment. The hall and the passages of the hospital were much confined, and so arranged as to render the cold of winter and the heat of summer equally intolerable and injurious. The chambers were exceedingly

small and inconvenient. Baths we had none, though I made repeated applications for them; nor had we extensive liberties for walking, gardening or other exercises. So destitute of accommodation, we found it impossible to class our patients according to the varieties and degrees of their respective maladies. On the other hand, the gentleman, to whom was committed the chief management of the hospital, exercised towards all that were placed under his protection, the vigilance of a kind and affectionate parent.* Accustomed to reflect, and possessed of great experience, he was not deficient either in the knowledge or execution of the duties of his office. He never lost sight of the principles of a most genuine philanthropy. He paid great attention to the diet of the house, and left no opportunity for murmur or discontent on the part of the fastidious. He exercised a strict discipline over the conduct of the domestics, and punished, with severity, every instance of ill treatment, and every act of violence, of which they were guilty towards those whom it was merely their duty to serve. He was both esteemed and feared by every maniac; for he was mild, and at the same time inflexibly firm. In a word, he was master of every branch of his art, from its simplest to its most complicated principles. Thus was I introduced to a man, whose friendship was an invaluable acquisition to me. . . .

The Advantages of Restraint upon
the Imagination of Maniacs Illustrated

A young religious enthusiast, who was exceedingly affected by the abolition of the catholic religion in France, became insane. After the usual treatment at the Hotel Dieu, he was transferred to the Asylum de Bicêtre.[†] His misanthropy was not to be equaled. His thoughts dwelled perpetually upon the torments of the other world; from which he founded his only chance of escaping, upon conscientious adoption of the abstinences and mortifications of the ancient anchorites. At length, he refused nourishment altogether; and on the fourth day after that unfortunate resolution was formed, a state of langour succeeded, which excited considerable apprehension for

---

*Editor's note: This was Jean-Baptiste Pussin (1745–1811), a tanner who himself had been a scrofula patient in the Bicêtre Asylum in 1771 and was later cured. He was thereafter employed by the hospital, and in 1784, he became the superintendent of the ward for incurable mental patients.

[†]Editor's note: Hôtel-Dieu is one of the oldest hospitals in Paris.

his life. Kind remonstrances and pressing invitations proved equally ineffectual. He repelled, with rudeness, the services of the attendants, rejected, with the utmost pernacity, some soup that was placed before him, and demolished his bed (which was of straw) in order that he might lie upon the boards. How was such a perverse train of ideas to be stemmed or counteracted? The excitement of terror presented itself as the only resource. For this purpose, Citizen Pussin appeared one night at the door of his chamber, and, with fire darting from his eyes, and thunder in his voice, commanded a group of domestics, who were armed with strong and loudly clanking chains, to do their duty. But the ceremony was artfully suspended;—the soup was placed before the maniac, and strict orders were left him to eat it in the course of the night, on pains of the severest punishment. He was left to his own reflections. The night was spent (as he afterwards informed me) in a state of most distressing hesitation, whether to incur the present punishment, or the distant but still more dreadful torments of the world to come. After an internal struggle of many hours, the idea of the present evil gained the ascendancy; and he determined to take the soup. From that time he submitted, without difficulty, to a restorative system of regimen. His sleep and strength gradually returned; his reason recovered its empire; and, after the manner above related, he escaped certain death. It was during his convalescence, that he mentioned to me the perplexities and agitations which he endured during the night of the experiment.

A Happy Expedient Employed in the Cure of a Mechanician

A celebrated watchmaker, at Paris, was infatuated with the chimera of perpetual motion, and to effect this discovery, he set to work with indefatigable ardour. From unremitting attention to the object of his enthusiasm coinciding with the influence of revolutionary disturbances, his imagination was greatly heated, his sleep was interrupted, and, at length, a complete mental derangement of the understanding took place. His case was marked by a most whimsical illusion of the imagination. He fancied that he had lost his head on the scaffold; that it had been thrown promiscuously among the heads of many other victims; that the judges, having repented of their cruel sentences, had ordered those heads to be restored to their respective owners, and placed upon their respective shoulders; but that, in consequence of an unfortunate mistake, the gentlemen, who had the management of that business, had placed upon his shoulder the head of one of his unhappy companions. The idea of this whimsical exchange of his head, occupied his thoughts night and day; which determined his relations to send him to the Hotel Dieu. Thence he was transferred to the Asylum de Bicêtre. Nothing could equal the extravagant overflowings of his heated brain. He sung, cried, or danced incessantly; and, as there appeared no propensity in him to commit acts of violence or disturbance, he was always allowed to go about the hospital without control, in order to expend, by evaporation, the effervescent excess of his spirits. "Look at these teeth," he constantly cried,— "Mine were exceedingly handsome;—these are rotten and decayed. My mouth was sound and healthy: this is foul and diseased. What difference between this hair and that of my own head. . . ."

A keen and unanswerable stroke of pleasantry seemed best adapted to correct this fantastic whim. Another convalescent of a gay and facetious humour, instructed in the part he should play in this comedy, adroitly turned the conversation to the subject of the famous miracle of Saint Denis.* Our mechanician strongly maintained the possibility of the fact, and sought to confirm it by an application of his own case. The other set up a loud laugh, and replied with a tone of the keenest ridicule: "Madman as thou art, how could Saint Denis kiss his own head? Was it with his heels?" This equally unexpected and unanswerable retort, forcibly struck the maniac. He retired confused amidst the peals of laughter, which were provoked at his expense, and never afterwards mentioned the exchange of his head. Close attention to his trade for some months, completed the restoration of his intellect. He was sent to his family in perfect health; and has, now for more than five years, pursued his business without a return of his complaint.

Maniacal Fury to be Repressed; but Not by Cruel Treatment

The lesions of the human intellect simply, embrace but part of the object of the present treatise. The active faculties of the mind are not less subject to serious lesions and changes, nor less deserving of ample consideration. The

---

*Editor's note: Saint Denis was a third-century Christian martyr and bishop of Paris. As legend has it, after Saint Denis was beheaded by opponents, he picked up his own head and continued to preach for several miles.

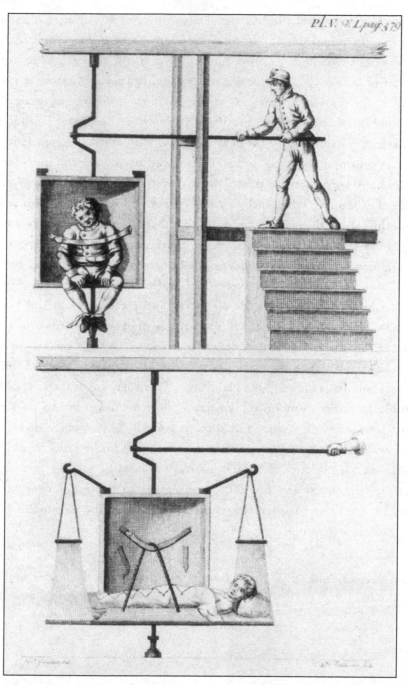

Two views of circulating swings for treating insanity. Devices like these were often used to calm acutely agitated patients. From William Saunders Hallaran, *Practical Observations of the Causes and Cure of Insanity* (Cork: Edwards and Savage, 1818), 95. Courtesy of the National Library of Medicine, Bethesda, MD.

diseased affections of the will—excessive or defective emotions, passion, &c. whether intermittent or continued, are sometimes associated with lesions of the intellect. At other times, however, the understanding is perfectly free in every department of its exercise. In all cases of excessive excitement of the passion, a method of treatment, simple enough in application, but highly calculated to render the disease incurable, has been adopted from time immemorial;—that of abandoning the patient to his melancholy fate, as an untameable being, to be immured in solitary durance, loaded with chains, or otherwise treated with extreme severity, until the natural close of a life so wretched shall rescue him from his misery, and convey him from the cells of the mad-house to the chambers of the grave. But this treatment convenient indeed to a governor, more remarkable for his indolence and ignorance than for his prudence or humanity, deserves, at the present day, to be held up to public execration, and classed with the other prejudices which have degraded the character and pretensions of the human species. To allow every maniac all the latitude of personal liberty consistent with safety; to proportion the degree of coercion to the demands upon it from his extravagance of behaviour; to use mildness of manners or firmness as occasion may require,—the bland arts of conciliation, or the tone of irresistible authority pronouncing an irreversible mandate, and to proscribe, most absolutely, all violence and ill treatment on the part of the domestics, are laws of fundamental importance, and essential to the prudent and successful management of all lunatic institutions. But how many great qualities, both of mind and body, it is necessary that the governor should possess, in order to meet the endless difficulties and exigencies of so responsible a situation!

From Philippe Pinel, A *Treatise on Insanity*, translated from the French by D. D. Davis (Sheffield: W. Todd, 1806), 1–6, 13–14, 16, 27–28, 52–54, 61–63, 68–72, 82–83.

Johann Christian August Heinroth
(1773–1843)
Textbook of Disturbances of Mental Life
(1818)

The German physician J.C.A. Heinroth was among the first generation of so-called mental doctors (*psychische Ärzte*), a group of physicians who combined the tradition of mad-doctoring with academic learning. Having studied theology for a time, he then took up medicine, working in military hospitals and a workhouse before becoming professor of psychotherapy (the first in Europe) at the University of Leipzig in 1811. Along with a host of other prominent asylum directors and physicians in Germany at the time, Heinroth was influenced by the intellectual movement of Romanticism, which emphasized values such as reason, the unity of mind and body, spiritual growth, and moral awakening. For him, madness was the result of an alienation from nature, a condition he believed was inherent to modern life. Although rarely acknowledged today, Heinroth and the other Romantic mental doctors were enormously influential in the nineteenth century, responsible for coining the term *psychosomatic* and developing the concept of the conflicted personality—notions that would later be taken up by Sigmund Freud. The following excerpt from Heinroth's textbook explains his general understanding of mental health and illness as well as the kind of role he believed the mental doctors needed to play in treating those in their care.

The Concept of Disturbed Mental Life or Disturbances of the Soul

The development of human life through all its ages may be considered as a journey made at a measured pace and aimed at the highest consciousness or life of reason; nay, one is forced to this conclusion or else to consider that man, with all the tendencies and forces which determine his life, is a creature which spends its existence in perpetual self-contradiction. The free creative force in man, his imagination, at first resembles the still amorphous sap of plants which rises by way of roots, stem, branches, and leaves, is purified and transformed into flowers and fruit. The mental life of a child is sensual, and the imagination of the child exercises itself in the sensual world in play. The play urge is the child's expression of love. The mental life of the age of youth is also wholly dedicated to the imagination and concentrates the entire activity of the creative force on one point, on one object, viz., beauty; the beauty urge is the expression of love in youth. Not necessity but love is also the mother of the arts which originate from the individual man and from the human race, inasmuch as the individual and society live and love in the way of the young. The mental life of the mature age extends all the accumulated and complete activities of the creative force into the broad spheres of life with the aid of reason, and it is the business of this age to understand and to bring order, to enlighten and to control, and to stand free and independent through reason or at least to strive for freedom and independence. The urge for freedom is the expression of love of mental life at its zenith. . . .

This is the way man ought to grow. We learn this through faithful observation of his developing urge for growth in a regular determined form. But man is not a plant, and natural necessity is not his all-powerful master. Even though his conscience, his supreme law, affects him with all the severity of a natural necessity, he is nevertheless free not to obey it. Thus he is the first and the only creature on this earth who is a free agent. . . .

The Divine intentions in man are frustrated by man himself in many different ways. The way to the highest development in world-consciousness and in self-consciousness leads through the senses, imagination, and reason, but human life must not become arrested at the lower stages of development and refuse the Divine summons to proceed to higher stages. The man who scorns this repeated summons and is content with and stays only in the non-Divine existence and life will become enslaved by the non-Divine and lose his free will; this loss will not be direct or immediate, but the only possible truly free condition of life, and with it the feeling of pure satisfaction and joy, will be lost to him. A prey to passions, madness, and vice, the creative processes will be impeded, halted, and forced back in many different ways. Thus, by observing such a disturbed process of the inner organization that should have served to sustain the complete life, that is, the free life, we arrive at the concept of a disturbed mental life, or, in short, disturbance of the soul.

This concept is as yet very general, and no definite meaning has so far been assigned to it. It means nothing more than a mental life impeded in some way in its normal growth. Thus, any diseased condition could be denoted as mental disturbance. However, it must be borne in mind that passion, madness, and even vice often assist the soul of a man who, admonished by the voice of his conscience heard through the dim fog of his condition, may gather his forces, break his chains, and rise to a freer, higher plan and pursue good with a greater will. Furthermore, in any soul which still retains its free will, that is, at least potentially free, and which is enslaved by some but not all relationships of life (for good seed often bears fruit in the midst of weeds), the condition of the disturbance, the whole interference with the inner life, is neither complete nor exhaustive. Therefore the concept of disturbance of the soul must be understood more precisely as a total halt, a total standstill, or else an innate desire of the creative force, which was originally intended to produce the highest development, for the opposite, that is, for self-destruction, and must be restricted to cases in which such signs are distinctly evident.

In this condition the free will exists no more and is replaced by complete and permanent loss of freedom. This condition prevails in diseases commonly known as mental breakdown, aberrations of reason, madness, disease of temperament, mental diseases in general, etc. All these diseases, however, much as their external manifestations may differ, have this one feature in common, namely, that not only is there no freedom but not even the capacity to regain freedom. The world-consciousness and the self-consciousness are to a greater or lesser extent disturbed, confused, or wholly extinct, while there is no room for the reasoned consciousness, since free will, which is the receptacle of this consciousness, has died. Thus, individuals in this condition exist no longer in the human domain, which is the domain of freedom, but follow the coercion of internal and external natural necessity. Rather than resembling animals, which are led by a wholesome instinct, they resemble machines and are maintained by vital laws in bodily life alone.

The Concept of Doctor of the Psyche

If we assume that it is possible to cure mental disturbances, or at least to cure some of them under certain conditions, there arises the following question. Since it is the degenerate mental life which must be led back to normal, since it is the humanly healthy condition which must be restored, would this be the task of a doctor? or perhaps of a cleric? of a philosopher? or of an educator? There are arguments which speak in favor of each of these four viewpoints, and each of these professions is at least apparently entitled to take possession of this curative task. . . .

Since we are speaking of medical art and science, we should think that nobody but a doctor should have a right to make mental distur-bance the object of his studies and treatment. Indeed, doctors have claimed this right in their compendia and practice. . . . Nevertheless, since we are claiming that mental disturbances are the opposite of human health and since this claim is not arbitrary but stems from a faithful observation of human nature, we must separate the entire sphere of manifestations from the forms of illness which have symptoms the doctors are accustomed to diagnose. We must transfer them to another domain, the domain of mental life, with which doctors (since they are only familiar with bodily nature) are not familiar with regard to both the recognition of the disease and its treatment. The medical studies to be indicated below testify to this complete ignorance; furthermore, the point of view and the sphere of activity for which doctors are trained and prepared at high schools of learning and at the sickbed are totally differ-ent from the legitimate and true ones given in the present textbook. Accordingly, since doctors are pupils and adepts of medicinal art and sci-ence in the field of disturbed bodily lives only, they are not directly and immediately suited, at least not in the present condition of both educa-tion and experience as practicants, to carry out the business of healing the psyche.

The clerics, as the recognized shepherds of the soul, are just as unfit for the tasks, owing to their point of view and the training and direction they have received. For their field of activity is the moral nature of man for as long as it exists and not after it has died or at least temporarily disappeared. Their business, their profession, is thus concerned with a sphere which is quite different from the one which the doctor of the soul must be familiar. Philosophers, especially psychologists, have at times ventured into the sphere of disturbed mental life, at least theoretically, but they cannot accomplish anything, even in the theory of mental disturbances alone, unless they apply themselves to a faithful observation of nature. This has not yet happened, as will be demonstrated later. Since their activity is confined to the writing desk, nothing in the nature of practical work can be expected of them, whereas the purpose of medicine of the psyche is precisely to take action in order to teach the art of guiding the disturbed mental life back to normal.

This science and art has much more in common with the art of an educator, even doctors agree that curing mentally disturbed individuals is at the same time a reeducation. But all will consent, at least, that this science and art was not invented by educators, even if it already existed; and educators, just like clerics, are at present trained and prepared to deal with free human force, but not to restore a freedom which has been lost. . . .

However, these requirements, or at least some of them, are such as can never be met by an educator or by a cleric or by a philosopher. For the doctor of the psyche must first be a physician, in the full ordinary meaning of the word. He must be learned in the medical traditions and versed in medical practice, partly because mental disturbances are often accompanied by bodily disturbances which they excite, maintain, and modify, partly because in very many instances it is possible to influence the mentally disturbed only through their bodies. It must therefore be concluded that the doctor of the psyche must indeed come forth from the class of physicians. We are purposely saying come forth, for he must not remain in this class, firstly because this class is sufficiently occupied in its own field, whereas the field of soul medicine is so large that the forces of an active man are fully engaged therein; secondly because a doctor of the psyche must undergo special training and must go in a direction which is altogether different from that of the doctor of the body.

For whoever takes upon himself to be a doctor of the psyche must be specially schooled by the psychologist, by the cleric, and by the educator; or rather, he must develop in himself the gift for psychological observation, must adopt a religious point of view, and must himself attempt to live the life of a cleric, or such a life as a pious man would live, that is, to lead a life of reason, or, in the words of the Holy Writ, a life in Christ, or must walk in light, all of which is the same thing. Finally, he must become proficient in the methods of the educator, transform them to his own ends, and carry them over into his own sphere. . . .

This is what a doctor of the psyche, or rather one who has committed himself to being one, must do. Reason is the organ of any recognition and ought to be developed not only by a physician but by all men. This in fact happens very seldom, which explains why our knowledge and our actions are so often blundering. Whoever does not live in light lives in darkness (and a deceptive light, say, the light of a false philosophy, is also darkness), and it is the purpose of the doctor of the soul to bring the mentally disturbed, whose inner life is totally darkened, back to light. But how can he do this if he himself does not live in light? It is necessary to sharply emphasize this point of view of the doctor of the soul. Whoever cannot make this point of view his own must give up the name and the power and the business of a doctor of the soul.

Thus, the doctor of the soul (or psyche) is a true man of reason. He has overcome his selfish interests and treats for purely humanitarian reasons. He considers his patients only as sufferers and not in relation to his own personality. Much is gained even by this attitude alone, since in this manner he obtains an unprejudiced, correct view. He does not hold the vulgar and limited view according to which it is the bodily relationships which determine both the disturbance and the cure, but will concentrate on the soul life and will view all diseased manifestations of the psyche in relation to the latter. From the very outset he influences the patient by virtue of his, one may be permitted to say, holy presence, by the sheer strength of his being, his glance and his will. The will exists in man as a force which is not cultivated; it is however the will which gives rise to all creation, and man, too, has his share of this creative force. The will is the principle of miracles, the principle of magnetism. The magnetic manipulation is only an ad hoc device, a kind of mechanical stimulant of the will. But will without spirit is blind, and will without temperament is barren. The man of reason combines all forces of his inner being for a full understanding and for the living deed. *Sapere aude!**

From Johann Christian August Heinroth, *Textbook of Disturbances of Mental Life; or, Disturbances of the Soul and Their Treatment*, translated by J. Schmorak, introduction by George Mora, vol. 1, *Theory* (Baltimore: Johns Hopkins University Press, 1975), 19–29. © The Johns Hopkins University Press. Reprinted with permission of The Johns Hopkins University Press.

---

*Editor's note: "Dare to know!"

Jean Etienne Esquirol
(1772–1840)
"Monomania"
(1838)

Esquirol was a student of Philippe Pinel, whom he succeeded as director at the Salpêtrière Hospital in Paris in 1811. Expanding on Pinel's thinking, Esquirol believed that dealing with madness required a host of social and legal reforms, and he eventually became the chief architect of France's modern asylum system. Enamored with nosology (the science of disease classification), one of his legacies was to develop the diagnosis of monomania. Up until the turn of the nineteenth century, physicians, legislators, and courts tended to see insanity as a defect of reason, namely, the problem rested in the individual's inability to rationally comprehend. Esquirol's innovation was to argue that a person's emotions or will power could be impaired, without affecting his or her ability to reason. The diagnosis of monomania was an attempt to come to grips with this possibility. In the decades that followed, it provided the inspiration for concepts such as obsession and psychopathy.

Monomania

After having set forth characteristics of lypemania (melancholy with delirium), it becomes my duty to describe that form of partial delirium, to which I have given the name monomania; but first, I will endeavor to point out the distinctive characteristics of those two forms of delirium. Monomania and lypemania, are chronic cerebral affections, unattended by fever, and characterized by a partial lesion of the intelligence, affections, or will. At one time, the intellectual disorder is confined to a single object, or a limited number of objects. The patients seize upon a false principle, which they pursue without deviating from logical reasonings, and from which they deduce legitimate consequences, which modify their affections, and the acts of their will. Aside from this partial delirium, they think, reason and act, like other men. Illusions, hallucinations, vicious associations of ideas, false and strange convictions, are the basis of this delirium, which I would denominate, *intellectual monomania*. At another; monomaniacs are not deprived of the use of their reason, but their affections and dispositions are perverted. By plausible motive, by very reasonable explanations, they justify the actual condition of their sentiments, and excuse the strangeness and inconsistency of their conduct. It is this, which authors have called *reasoning mania*, but which I would name *affective monomania*.

In a third class of cases, a lesion of the will exists. The patient is drawn away from his accustomed course, to the commission of acts, to which neither reason nor sentiment determine, which conscience rebukes, and which the will has no longer the power to restrain. The actions are involuntary, instinctive, irresistible. This is *monomania without delirium*, or, *instinctive monomania*. . . .

M. H., forty-five years of age, a bachelor, and counsellor-at-law, is of a medium stature, bilious-sanguine temperament, of an excellent constitution, and has a remarkably voluminous head. His forehead is uncovered to a very considerable extent, his hair black, his eyes full of vivacity, and his complexion swarthy. He has always led a regular life, and conducted his affairs with system and integrity. He resided for some time at Guadeloupe, was sick for a year after a struggle with the climate, in connection with reverses of fortune, was sent back to Paris, and admitted to Charenton, Nov. 20th, 1832. During the first months of his sojourn at this establishment, he appears composed, walking in the garden, reading much, and conversing with spirit. He would have been regarded as rational, if, from time to time, his delirium did not make itself manifest. He called himself the son of Louis XVI, and was accustomed to add, that an attempt had been made to poison him, for political purpose. After some months, the delirium manifests itself more habitually, and at length reaches a state of fury. He is king, and as such, expects to command and to be obeyed. Those who surround him are his slaves, and their right to life and death is vested in him. Wo to the man who accosts him, without recognizing his kingly power. A doubt on this point, is high treason. The domestics who serve him, know full well the precautions which it is necessary to take, in presenting themselves to him. In several instances, his threats and transports of passion, on my endeavoring to combat his error, have put me on my guard.

In his case, every circumstance comports with his conviction. His lofty carriage, his attitude and look; the imperious tone of his voice and gestures, most clearly express the vain prejudices that occupy his mind. He does not adorn himself with the insignia of his rank, and with ribbons, after the manner of monomaniac *kings* with whom we meet among assemblages of the insane; but the walls of his cell, which he regards as a dungeon, present, written in large characters, both words and phrases, which disclose his mental condition. Observe some of the inscriptions, which he has traced in the form of letters, as they stand upon the walls:

I have–. Tuesday–. *A rabble of Frenchmen*–. Farther on: *Mortal hatred to the French Nation*,– to the people, to the Nobility–by S.A.R., Prince of Bourbon, etc. April 1st, 1837: Son of Louis XVI.– King. Below: I am not a Man—but a Prince—King—MONARCH.

This hatred of the French, and these titles which he proclaims with pride, constitute the subject of all his letters and writings. He feels indignant at the injustice that restrains him by prison bolts; so great and powerful as he is. He pretends that they have taken possession of him by supernatural means, which spies,—selected from the most degraded of the French people—employ; *by pouring upon his majesty, torrents of electricity, in order to annihilate him.* Sometimes he refuses food, not wishing to be nourished like the clowns of his corridor. His food ought to be prepared in royal kitchens. His grandeur and power permit him to recognize, as his relatives and friends, none other than the Bourbons, Ferdinands, Nicholases, etc. . . .

Monomaniacs, like other insane persons, are subject to illusions and hallucinations, which often alone characterize their delirium, and are the causes of the perversion of their affections, and the disorder of their actions. Numerous facts justify this statement. Transported by enthusiasm, by religious or political fanaticism, warmed by erotic passions, blinded by notions of an imaginary good fortune, flattered by sentiments of a felicity of which they deem themselves alone worthy, monomaniacs entertain little affection for their relatives and friends, or their tenderness is exaggerated. They often disdain persons whom they are accustomed to love most tenderly, and feel a sort of pity for them, in consequence of their pretended ignorance, or supposed poverty, or because they are unworthy of understanding the good fortune of the monomaniac, or of participating in it. Like all insane persons, these patients neglect their own interest and affairs, and treat with contempt the usages of society. There are insane persons in conformity with the strictest principles, remarkable for the rectitude of their understanding, for the delicacy of their sentiments, for the mildness of their dispositions, and for a uniformly sober and moral life; who, in consequence of some physical or moral causes, change their disposition and habits of conduct, become turbulent and unsociable, and perform odd, singular, culpable, and sometimes dangerous acts, in opposition to their affections and interests. A partial lesion of the understanding causes these changes, and perverts the sentiments and actions of this class of patients. Thus, the old man, who believes that he hears the voice of an angel, who commands him to offer up his son, after the example of Abraham, and perform this sacrifice, is a monomaniac. . . .

The causes which predispose and produce monomania, are the same with those which produce insanity in general. Sanguine and nervous-sanguine temperaments, and persons endowed with a brilliant, warm and vivid imagination; minds of a meditative and exclusive cast, which seem to be susceptible only of a series of thoughts and emotions; individuals who, through self-love, vanity, pride and ambition, abandon themselves to their reflections, to exaggerated projects and unwarrantable pretensions, are especially disposed to monomania. It is remarkable, that these individuals almost invariably beguile themselves with the hope of a happy fortune, when, stricken by some reverse, or disappointed in their lofty expectations, they fall sick. Thus, a man who is actually happy, and moderate in his desires, and who, by some exciting cause, becomes insane, will not be a monomaniac; whilst an ambitious, proud, or amorous man, who shall have become unfortunate, or have lost the object of his affections, will. It would seem as if monomania were only an exaggeration of the thoughts, desires and illusions with respect to the future, with which these unfortunate beings amuse their fancy, previous to their illness.

A weak understanding, little cultivated or developed; and the want, or vices of education, also predispose to monomania. The exciting causes are; errors of regimen, strong passions, and especially reverses of fortune, disappointed self-love, or ambition. Religious excitement also, ascetic meditations and the reading of romances, often produce this disease among those who are essentially controlled by pride and vanity. . . . Monomania is remittent or intermittent; and the symptoms are exasperated, particularly at the menstrual periods. It is sometimes preceded by melancholy and lypemania, and is complicated with epilepsy, hysteria, hypochondria, and very frequently with paralysis. The progress of monomania is rapid and violent. Its termination is often unexpected, and is effected like other forms of mental alienation, by crises, more or less sensible. But it not unfrequently terminates suddenly, without cause, or perceptible crisis, or by a vivid moral impression. Monomania sometimes passes into mania, and sometimes alternates with lypemania. When prolonged, it degenerates into dementia. . . . But when the disease degenerates into a chronic state, the monomaniac is not only irrational in his hypothesis, but his reasonings, affections and acts, which were previously, the proper consequences of the idea or controlling affection of his mind, no longer maintain their logical and natural connection. . . . The treatment of monomania should, as in other forms of mental alienation, be directed with a special reference to the predisposing and exciting causes of the disease, and to the physical disorders. The intellectual and moral symptoms should have great weight in the therapeutic views of the physician. In this malady, which is characterized by a peculiarly nervous condition of the system, antispasmodics are very useful. While we may, with advantage, have recourse to hygienic agents, it is proper also, to hope for success from moral treatment. Here, more than in other forms of mental disease, and with better hopes of success, we apply to the understanding and passions of the patient, with a view to effect his cure. We have recourse to surprises, subterfuges, and oppositions, ingeniously managed, as circumstances suggest, the genius of the physician gives birth to, and as experience may hit upon, and appropriately pursue.

From E. Esquirol, *Mental Maladies: A Treatise on Insanity* (Philadelphia: Lea and Blanchard, 1845), 320, 327–328, 333–334.

Dorothea Dix
(1802–1887)

Memorial to the Legislature
of Massachusetts
(1843)

Dorothea Dix was one of the early American activists for prisoners and the insane poor. The daughter of an itinerant preacher, she had the opportunity in 1836 to travel to England, where she became familiar with the ideas of the prison reformer Elizabeth Frye (1780–1845) and the reform-minded asylum director Samuel Tuke (1784–1857). After returning to the United States, she happened to examine accommodations for the insane at the Cambridge, Massachusetts, jail and was appalled to find the inmates there chained up in dungeon cells. She then set about touring poorhouses, jails, and prisons to investigate conditions elsewhere, first traveling from county to county, then from state to state. Her findings led her to publicly advocate for the reform of state institutions of confinement. In the 1850s, she took her mission overseas to Britain, France, Greece, Russia, and Japan. All in all, Dix proved to be one of the most internationally respected and effective reformers of the nineteenth century. The following excerpt comes from her 1843 appeal to the state legislature of Massachusetts.

GENTLEMEN.

I respectfully ask to present this Memorial, believing that the *cause*, which actuates to and sanctions so unusual a movement, presents no equivocal claim to public consideration and sympathy. Surrendering to calm and deep convictions of duty my habitual views of what is womanly and becoming, I proceed briefly to explain what has conducted me before you unsolicited and unsustained, trusting, while I do so, that the memorialist will be speedily forgotten in the memorial.

About two years since leisure afforded opportunity, and duty prompted me to visit several prisons and alms-houses in the vicinity of this metropolis. I found, near Boston, in the Jails and Asylums for the poor, a numerous class brought into unsuitable connexion with criminals and the general mass of Paupers. I refer to Idiots and Insane persons, dwelling in circumstances not only adverse to their own physical and moral improvement, but productive of extreme disadvantages to all other persons brought into association with them. I applied myself diligently to trace the causes of these evils, and sought to supply remedies. As one obstacle was surmounted, fresh difficulties appeared. Every new investigation has given depth to the conviction that it is only by decided, prompt, and vigorous legislation the evils to which I refer, and which I shall proceed more fully to illustrate, can be remedied. I shall be obliged to speak with great plainness, and to reveal many things revolting to the taste, and from which my woman's nature shrinks with peculiar sensitiveness. But truth is the highest consideration. *I tell what I have seen*—painful and shocking as the details often are—that from them you may feel more deeply the imperative obligation which lies upon you to prevent the possibility of a repetition or continuance of such outrages upon humanity. If I inflict pain upon you, and move you to horror, it is to acquaint you with sufferings which you have the power to alleviate, and make you hasten to the relief of the victims of legalized barbarity.

I come to present the strong claims of suffering humanity. I come to place before the Legislature of Massachusetts the condition of the miserable, the desolate, the outcast. I come as the advocate of helpless, forgotten, insane and idiotic men and women, sunk to a condition from which the most unconcerned would start with real horror; of beings wretched in our Prisons, and more wretched in our Alms-Houses. And I cannot suppose it needful to employ earnest persuasion, or stubborn argument, in order to attest and fix attention upon a subject, only the more strongly pressing in its claims, because it is revolting and disgusting in its details.

I must confine myself to few examples, but am ready to furnish other and more complete details, if required. If my pictures are displeasing, coarse, and severe, my subjects, it must be recollected, offer no tranquil, refined, or composing features. The condition of human beings, reduced to the extremest states of degradation and misery, cannot be exhibited in softened language, or adorn a polished page.

I proceed, Gentlemen, briefly to call your attention, to the *present* state of Insane Persons confined within this Commonwealth, in *cages, closets, cellars, stalls, pens! Chained, naked, beaten with rods,* and *lashed* into obedience!

As I state cold, severe *facts,* I feel obliged to refer to persons, and definitely to indicate localities. But it is upon my subject, not upon localities or individuals, I desire to fix attention; and I would speak as kindly as possible of all Wardens, Keepers, and other responsible officers, believing that *most* of these have erred not through hardness of heart and willful cruelty, so much as want of skill and knowledge, and want of consideration. Familiarity with suffering, it is said, blunts the sensibilities, and where neglect once finds a footing other injuries are multiplied. This is not all, for it may justly and strongly be added that, from the deficiency of adequate means to meet the wants of these cases, it has been an absolute impossibility to do justice in this matter. Prisons are not constructed in view of being converted into County Hospitals, and Alms-Houses are not constructed as receptacles for the Insane. And yet, in the face of justice and common sense, Wardens are by law compelled to receive, and the Masters of Alms-Houses not to refuse, Insane and Idiotic subjects in all stages of mental disease and privation.

It is the Commonwealth, not its integral parts, that is accountable for most of the abuses which have lately, and do still exist. I repeat it, it is defective legislation which perpetuates and multiplies these abuses.

In illustration of my subject, I offer the following extracts from my Note-Book and Journal. . . .

The use of cages all but universal; hardly a town but can refer to some not distant period of using them; chains are less common; negligences frequent; willful abuse less frequent than sufferings proceeding from ignorance, or want of consideration. I encountered during the last three months many poor creatures wandering reckless and unprotected through the country. Innumerable accounts have been sent me of persons who had roved away unwatched and unsearched after; and I have heard that responsible persons, controlling the almshouses, have not thought themselves culpable in sending away from their shelter, to cast upon the chances of remote relief, insane men and women. These, left on the highways, unfriended and incompetent to control or direct their own movements, sometimes have found refuge in the hospital, and others have not been traced. But I cannot particularize; in traversing the state I have found hundreds of insane person in every variety of circumstance and condition;

many whose situation could not and need not be improved; a less number, but very large, whose lives are the saddest pictures of human suffering and degradation. I give a few illustrations; but description fades before reality.

Danvers. November; visited the almshouse; a large building, much out of repair; understand a new one is in contemplation. Here are fifty-six to sixty inmates; one idiotic; three insane; one of the latter in close confinement at all times.

Long before reaching the house, wild shouts, snatches of rude songs, imprecations, and obscene language, fell upon the ear, proceeding from the occupant of a low building, rather remote from the principal building to which my course was directed. Found the mistress, and was conducted to the place, which was called *"the home"* of the *forlorn* maniac, a young woman, exhibiting a condition of neglect and misery blotting out the faintest idea of comfort, and outraging every sentiment of decency. She had been, I learnt, "a respectable person; industrious and worthy; disappointments and trials shook her mind, and finally laid prostrate reason and self-control; she became a maniac for life! She had been at Worcester Hospital for a considerable time, and had been returned as incurable." The mistress told me she understood that, while there, she was "comfortable and decent." Alas! what a change was here exhibited! She had passed from one degree of violence and degradation to another, in swift progress; there she stood, clinging to, or beating upon, the bars of her caged apartment, the contracted size of which afforded space only for increasing accumulations of filth, a *foul* spectacle; there she stood with naked arms and disheveled hair; the unwashed frame invested with fragments of unclean garments, the air so extremely offensive, though ventilation was afforded on all sides save one, that it was not possible to remain beyond a few moments without retreating for recovery to the outward air. Irritation of body, produced by utter filth and exposure, incited her to the horrid process of tearing off her skin by inches; her face, neck, and person, were thus disfigured to hideousness; she held up a fragment just rent off; to my exclamation of horror, the mistress replied, "Oh, we can't help it; half the skin is off sometimes; we can do nothing with her; and it makes no difference what she eats, for she consumes her own filth as readily as the food which is brought her."

It is now January; a fortnight since, two visitors reported that most wretched outcast as "wallowing in dirty straw, in a place yet more dirty, and without clothing, without fire. Worse cared for than the brutes, and wholly lost to consciousness of decency!" Is the whole story told? What was seen is; what is reported is not. These gross exposures are not for the pained sight of one alone; all, all, coarse, brutal men, wondering, neglected children, old and young, each and all, witness the lowest, foulest state of miserable humanity. And who protects her, that worse than Paria outcast, from other wrongs and blacker outrages? I do not *know* that such *have been*. I do know that they are to be dreaded, and that they are not guarded against.

Some may say these things cannot be remedied; these furious maniacs are not to be raised from these base conditions. I *know* they are; could give *many* examples; let *one* suffice. A young woman, a pauper, in a distant town, *Sandisfield*, was for years a raging maniac. A cage, chain, and *the whip*, were the agents for controlling her, united with harsh tones and profane language. Annually, with others (the town's poor) she was put up at auction, and bid off at the lowest price which was declared for her. One year, not long past, an old man came forward in the number of applicants for the poor wretch; he was taunted and ridiculed; "what would he and his old wife do with such a mere beast?" "My wife says yes," replied he, "and I shall take her." She was given to his charge; he conveyed her home; she was washed, neatly dressed, and placed in a decent bed-room, furnished for comfort and opening into the kitchen. How altered her condition! As yet *the chains* were not off. The first week she was somewhat restless, at times violent, but the quiet kind ways of the old people wrought a change; she received her food decently; forsook acts of violence, and no longer uttered blasphemous or indecent language; after a week, the chain was lengthened, and she was received as a companion into the kitchen. Soon she engaged in trivial employments. "After a fortnight," said the old man, "I knocked off the chains and made her a free woman." She is at times excited, but not violently; they are careful of her diet; they keep her very clean; she calls them "father" and "mother." Go there now and you will find her "clothed," and though not perfectly in her "right mind," so far restored as to be a safe and comfortable inmate.

Newburyport. Visited the almshouse in June last; eighty inmates; seven insane, one idiotic. Commodious and neat house; several of the partially insane apparently very comfortable; two very improperly situated, namely, an insane man, not considered incurable, in an out-building, whose room opened upon what was called "the dead room," affording in lieu of companionship with the living, a contemplation of corpses! The other subject was a woman in a *cellar*. I desired to see her; much reluctance was shown. I pressed the request; the Master of the House stated that she was *in the cellar*; that she was *dangerous to be approached*; that "she had lately attacked his wife"; and *was often naked*. I persisted: "if you will not go with me, give me the keys and I will go alone." Thus importuned, the outer doors were opened. I descended the stairs from within; a strange, unnatural noise seemed to proceed from beneath our feet; at the moment I did not much regard it. My conductor proceeded to remove a padlock while my eye explored the wide space in quest of the poor woman. All for a moment was still. But judge my horror and amazement, when a door to a closet *beneath* the *staircase* was opened, revealing in the imperfect light a female apparently wasted to a skeleton, partially wrapped in blankets, furnished for the narrow bed on which she was sitting; her countenance furrowed, not by age, but suffering, was the image of distress; in that contracted space, unlighted, unventilated, she poured forth the wailings of despair; mournfully she extended her arms and appealed to me, "why am I consigned to hell? dark—dark—I used to pray, I used to read the Bible—I have done no crime in my heart; I had friends, why have all forsaken me!—my God! my God! why hast *thou* forsaken me!" Those groans, those wailings come up daily, mingling with how many others, a perpetual and sad memorial. When the good Lord shall require an account of stewardship, what shall all and each answer!

Perhaps it will be inquired how long, how many days or hours she was imprisoned in these confined limits? *For years!* In another part of the cellar were other small closets, only better, because higher through the entire length, into one of which she by turns was transferred, so as to afford opportunity for fresh whitewashing, &c. . . .

Violence and severity do but exasperate the Insane: the only availing influence is kindness and firmness. It is amazing what these will produce. How many examples might illustrate this position: I refer to one recently exhibited in Barre. The town Paupers are disposed of annually to some family who, for a stipulated sum agree to take charge of them. One of them, a young woman, was shown to me well clothed, neat, quiet, and employed at needle-work. It is possible that this is the same being who, but last year, was a raving madwoman, exhibiting every degree of violence in action and speech; a very tigress wrought by fury; caged, chained, beaten, loaded with injuries, and exhibiting the passions which an iron rule might be expected to stimulate and sustain. It is the same person; another family hold her in charge who better understand human nature and human influences; she is no longer chained, caged, and beaten; but if excited, a pair of mittens drawn over the hands secures from mischief. Where will she be next year, after the annual sale?

. . . I may here remark that severe measures, in enforcing rule, have in many places been openly revealed. I have not seen chastisement administered by stripes, and in but few instances have I seen the *rods* and *whips*, but I have seen blows inflicted, both passionately and repeatedly.

I have been asked if I have investigated the causes of insanity? I have not; but I have been told that this most calamitous overthrow of reason, often is the result of a life of sin; it is sometimes, but rarely added, they must take the consequences; they deserve no better care! Shall man be more just than God; he who causes his sun, and refreshing rains, and lifegiving influence, to fall alike on the good and the evil? Is not the total wreck of reason, a state of distraction, and the loss of all that makes life cherished a retribution, sufficiently heavy, without adding to consequences so appalling, every indignity that can bring still lower the wretched sufferer? Have pity upon those who, while they were supposed to lie hid in secret sins, "have been scattered under *a dark veil of forgetfulness*; over whom is spread a heavy night, and who unto themselves are more grievous than the darkness."

. . . We need an Asylum for this class, the incurable, where conflicting duties shall not admit of such examples of privations and misery.

One is continually amazed as the tenacity of life in these persons. In conditions that wring the heart to behold, it is hard to comprehend that days rather than years should not conclude the measure of their griefs and miseries. Picture her condition! place yourselves in that dreary cage, remote from the inhabited dwelling, alone by day and night, without fire, without clothes, *except when remembered*; without object or employment; weeks and months passing on in drear succession, not a blank, but with keen life to suffering; with kindred, but deserted by them; and you shall not lose the memory of that time when they loved you, and you in turn loved them, but now no act or voice of kindness makes sunshine in the heart. Has fancy realized this to you? It *may* be the state of some of those you cherish! Who shall be sure his own hearth-stone shall not be desolate? nay, who shall say his own mountain stands strong, his lamp of reason shall not go out in darkness! To show how many has this become a heart-rending reality! If for selfish ends only, should not effectual Legislation here interpose?

... Men of Massachusetts, I beg, I implore, I demand, pity and protection, for these of my suffering, outraged sex!—Fathers, Husbands, Brothers, I would supplicate you for this boon—but what do I say? I dishonor you, divest you at once of christianity and humanity—does this appeal imply distrust. If it comes burthened with a doubt of your righteousness in this Legislation, then blot it out; while I declare confidence in your honor, not less than your humanity. Here you will put away the cold, calculated spirit of selfishness and self-seeking; lay off the armor of local strife and political opposition; here and now, for once, forgetful of the earthly and perishable, come up to these halls and consecrate them with one heart and one mind to works of righteousness and just judgment. Become the benefactors of your race, the just guardians of the solemn rights you hold in trust. Raise up the fallen; succor the desolate; restore the outcast; defend the helpless; and for your eternal and great reward, receive the benediction . . . "Well done, good and faithful servants, become rulers over many things!"

From Dorothea Dix, *Memorial* (Boston: Munroe & Francis, 1843), 3–9, 12, 17–18, 20–21, 24–25.

The M'Naughten Rules
(1843)

Up until the early nineteenth century, British and American courts had no universally accepted standard for defining mental incompetence in criminal cases. In general, judges tended to focus on the accused's intellectual capacity for understanding right and wrong. The growing emphasis in psychiatry on impairments of emotion and will, however, seemed to challenge this more or less cognitive notion of insanity.

Daniel M'Naughten (1813–1865) was a Scottish craftsman, active in the early workers' movement in Great Britain. On 20

January 1843, believing that conservatives were intent on murder-ing him, M'Naughten set out to stalk and kill the sitting prime min-ister, Robert Peel. Mistaking Peel's secretary Edward Drummond for the government leader, M'Naughten shot Drummond with a pistol at point-blank range. Drummond later died. At his trial in March, M'Naughten pleaded not guilty, his legal counsel enlisting the expert testimony of physicians, who argued that M'Naughten suffered from a "moral insanity" in the form of monomania. The strategy succeeded, and M'Naughten was found not guilty by rea-son of insanity and confined to an asylum for the rest of his life.

Queen Victoria, displeased with the verdict, asked the House of Lords to review the decision with a panel of judges. In June 1843, the House of Lords demanded that the judges answer several abstract questions involving issues raised by the case. The judges' responses have since become known as the M'Naughten Rules, and they have served as the basis for determining legal insanity through-out many parts of England and the United States to this very day.

Notwithstanding a party accused did an act, which was in itself criminal, under the influence of insane delusion, with a view of redressing or reveng-ing some supposed grievance or injury, or of producing some public bene-fit, he is nevertheless punishable if he knew at the time that he was acting contrary to law.

That if the accused was conscious that the act was one which he ought not to do; and if the act was at the same time contrary to law, he is pun-ishable. In all cases of this kind the jurors ought to be told that every man is presumed to be sane, and to possess a sufficient degree of reason to be responsible for his crimes, until the contrary be proved to their satisfaction: and that to establish a defence on the ground of insanity, it must be clearly proved that at the time of commiting the act the party accused was labour-ing under such a defect of reason, from disease of the mind, as not to know the nature and quality of the act he was doing, or as not to know that what he was doing was wrong.

That a party labouring under a partial delusion must be considered in the same situation, as to responsibility, as if the facts, in respect to which the delusion exists, were real.

That where an accused person is supposed to be insane, a medical man, who has been present in Court and heard the evidence, may be asked, as a matter of science, whether the facts stated by the witnesses, supposing them to be true, show a state of mind incapable of distinguishing between right and wrong.

The prisoner had been indicted for that he, on the 20th day of January 1843, at the parish of Saint Martin in the Fields, in the county of Middlesex, and within the jurisdiction of the Central Criminal Court, in and upon one Edward Drummond, feloniously, wilfully, and of his malice aforethought, did make an assault; and that the said Daniel M'Naghten,* a certain pistol of the value of 20s, loaded and charged with gunpowder and a leaden bullet (which pistol he in his right hand had and held), to, against and upon the said Edward Drummond, feloniously, wilfully, and of his malice aforethought, did shoot and discharge; and that the said Daniel M'Naghten, with the leaden bullet aforesaid, out of the pistol aforesaid, by force of the gunpowder, etc., the said Edward Drummond, in and upon the back of him the said Edward Drummond, feloniously, etc. did strike, penetrate and wound, giving to the said Edward Drummond, in and upon the back of the said Edward Drummond, one mortal wound, etc., of which mortal wound the said E. Drummond languished until the 25th of April and then died; and that by the means aforesaid, he the prisoner did kill and murder the said Edward Drummond. The prisoner pleaded Not guilty.

Evidence having been given of the fact of the shooting of Mr. Drummond, and of his death in consequence thereof, witnesses were called on the part of the prisoner, to prove that he was not, at the time of committing the act, in a sound state of mind. The medical evidence was in substance this: That persons of otherwise sound mind, might be affected by morbid delusions: that the prisoner was in that condition: that a person so labouring under a morbid delusion, might have a moral perception of right and wrong, but that in the case of the prisoner it was a delusion which carried him away beyond the power of his own control, and left him no such perception; and that he was not capable of exercising any control over acts which had connexion with his delusion: that it was of the nature of the disease with which the prisoner was affected, to go on gradually until it had

---

*Editor's note: M'Naughten's surname was spelled a variety of ways in public documents.

reached a climax, when it burst forth with irresistible intensity: that a man might go on for years quietly, though at the same time under its influence, but would all at once break out into the most extravagant and violent paroxysms.

Some of the witnesses who gave this evidence, had previously examined the prisoner: others had never seen him till he appeared in Court, and they formed their opinions on hearing the evidence given by the other witnesses.

Lord Chief Justice Tindal (in his charge): The question to be determined is, whether at the time the act in question was committed, the prisoner had or had not the use of his understanding, so as to know that he was doing a wrong or wicked act. If the jurors should be of opinion that the prisoner was not sensible, at the time he committed it, that he was violating the laws both of God and man, then he would be entitled to a verdict in his favour: but if, on the contrary, they were of opinion that when he committed the act he was in a sound state of mind, then their verdict must be against him.

Verdict, Not guilty, on the ground of insanity.

This verdict, and the question of the nature and extent of the unsoundness of mind which would excuse the commission of a felony of this sort, having been made the subject of debate in the House of Lords (the 6th and 13th March 1843; see Hansard's Debates, vol. 67, pp. 288, 714), it was determined to take the opinion of the Judges on the law governing such cases. Accordingly, on the 26th of May, all the Judges attended their Lordships, but no questions were then put.

On the nineteenth of June, the Judges again attended the House of Lords; when (no argument having been had) the following questions of law were propounded to them:

1st. What is the law respecting alleged crimes committed by persons afflicted with insane delusion, in respect of one or more particular subjects or persons: as, for instance, where at the time of the commission of the alleged crime, the accused knew he was acting contrary to law, but did the act complained of with a view, under the influence of insane delusion, of redressing or revenging some supposed grievance or injury, or of producing some supposed public benefit?

2d. What are the proper questions to be submitted to the jury, when a person alleged to be afflicted with insane delusion respecting one or more particular subjects or persons, is charged with the commission of a crime (murder, for example), and insanity is set up as a defence?

3d. In what terms ought the question to be left to the jury, as to the prisoner's state of mind at the time when the act was committed?

4th. If a person under an insane delusion, as to existing facts, commits an offence in consequence thereof, is he thereby excused?

5th. Can a medical man conversant with the disease of insanity, who never saw the prisoner previously to the trial, but who was present during the whole trial and the examination of all the witnesses, be asked his opinion as to the state of the prisoner's mind at the time of the commission of the alleged crime, or his opinion whether the prisoner was conscious at the time of doing the act, that he was acting contrary to law, or whether he was labouring under any and what delusion at the time?

Mr. Justice Maule: I feel great difficulty in answering the questions put by your Lordships on this occasion: First, because they do not appear to arise out of and are not put with reference to a particular case, or for a particular purpose, which might explain or limit the generality of their terms, so that full answers to them ought to be applicable to every possible state of facts, not inconsistent with those assumed in the questions: this difficulty is the greater, from the practical experience both of the bar and the Court being confined to questions arising out of the facts of particular cases: Secondly, because I have heard no argument at your Lordships' bar or elsewhere, on the subject of these questions; the want of which I feel the more, the greater are the number and extent of questions which might be raised in argument: and Thirdly, from a fear of which I cannot divest myself, that as these questions relate to matters of criminal law of great importance and frequent occurrence, the answers to them by the Judges may embarrass the administration of justice, when they are cited in criminal trials. For these reasons I should have been glad if my learned brethren would have joined me in praying your Lordships to excuse us from answering these questions; but as I do not think they ought to induce me to ask that indulgence for myself individually, I shall proceed to give such answers as I can, after the very short time which I have had to consider the questions, and under the difficulties I have mentioned; fearing that my answers may be as little satisfactory to others as they are to myself.

The first question, as I understand it, is, in effect, What is the law respecting the alleged crime, when at the time of the commission of it, the accused knew he was acting contrary to the law, but did the act with a view, under the influence of insane delusion, of redressing or revenging some supposed grievance or injury, or of producing some supposed public bene-fit? If I were to understand this question according to the strict meaning of its terms, it would require, in order to answer it, a solution of all questions of law which could arise on the circumstances stated in the question, either by explicitly stating and answering such questions, or by stating some prin-ciples or rules which would suffice for their solution. I am quite unable to do so, and, indeed, doubt whether it be possible to be done; and therefore request to be permitted to answer the question only so far as it compre-hends the question, whether a person, circumstanced as stated in the ques-tion, is, for that reason only, to be found not guilty of a crime respecting which the question of his guilt has been duly raised in a criminal proceed-ing, and I am of opinion that he is not. There is no law, that I am aware of, that makes persons in the state described in the question not responsible for their criminal acts. To render a person irresponsible for crime on account of unsoundness of mind, the unsoundness should, according to the law as it has long been understood and held, be such as rendered him incapable of knowing right from wrong. The terms used in the question cannot be said (with reference only to the usage of language) to be equiva-lent to a description of this kind and degree of unsoundness of mind. If the state described in the question be one which involves or is necessarily con-nected with such an unsoundness, this is not a matter of law but of physi-ology, and not of that obvious and familiar kind as to be inferred without proof.

Second, the questions necessarily to be submitted to the jury, are those questions of fact, which are raised on the record. In a criminal trial, the question commonly is, whether the accused be guilty or not guilty: but, in order to assist the jury in coming to a right conclusion on this necessary and ultimate question, it is usual and proper to submit such subordinate or intermediate questions, as the course which the trial has taken may have made it convenient to direct their attention to. What those questions are, and the manner of submitting them, is a matter of discretion for the Judge: a discretion to be guided, by a consideration of all the circumstances attend-ing the inquiry. In performing this duty, it is sometimes necessary or con-venient to inform the jury as to the law; and if, on a trial such as is suggested in the question, he should have occasion to state what kind and degree of insanity would amount to a defence, it should be stated conformably to what I have mentioned in my answer to the first question, as being, in my opinion, the law on this subject.

Third, there are no terms which the Judge is by law required to use. They should not be inconsistent with the law as above stated, but should be such as, in the discretion of the Judge, are proper to assist the jury in coming to a right conclusion as to the guilt of the accused.

Fourth, the answer which I have given to the first question, is applicable to this.

Fifth, whether a question can be asked depends not merely on the questions of fact raised on the record, but on the course of the cause at the time it is proposed to ask it; and the state of an inquiry as to the guilt of a person charged with a crime, and defended on the ground of insanity, may be such, that such a question as either of those suggested, is proper to be asked and answered, though the witness has never seen the person before the trial, and though he has merely been present and heard the witnesses: these circumstances, of his never having seen the person before, and of his having merely been present at the trial, not being necessarily sufficient, as it seems to me, to exclude the lawfulness of a question which is otherwise lawful; though I will not say that an inquiry might not be in such a state, as that these circumstances should have such an effect.

Supposing there is nothing else in the state of the trial to make the questions suggested proper to be asked and answered, except that the witness had been present and heard the evidence; it is to be considered whether that is enough to sustain the question. In principle it is open to this objection, that as the opinion of the witness is founded on those conclusions of fact which he forms from the evidence, and as it does not appear what those conclusions are, it may be that the evidence he gives is on such an assumption of facts, as makes it irrelevant to the inquiry. But such questions have been very frequently asked, and the evidence to which they are directed has been given, and has never, that I am aware of, been successfully objected to. Evidence, most clearly open to this objection, and on the admission of which the event of a most important trial probably turned, was received in the case of The Queen v. M'Naghten, tried at the Central Criminal Court in March last, before the Lord Chief Justice, Mr. Justice Williams, and Mr. Justice Coleridge, in which counsel of the highest eminence were engaged on both sides; and I think the course and practice of receiving such evidence, confirmed by the very high authority of these Judges, who not only received it, but left it, as I understand, to the jury, without any remark derogating from its weight, ought to be held to warrant its reception, notwithstanding the objection in principle to which it may be open. In cases even where the course of practice in criminal law has been unfavourable to parties accused, and entirely contrary to the most obvious principles of justice and humanity, as well as those of law, it has been held that such practice constituted the law, and could not be altered without the authority of Parliament.

Lord Chief Justice Tindal: My Lords, Her Majesty's Judges (with the exception of Mr. Justice Maule, who has stated his opinion to your Lordships), in answering the questions proposed to them by your Lordships' House, think it right, in the first place, to state that they have forborne entering into any particular discussion upon these questions, from the extreme and almost insuperable difficulty of applying those answers to cases in which the facts are not brought judicially before them. The facts of each particular case must of necessity present themselves with endless variety, and with every shade of difference in each case; and as it is their duty to declare the law upon each particular case, on facts proved before them, and after hearing argument of counsel thereon, they deem it at once impracticable, and at the same time dangerous to the administration of justice, if it were practicable, to attempt to make minute applications of the principles involved in the answers given by them to your Lordships' questions.

They have therefore confined their answers to the statement of that which they hold to be the law upon the abstract questions proposed by your Lordships; and as they deem it unnecessary, in this peculiar case, to deliver their opinions seriatim, and as all concur in the same opinion, they desire me to express such their unanimous opinion to your Lordships.

The first question proposed by your Lordships is this: "What is the law respecting alleged crimes committed by persons afflicted with insane delusion in respect of one or more particular subjects or persons: as, for instance, where at the time of the commission of the alleged crime the accused knew he was acting contrary to law, but did the act complained of with a view, under the influence of insane delusion, of redressing or revenging some supposed grievance or injury, or of producing some supposed public benefit?"

In answer to which question, assuming that your Lordships' inquiries are confined to those persons who, labour under such partial delusions only, and are not in other respects insane, we are of opinion that, notwithstanding the party accused did the act complained of with a view, under the influence of insane delusion, of redressing or revenging some supposed grievance or injury, or of producing some public benefit, he is nevertheless punishable according to the nature of the crime committed, if he knew at the time of committing such crime that he was acting contrary to law; by which expression we understand your Lordships to mean the law of the land.

Your Lordships are pleased to inquire of us, secondly, "What are the proper questions to be submitted to the jury, where a person alleged to be afflicted with insane delusion respecting one or more particular subjects or persons, is charged with the commission of a crime (murder, for example), and insanity is set up as a defence?" And, thirdly, "In what terms ought the question to be left to the jury as to the prisoner's state of mind at the time when the act was committed?" And as these two questions appear to us to be more conveniently answered together, we have to submit our opinion to be, that the jurors ought to be told in all cases that every man is to be presumed to be sane, and to possess a sufficient degree of reason to be responsible for his crimes, until the contrary be proved to their satisfaction; and that to establish a defence on the ground of insanity, it must be clearly proved that, at the time of the committing of the act, the party accused was labouring under such a defect of reason, from disease of the mind, as not to know the nature and quality of the act he was doing; or, if he did know it, that he did not know he was doing what was wrong. The mode of putting the latter part of the question to the jury on these occasions has generally been, whether the accused at the time of doing the act knew the difference between, right and wrong: which mode, though rarely; if ever, leading to any mistake with the jury, is not, as we conceive, so accurate when put generally and in the abstract, as when put with reference to the party's knowledge of right and wrong in respect to the very act with which he is charged. If the question were to be put as to the knowledge of the accused solely and exclusively with reference to the law of the land, it might tend to confound the jury, by inducing them to believe that an actual knowledge of the law of the land was essential in order to lead to a conviction; whereas the law is administered upon the principle that every one must be taken conclusively to know it, without proof that he does know it. If the accused was conscious that the act was one which he ought not to do, and if that act was at the same time contrary to the law of the land, he is punishable; and the usual course therefore has been to leave the question to the jury, whether the party accused had a sufficient degree of reason to know that he was doing an act that was wrong: and this course we think is correct, accompanied with such observations and explanations as the circumstances of each particular case may require.

The fourth question which your Lordships have proposed to us is this: "If a person under an insane delusion as to existing facts, commits an offence in consequence thereof, is he thereby excused?" To which question the answer must of course depend on the nature of the delusion: but, making the same assumption as we did before, namely, that he labours under such partial delusion only, and is not in other respects insane, we think he must be considered in the same situation as to responsibility as if the facts with respect to which the delusion exists were real. For example, if under the influence of his delusion he supposes another man to be in the act of attempting to take away his life, and he kills that man, as he supposes, in self-defence, he would be exempt from punishment. If his delusion was that the deceased had inflicted a serious injury to his character and fortune, and he killed him in revenge for such supposed injury, he would be liable to punishment.

The question lastly proposed by your Lordships is: "Can a medical man conversant with the disease of insanity, who never saw the prisoner previously to the trial, but who was present during the whole trial and the examination of all the witnesses, be asked his opinion as to the state of the prisoner's mind at the time of the commission of the alleged crime, or his opinion whether the prisoner was conscious at the time of doing the act that he was acting contrary to law, or whether he was labouring under any and what delusion at the time?" In answer thereto, we state to your Lordships, that we think the medical man, under the circumstances supposed, cannot in strictness be asked his opinion in the terms above stated, because each of those questions involves the determination of the truth of the facts deposed to, which it is for the jury to decide, and the questions are not mere questions upon a matter of science, in which case such evidence is admissible. But where the facts are admitted or not disputed, and the question becomes substantially one of science only, it may be convenient to allow the question to be put in that general form, though the same cannot be insisted on as a matter of right.

From 8ER 718, [1843] UKHL J16 British and Irish Legal Information Institute, United Kingdom House of Lords Decisions, http://www.bailii.org/uk/cases/UKHL/1843/J16.html.

The Asylum

The Opal: A Monthly Periodical of the State Lunatic Asylum, Devoted to Usefulness, Edited by the Patients of the Utica State Lunatic Asylum

(1850–1860)

Beginning in November 1850, the patients at the Utica State Lunatic Asylum in upstate New York began writing, editing, and publishing a monthly newsletter, the *Opal*. Dedicating their effort to "usefulness," patients and ex-patients were given remarkable license to pen essays, poems, and reflections. Proceeds from subscriptions were used to stock the patient library collection. The monthly was eventually discontinued in 1860. Since the *Opal* was directed at readers both inside and outside the asylum, its stories and articles provide a glimpse into not only how patients viewed insanity and themselves, but also how they perceived staff, treatment, and the outside world.

Truthfulness with the Insane (1852)

The most numerous by far of all cases of conscience brought constantly into the casuistical court are those which relate to the duties of Truth. "Are

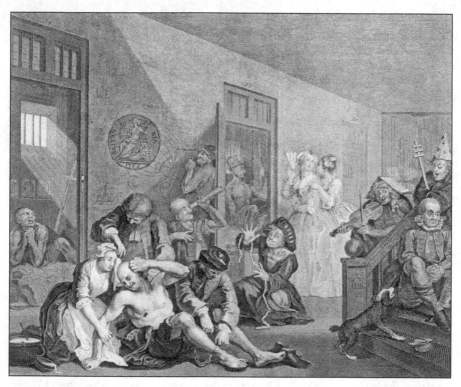

William Hogarth (1697–1764), *Scene in Bedlam* (1735), from *A Rake's Progress* (plate 8). Bedlam, or Bethlem (medieval variations of "Bethlehem"), Hospital in London began specializing in the care of the insane in 1403. Well into the nineteenth century, it was possible for locals and travelers to tour madhouses, much like the two women portrayed here. Etching and engraving on paper. Tate Gallery, London, Great Britain. © Tate, London/Art Resource, NY.

we bound to speak the truth at all times?" Who has not, at some periods of his experience, been perplexed with this question, and longed to know in what way to resolve it. . . .

Now, we venture to say, there is no one case of conscience more commonly deemed easy of solution, than that which has regard to the duty of *truthfulness with the sick and the insane*. We put both of these classes of persons together, because, for our purpose, the question is substantially the same with respect to both. An insane man is a man under the influence, commonly, of some bodily weakness or disease, and it is a very common effect of bodily sickness to produce, in greater or lesser degree, mental derangement.

We say there is no case of conscience more easily solved, according to the popular estimation, than this one with reference to truth-telling towards the sick and insane. In fact, it has become hardly a question at all, with the great majority. Leaving the insane out of the question, who does not know how common is the practice of equivocation and deceit towards the sick? Who does not know how often *physicians* lead the way in this sort of dealing? It is not an unfrequent thing—we speak from our own observation—that physicians conduct themselves in this particular, as if they were absolved from all obligation to the rules of veracity by virtue of their profession. How often does it occur that they flatter their patients with speedy, or, at least, ultimate recovery, when they have already judged the case to be hopeless, and the sufferer is already lying upon the verge of the grave. We have known the sick, and the family that watched around the bed-side, kept in utter ignorance of the true state of the progress of the disease, at the same time that the patient was rapidly sinking into the arms of death, and the physician who had spoken only words of assurance and hope in his ear, was telling to all *without* the household that recovery was impossible! We trust that such a course is not characteristic of the profession in general. We are glad to know that by the best medical authorities, and by our most scientific and distinguished practitioners, it is entirely disapproved. We hesitate not, to brand such conduct on the part of the appointed guardians of the sick-bed, to be as uncalled for and cruel as it is treacherous and wicked.

There are many who will assent to the justness of the views stated above, who will very likely dissent from us when we come to speak of the expediency and duty of *truthfulness towards the insane*. There are multitudes who, doubtless, consider it neither expedient nor a duty to observe strict veracity with this unfortunate class of persons. It is, we believe, a general impression that those who have to do with the insane in our Asylums are governed by no rules upon the subject, unless it be the rule of employing both truth and falsehood, according as one or the other shall be best suited to the particular exigency. This, in fact, was our own impression, until our residence and entrance as a patient within the walls of the N.Y. State Asylum gave us an opportunity to ascertain the policy actually adopted. . . . It will, perhaps, be presuming too much, but we will venture one or two suggestions upon this subject. . . .

First then, Insanity is but another word for delusion, the *delusion* of falsehood, and falsehood manifestly, therefore, is not the proper cure for a disease of which it is, in itself, the essence. The thing which needs to be expelled from the mind of an insane person, before it can be recovered to soundness, is the falsehood under which it labors, and how this can be best done by injecting new falsehood into the mind, we may well be at a loss to know. If a child has been fed upon sweetmeats until it has become pale and thin like a skeleton, is it best, in order to its recovery, to continue the sweetmeats or to endeavor to neutralize and overcome their already hurtful effect by a new and nourishing diet? There is but one answer to this question, an answer suggested by the very nature of the case, as we should say. Now as with the emaciated body, so with the deranged mind. No mind can be in a health condition that feeds upon falsehood. It must, of course, be diseased and hastening to decay. What it needs is something different and opposite to that which it has fed upon, and that something is TRUTH.

It is certain, furthermore, that the insane are more or less susceptible to all influences exerted in consistency with the requirements of veracity. It no uncommon thing in the experience of those who have charge of institutions for the insane to find the delusion of their patients giving way before a continual representation of the truth. Nor is it unfrequent that the recovered patient is able to call to mind, how the truthful declarations of his physician first broke in upon his delusions with persuasive power, and how from this source the first ray of light shone upon the brooding darkness. We can speak from experience, how much it contributed to the rest of a mind tossed upon the billows of phrenzy and despair, when we had gained the conviction that those who were placed in charge of us were men in whose slightest utterance we could have confidence; men who made it a sacred principle not to deceive their patients in any particular. There is a certain point of recovery when the disordered mind seeks to discriminate between that which is true and that which is false in its condition. It has delusions which it would gladly rid itself of, if it might dare to do so; but it has others, equally hurtful, to which it would as gladly hold fast. Then also, there are some of which are pleasant, and others, it may be disagreeable to contemplate; but now, as he finds his delusions beginning to dissipate, what shall he do with these? Ought he to retain his confidence in them while he dismisses it in the others? In such circumstances what can be more grateful to the tempest-tost soul than to have at hand a faithful counsellor, whose every word is truth, and who may be relied on to guide his trembling steps through the maze he is treading.

Editor's Table (1852)

Considerable anxiety is sometimes expressed by persons who derive a morbid satisfaction from looking on scenes of human misery, as to the propriety, safety, &c., of their visiting the Asylum. This diseased state of the sentiments is most incident to those who have been badly educated, and who, especially, have not been taught to follow up feeling by the corresponding actions. They are mightily stirred by a story of distress, but never think of an effort to relieve it. The natural tie between emotion and conduct has suffered a violent disruption.—We do not like to see such people passing through the halls. The authoress of the following letter belongs to the class we have been describing, and a decent respect for her sex demands that we should not pass it by unnoticed.

> To the Editor of The Opal:
> Sir,— My father is a citizen of the State of New York, and a voter in regular standing, and he has told me that by reason of these things he and his family have free admission to the Asylum. As I have not much to do at home, (mother and the help doing all the work), I proposed a few days ago that we should have a good sleigh-ride and fetch up at the Asylum. We were a merry party. When we got up on the big stoop and among the stone pillars, we were surprised to have a man say to us, that "it was past the hour for visitors." We were indignant of course, and told him that we had come to go through the Asylum, and not to learn the time of day. He said that he would have to speak to some one; and soon a man came to us, (a mighty handsome one by the way) and fixing a great searching black eye upon us, said to us that we might go through; but he scared us all by cautioning us with a tone and look, which I shall never forget, to bear in mind that we were in a Hospital for the Insane. So we went around. Every thing was as clean as clean can be. (I hope mother wont go there; for she is forever dinging at me about dirt in my room): We were all disappointed. For all we could see, the patients look and act like other people. We asked our guide, who was civil enough, if he wouldn't take us where we could see *something*. He politely bowed us away to the sleigh.
> Now, Sir, if this is all that one can see in your place, I beg leave to tell you that I shall not visit it again, and shall dissuade all my friends from doing so.

This is all at present from
Yours to command,
Araminta C. Stubbs
P.S.—Pray, is not the young man who went round with us a bit of a
wag, or is he one of the patients? A.C. S.

Miss Araminta C. complains that "for all she could see, the patients look and act like other people." Ah—could she look into the inner soul of those whose apparent composure has so disappointed her sickly and vulgar anticipations! Could she see the heart aching with a grief which will not and cannot be comforted—or withered by long and solitary indulgence in thoughts of the neglect or scorn of the world, which, whether real or imaginary, cannot be removed by the sympathising tones nor cheering smiles of that love which always soothes and animates a mind in trouble—or torn and racked by passions which are always contending with each other, and, having no reality for their object, may never give any outward manifestation of the agonizing tumult which reigns within!

But Araminta complains, that she was not taken where she could "see something."—What does she mean by something? Is it slam-bang, kick, rear up, smash windows, make fun, and yell? Such things are to be seen outside of, as well as within the Asylum; but however entertaining they might be to the lady, the performance of them might hazard her safety. There are, we own, many queer cases amongst us, whose idiosyncrasies, while they are very funny, never endanger the safety of the most timid or the most pure. There is especially one little fellow whose ideas run incessantly on osculation. An uncontrollable desire to kiss every thing he sees is his failing. And the dreadful looks of the objects he sometimes selects for this pastime are the chief grounds for declaring him insane. . . .

Editor's Table (1855)

"An Hour with the Insane," says the courteous editor of the N.Y. *Commercial Advertiser*, "we spent the other day." Not that the editor was really here, in *propria persona*, but in perusing the pages of the OPAL, his mind and kind sympathies were here. Well, others, we trust, have in like manner, "spent an instructive hour," and others, still, might find the perusal of its unpretending pages instructive and pleasing, were they to receive it. The fragrance of the rose is not diminished by its seclusion from the embellished floral bower—nor are the thoughts of truth and beauty which find utterance here, less fraught with the aroma of wisdom because they emanate from the seclusive quite of Asylumia.

If not our gratitude, certainly our pride is awakened by the fraternal etiquette of the *Advertiser*—somewhat critical though it is, since by having nearly now reached its half century, it deserves, as it surely has, our need of veneration—and the manner of its allusion to our opalescent gems is in nowise unappreciated. But we deem it proper to say, here, that its articles are all written by patients, and under no other "supervision" or restraint than their own *genii*. The beloved and honored Superintendent, nor either of his estimable Assistants interpose any control or direction in the productions of the brains or pens of the contributors to the OPAL—that is, they do not advise or supervise in the matter, farther than to express their decisions that such and such individuals, thus desiring—and many are *here*, somehow seized with *author-mania*, who before never thought of the thing—may be furnished with writing materials and opportunities to "improve their gifts." Every one thus furnished, writes "what is written;" and as written, each article appears, with such alterations only, as the principal editor, or the printer, might properly make in similar cases, regarding punctuation, &c. And when we reflect that many of our most approved articles are written by patients occupying halls where there is little to superinduce that elasticity of mind, and that gaiety of feeling indicated by their compositions—but where, on the contrary, they are often unavoidably subjected to annoyances from insane singing, talking, laughing, weeping, walking, etc, etc.— scenes ever to be found among a company of insane persons—we think we have reason to feel a degree of satisfaction with, if not literary pride of our productions. And what encouragement doth this one thought of itself afford the Superintendent and his Assistants, that they do not "labor in vain," in a most humane and important department of society, while laboring to restore their unfortunate fellow-beings to health, usefulness and happiness.

And what higher incentive can be presented to the enlightened legislator or to the statesman, in favor of a liberal appropriation of the public funds for supplying the Institution with all needful facilities for the care and restoration to active usefulness the men and women who, for various reasons, it becomes necessary, for a time, to isolate from the associations and responsibilities of life at large, in the halls of the Asylum?

Views of Insanity by an Ex-patient (1859)

As far as any personal experience goes, we are rather at a loss to convey to the mind of the sane reader a definite idea of insanity. We were going to say we never had a spectral vision; but a perhaps Quixotic desire to stick to the truth, leads us to record the following incident: when a youngster we once fell asleep on the kitchen floor: being suddenly aroused to consciousness, we for but an instant of time—hardly that, fancied we saw a *gray cat* in the very act of falling upon us: this was our first and last apparition. During a period antecedent to the last ten years our physical frame was subject to some disturbances; therefore in giving any opinion as to the essence of insanity—excepting what we make *inferentially* from witnessing or hearing of diseased mentality in others, we draw upon our memory of what we were at that period.

Without pretending to a very accurate knowledge of metaphysical or medical science, our knowledge enables us to make these two classifications of insanity—diseased will; diseased perception. Under the first class, we are forced to enroll ourselves; in the second, not at all; yet, ten years ago, we might have properly been under that other classification.

Previous to the time in question, *we dreamed* (perhaps in a secondary sense the observation applied to the day as well as the night): *during* that time our slumbers have been dreamless. To this assertion we add the following qualification: we have sometimes awakened from an apparently unbroken rest and been told that we had talked in our sleep. Nevertheless we believe that during the period specified, unbroken rest has been the rule, and dreaming the momentary exception.

Let us without making open war against the dogmas of science, in making our *classification*, record our *impression* that the first has (in a great measure) but an existence in the imagination of men—that the proper nomenclature of moral insanity is wicked will. Acting under the conviction to a great extent, we state our opinions. *Insanity is the stuff that dreams are made of.* We fancy it closely allied to somnambulism. In some temperaments, under severe exertion of the mental and physical powers, the mind is withdrawn from contact with surrounding objects, while the body continues mechanically to perform its customary actions—to exemplify which, a canal-driver, I think, told me that he had, when on foot, following his horse in the night-time, fallen asleep, yet continuing to follow his horse. We mention also that after the toil of a summer's day (during the period when our physical frame was not what it is now) playing on an instrument of music, we have fallen asleep and awakened, without, as we believed, disturbing the progress of the music.

Insanity, dreams, clairvoyance, somnambulism, and catalepsy—all, we have an opinion, are links between the terrestrial and spirit world. This last is the region or regions where the spirit, disembodied, betakes itself after death—and, under abnormal conditions, before. In these abnormal states the mind has *gone*, partially or wholly. Where a slight degree of exterior (physical) perception remains, an insane person seems to have his physical senses, seeing, etc.,—while he is in most respects like one in a fit or cataleptic trance. That insanity is but a waking-day-sleep, is gathered not from our own experience, but that of lunatics with whom we conversed after they had become sound.

From *Opal: A Monthly Periodical of the State Lunatic Asylum, Devoted to Usefulness, Edited by the Patients of the Utica State Lunatic Asylum* (Utica, NY: Utica State Lunatic Asylum), 1851–1860; excerpts are from the following: 1852, vol. 2, 33–35, 121–122; 1855, vol. 5, 188–189; 1859, vol. 9, 32–33.

Limerick District Lunatic Asylum
Report of the Limerick District Lunatic Asylum for the Year Ending December 31st, 1866

(1867)

Superintendents of asylums were generally obligated to submit an annual report to those organizations and authorities in charge of supporting and supervising the facility. These reports provide fairly detailed information about matters such as the number of admissions and discharges, patient behavior and treatment, staff, and the status of buildings and grounds. The following is an excerpt from an annual report submitted by the physician Robert Fitzgerald, resident medical superintendent of the Limerick District Lunatic Asylum in Ireland, to local political and church authorities. What appear at first glance to be rather mundane statistical tables reveal a great deal about the kinds of individuals institutionalized, how life in the asylum was organized, and how administrators categorized patients and disorders. Note that the abbreviation "Do." below stands for "ditto."

Return of the Number of Patients Admitted,
Discharged, Died, and Escaped within the Year

	Males	Females	TOTAL
Number of patients remaining in Asylum on 31 December 1865	224	219	443
Do. Patients admitted to 31 Dec 1866	31	39	70
TOTAL	255	258	513
Number Discharged Recovered during the year . . .	20	17	
Do. Improved	4	10	
Do. Unimproved	2	3	
Do. Escaped	1	0	
Do. Deaths	2	9	
TOTAL			68
Remaining in Asylum on 31 Dec 1866	226	219	445
Distribution by Counties			
City of Limerick	21	31	52
County of Limerick	110	103	213
County of Clare	95	85	180
TOTAL	226	219	445
State as to Probability of Recovery of those in Asylum on 31 December 1866			
Lunatics Probably Curable	49	46	95
Lunatics Probably Incurable	154	149	303
Lunatics, Idiots	9	10	19
Lunatics, Epileptics	14	14	28
TOTAL	226	219	445
Classification of Patients according to Physician's Abstract of Cases			
Mania—Probably Curable	49	46	95
Do. Do. Incurable	154	149	303
Do. Idiots	9	10	19
Do. Epileptics	14	14	28
TOTAL	226	219	445
Daily Average Number of Patients			443

Daily Average Number of Patients Employed during the Year Ended 31st December, 1866

Male		Female	
Garden Labour	2	Needle Work	35
Agricultural Labour	30	Knitting	34
Tailoring Work	1	Assisting in Laundry	18
Carpentry	1	Cleaning House	18
Cleaning House	14	Miscellaneous	23
Miscellaneous	8		
TOTAL EMPLOYED	**56**	**TOTAL EMPLOYED**	**128**

Work Done by Female Patients

Made: 400 shirts, 240 sheets, 364 chemises, 180 gowns, 162 petticoats, 310 caps, 498 aprons, 89 bed ticks, 124 bolsters, 24 table cloths, 12 bath towels, 13 rollers, 604 pairs of stockings, and 623 pairs of socks.

Repaired: 500 jackets, 601 pairs of trousers, 276 waist coats, 571 shirts, 244 sheets, 167 blankets, 134 bed ticks, 149 bolsters, 800 gowns, 921 chemises, 621 petticoats, 214 caps, 281 aprons, 10 table cloths, 47 shawls, 3814 pairs of stockings, and 4124 pairs of socks.

Authority for Admissions

Authority for Admission of Patients, and Number Admitted
during the Year ended 31st December, 1866

	Males	Females	TOTAL
Ordinary cases admitted by order of the Board	4	7	11
Ordinary cases admitted as urgent by the Physicians	16	23	39
Dangerous Lunatics, by Warrant of the Lord Lieutenant	9	6	15
Lunatics charged with offences, by Warrant of the Lord Lieutenant	2	3	5
TOTAL	31	39	70

Age of Patients

Age of Patients Admitted and Discharged Recovered
during the Year ended 31st December, 1866

	Admitted Male	Admitted Female	Admitted TOTAL	Discharged Cured Male	Discharged Cured Female	Discharged Cured TOTAL
Under 10	1	1	2	0	1	1
10–20	17	4	21	0	2	2
20–30	5	8	13	11	8	19
30–40	6	9	15	3	2	5
40–50	0	11	11	4	3	7
50–60	0	5	5	0	1	1
60–70	1	1	2	1	0	1
70 and upwards	1	0	1	1	0	1
TOTAL	31	39	70	20	17	37

Duration of Illness

Duration of Disease previous to Admission in those
Discharged Recovered during the Year ended 31st December, 1866

	Males	Females	TOTAL
Under 1 month	5	3	8
Under 3 months	3	1	4
Under 6 months	2	1	3
Under 9 months	1	1	2
Under 1 year	2	1	3
Under 2 years	1	1	2
Under 3 years		2	2
Under 4 years		2	2
Under 5 years	1	2	3
Under 6 years			
Under 8 years			
Under 10 years and upwards			
Unknown	5	3	8
TOTAL	20	17	37

Length of Stay

Length of Residence in Asylum of those Discharged, Recovered,
and Improved during the Year ended 31st December, 1866

	Recovered Male	Recovered Female	Recovered TOTAL	Improved Male	Improved Female	Improved TOTAL
Under 2 months	7	2	9	2	1	3
Under 4 months	2	2	4			
Under 6 months	2	2	4		1	1
Under 8 months		2	2			
Under 12 months	2	6	8	1	3	4
Under 18 months	3		3			
Under 2 years	1	2	3	1		1
Under 3 years	3	1	4	1		1
Under 4 years					1	1
Under 5 years					1	1
Under 6 years					1	1
Under 10 years					2	2
TOTAL	20	17	37	5	10	15

Form of Illness (Admittees)

Form of Disease in those Admitted during the Year ended 31st December, 1866

	Male	Female	TOTAL
Acute Mania	15	20	35
Chronic Mania	13	12	25
Melancholia		1	1
Melancholia Religious	1	2	3
Hereditary	2	3	5
Imbecility		1	1
TOTAL	31	39	70

Form of Illness (Those Remaining)

Form of Disease in those Remaining in Asylum on 31st December, 1866

	Male	Female	TOTAL
Mania Acute and Chronic	137	111	248
Melancholia Religious	39	47	86
Dementia	26	35	61
Monomania	1		1
Imbecility		2	2
Idiocy	9	10	19
Mental Affection	14	14	28
TOTAL	226	219	445

Education

Educational Condition of Patients in Asylum on 31st December, 1866

	Male	Female	TOTAL
Well Educated	21	14	35
Can Read and Write Well	24	28	52
Can Read and Write Indifferently	70	37	107
Can Read Only	48	49	97
Cannot Read or Write	50	81	131
Unknown	13	10	23
TOTAL	226	219	445

Marital Status

Social Condition of Patients in Asylum on 31st December, 1866

	Male	Female	TOTAL
Married	35	57	92
Single	187	130	317
Widowers and Widows	4	26	30
Unknown		6	6
TOTAL	226	219	445

Conduct

Classification of Patients in Asylum on 31st December, 1866

	Male	Female	TOTAL
Convalescent	18	9	27
Quiet and Orderly, but Insane	90	73	163
Moderately Tranquil	70	58	128
Noisy and Refractory	48	79	127
Imbecile and Epileptic	14	16	30
Suicidal		4	4
TOTAL	226	219	445

Previous Occupation

Previous Occupation of those in Asylum 31st December, 1866

	Male	Female	TOTAL
Labouring Class	145	44	189
Farming	9		9
Domestic Servants	1	38	39
Clerks	2		2
Shopkeepers	5	4	9
Tailors and Seamstresses	4	5	9
Artisans	2		2
Painters and Glaziers	1		1
Smiths and Workers in Metals	1		1
Masons and Bricklayers	1		1
Carpenters	4		4
Shoemakers	3		3
Hatters	1		1
Factory Workers	1		1
Vicutallers	3		3
Pedlars and Hucksters	1	5	6
Lawyers			
Medical Men	2		2
Members of Religious Communities	1		1
Students and Teachers	5	2	7
Soldiers and Pensioners	10		10
Police	2		2
Revenue Officers	2		2
Sailors	1		1
Publicans	1		1
Various Employments			
TOTAL	208	98	306
No Occupation or Unknown	18	121	139
TOTAL	226	219	445

Causes of Death

Causes of Death during the Year ended 31st December, 1866

	Male	Female	TOTAL
Debility		3	3
Congestion of Brain		2	2
Senile Insanity	1	1	2
Marasmus		1	1
Consumption		1	1
Exhaustion from Epilepsy	1	1	2
TOTAL	2	9	11

Escapes and Escape Attempts

Male	Female	TOTAL	Observations
	1	1	Attempted to get away but was caught inside the walls
1		1	Climbed over the front gate but was caught immediately
1		1	Attempted to get out through the Window of his Cell at Night
1		1	Effected his Escape, and his Friends kept him at home, where he ultimately became quite well

Supposed Cause of Mental Illness

Supposed Cause of Mental Disease of Patients
in Asylum on 31st December, 1866

	Males	Females	TOTAL
MORAL CAUSES			
Poverty and Reverse of Fortune	13	15	28
Grief, Fear, and Anxiety	15	12	27
Love, Jealousy, and Seduction	3	9	12
Domestic Quarrels and Afflictions	2	4	6
Religious Excitement	5	8	13
Study and Mental Excitement	5	3	8
Ill-Treatment		7	7
Pride		1	1
Anger		1	1
Kleptomania	1	1	2
TOTAL MORAL CAUSES	44	61	105
PHYSICAL CAUSES			
Intemperance and Irregularity of Life	10	5	15
Cerebral Diseases or Affections	24	21	45
Congenital Idiocy, Etc.		1	1
Febrile Affections		9	9
Effects of Climate and Sunstroke	5	1	6
Bodily Injuries and Disorders	7		7
Abuse of Medicine	2		2
Sedentary Habits	3	3	6
TOTAL PHYSICAL CAUSES	51	40	91
Hereditary	29	28	57
Not Known	102	90	192
TOTAL	226	219	445

Patients under Restraints

Number of Patients Placed under Mechanical Restraint or Seclusion
during the Year ended 31st December, 1866

Male: 0

Female: 14 (all with application of straight Waistcoat)

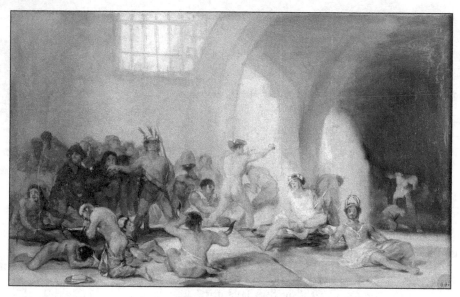

Francisco José de Goya y Lucientes, *Lunatic Asylum* (ca. 1812–1819). It is known that Goya visited an asylum around the area of Sargasso. The Sargasso asylum was part of a hospital complex first built in 1425, and, similar to what Goya depicts here, patients at the asylum were given tent cloth to wear, violent patients were kept in cells of wood or limestone, and the floor was covered with straw. The Sargasso asylum was also noteworthy, however, in that the inmates put on regular theatrical performances for visitors. Canvas. Real Academia de Bellas Artes de San Fernando, Madrid, Spain. © Erich Lessing/ Art Resource, NY.

Amusements, Games, Books, &c.

Description of Amusement and Games	Class of Books and Periodical supplied to Patients	Male	Female	TOTAL
Ball playing	Newspapers and periodicals	24		24
Card playing	"	36	36	72
Foot Ball	"	50		50
Instrumental Music	"	6		6
Music and Dancing	"	20	40	60

Patients' Dietary

Meals	Dietary	Male	Female	TOTAL
ORDINARY				
Breakfast	7 oz. of Indian Meal and Cutlins made into Stirabout	155	90	245
	12 oz. of Bread for Males and 8 oz. for Females	71	129	200
	1 pint of New Milk	200	120	320
	1 pint of Tea	26	99	125
Dinner	12 oz. of Bread, or a 1/4 stone of Potatoes for Males, 8 oz. of Bread or 3 lbs. of Potatoes for Females	226	219	445
	12 oz. of Beef on Sundays and Thursdays, 8 oz. on Mondays and Tuesdays, Ox Head soup on Saturdays,1 pint of Milk or Coffee on Wednesays and Fridays	219	213	432
Supper	6 oz. of Bread and 1/2 pint of Milk	226	219	445
	Tea		6	6
EXTRA				
Breakfast	Butter			
Dinner	Roast Beef and Mutton			
HOSPITAL DIET				
	Porter, Wine, Whiskey, Rice, and Brandy			

From Limerick District Lunatic Asylum, *Report of the Limerick District Lunatic Asylum for the Year Ending December 31st, 1866* (Limerick: G. M'Kern & Sons, 1867).

Office of Superintendent Government, Great Britain

Annual Report of the Insane Asylums in Bengal for the Year 1867

(1868)

Lunatic asylums first appeared in India toward the end of the eighteenth century. What began as an attempt by the East India Company to build replicas of British asylums on Indian soil was maintained by the British Crown after it formally established its rule in 1858. The spread of British asylums throughout India was justified on the same humanitarian grounds touted earlier by the likes of Pinel, Esquirol, and Tuke: a colonial obligation to advance and civilize backward people and institutions.

Since British colonials and authorities considered themselves superior to their colonized subjects, however, they were unwilling to compel British nationals to share facilities with native Indians. Thus, a segregated system was established. Insane Indians were confined in shabby, public institutions, while their European counterparts were accommodated in a private asylum, given time to recuperate, and then returned to their homeland. The following annual report describes conditions in the public asylum in Patna.

From Surgeon R. F. Hutchinson, M.D. (Superintendent, Patna Lunatic Asylum) to Surgeon-Major H. M. Macpherson (Secretary, Inspector General, Medical Department, Lower Provinces). Patna, 1 January 1868

Sir,

I have the honor of submitting the usual Asylum Report for the year 1867, and before entering upon the history of the year, I would draw special attention to the following objects of importance: —I. The necessity for increased accommodation in the Asylum buildings; and

II. The necessity of adapting the present erection to the present advanced condition of sanitary sciences.

But then the question may be put, *in limine*, why interfere with either? the Asylum has jogged on very well in the years that are past; let it do so equally in the years to come. I think, however, that, with the improvements I am about to suggest, it will be allowed that matters would progress still more favourably: that the present rate of sickness and mortality would be still further diminished, and the general comfort and happiness of the inmates still better maintained.

I. In May 1866, I reported on the crowded state of the Asylum, and suggested a mode of relief. It was then overcrowded with 138 patients. How much more so it is now with 151! The general form and proportions of the Asylum are known to the authorities; so I shall merely observe that the main building has accommodation for 59 insanes; the old Civil Jail holds 25; and the female side has 20 cells. Thus the maximum accommodation is for 104 patients, not taking into consideration the deep verandahs in both Asylums; but with cell accommodation for 104 patients, we have a total of 151 (113 males and 38 females), or 47 beyond our capacity. Such being the case, (and we are receiving weekly additions to our strength) some means should be devised for relieving the pressure before a dire epidemic of cholera sweeps away the surplus, as it did in 1866.

II. The sanitary improvements necessary. The drainage everywhere is excellent; but then the building is situated on low ground, which every year is subject to inundation. Last year the flood was so high that all the drains were full of backwater, and in 1861 the water was knee-deep at the south end of the Asylum enclosure. The buildings have not yet recovered from the effects of last year's flood; so great was the saturation of the soil, and the attendant percolation, that the mud floors of the manufacturing sheds, though a foot above the ground, were puddles, and the foot holes of the looms were little wells.

The south end of the main building was untenable from the damp which showed on the walls three feet from the floor; and from having a northern aspect, and never being reached by the sun, it remains damp and disagreeable, and unfit for occupation.

The sickness might have been considerable, had it not been for the large quantities of straw which I laid in for the insanes to lie upon.

This evil cannot, of course, be remedied without either raising the plinth or removing the Asylum bodily to a higher site.

The ventilation of the main block of the Asylum is very defective, and necessarily so from its shape, which, being that of a large quadrangle running North and South, can only receive ventilation from the prevailing eastern and western winds. Therefore the north and south ranges of cells rarely, if even, have a breath of air through them, as their doors and windows are all north and south, and they have dead walls to the East and west. These remarks only apply to the main block, the rest of the Asylum being admirably ventilated.

To increase the accommodation, and throw open the whole building to air and sunshine, I would suggest the following alterations, illustrating them by a plan of the main block. Remove entirely the northern and two southern rows of cells, and extend to the northern the eastern and western rows of cells. This extension would exactly compensate for the removals, and we should thus have two long rows of airy and well ventilated cells, accommodating 60 patients; and from there being no enclosing walls, there would be less risk of damp. To the north of the old Dewani Jail, I would erect two parallel blocks for 40 patients, and in the same manner extend the female block to the south, allowing accommodation for 40 patients, instead of 20, as at present. Thus the Asylum would be capable of separately accommodating 165 patients as follows:

Main block	60 patients
New block	40 patients
Dewani block	25 patients
Female block	40 patients
Total	165 patients

Our present strength being 150.

IV. On the whole, the health of the Asylum has been very good, considering the risk and discomfort to which the insanes were exposed by the inundation. The mortality was greater than in the previous year, but then our numbers were considerably increased; so that the balance is rather in favor of 1867.

As usual, dysentery and diarrhea carried off the majority of the fatal cases, there being ten cases of both. Of the nine dysentery cases, not one was struck down in robust health; four were cases of old age; and the other five were admitted feeble and emaciated.

V. The conservancy of the Asylum has been carefully attended to, the dry-earth system being enforced as strictly as possible. I have largely used McDougall's Disinfecting Powder, and find it very valuable as a deodoriser. Until the inundation, the cells were regularly leeped, and are so now, except in the south end of the male Asylum, where the damp still prevails so greatly.*

VI. The food of the insane has, on the whole, been good. Tricks have at times been played with the ata; and to prevent their occurrence, I am anxious to grind our own flour on the premises.†

VII. The clothing has been ample, and of good quality, every part of it manufactured in the Asylum; and its regular washing has been strictly attended to. But we have suffered a good deal at the hands of unruly patients, male and female, whole tháns of dosotee having been torn into shreds, and numerous blankets consigned to the same fate.‡

VIII. The manufactures are carried on steadily within certain limits. Insanes will work steadily in the beaten paths; but it is rather difficult to lead them across country by teaching them arts entirely new for they are by no means sharp in picking up knowledge, and Return N. 6 [data not included here] will show that we have not a very large stock of workmen to draw upon.

However, we manage, in considerable degree, to pay our way, and have a nice balance to our credit as well.

IX. I have repeatedly had occasion to draw attention to the unsatisfactory, if not illegal, manner in which alleged insanes are sent to the Asylum.

---

*Editor's note: Leeping involves washing something with cow dung and water.

†Editor's note: *Ata* is whole wheat flour typically used to make flatbread.

‡Editor's note: *Thans* refers to lengths of cloth; *dosotee* refers to a particular type of fabric.

In many instances patients have been sent in with merely a scrap of vernacular writing; in others no proper descriptive roll is sent; or if it is, the information is most meagre, and at times contradictory. Rarely, if ever, is the strict order requiring personal examination by a Magistrate carried out, and the consequence is that many a man, reeling about the bazaar intoxicated with ganjah or spirit, finds himself, on coming to his senses, an inmate of a Lunatic Asylum.*

And this incarceration, however temporary, is by no means a trifling matter; for let the man ever thereafter religiously eschew ganjah or spirit, he will never remove the stigma from his name that he once was págul, and once an inmate of a págul-khána.†

Return No. 4 [data not shown] shows how large a proportion of the admissions is due to ganjah and bháng.‡ Under the seduction and maddening influence of these poisons, so openly sold and easily procured, many a career, opening hopefully and prosperously, has terminated in sorrow and gloom. How bitterly the first, and perhaps only, whiff of that deadly chelum is lamented; how hopelessly the first, and perhaps solitary, draught of bháng is deplored!**

We must give the native credit for having feelings like ourselves. We must allow him a conscience which, though it be frequently dormant, is still open to the chidings of remorse.

And it is a sad, though interesting, study to watch the workings of the mind in many a poor patient. The reply with difficulty extracted,—the face hung down and averted,—the love of silence and solitude,—all indicate the smitings of conscience and gnawings of remorse, and excite a sincere pity for the unhappy victim to such seductions.

I have now in the Asylum two or three such cases; one in particular, where the patient, a Bengali lad, seems overwhelmed with a sense of his disgrace and degradation.

X. While noticing one undoubtedly powerful agent in creating insanity, we may fitly examine the pretensions of another supposed to be equally

---

*Editor's note: *Ganjah* is also known as cannabis and hashish.

†Editor's note: *Págul* means "insane" or "mad"; a *págul*-khána is an insane asylum or madhouse.

‡Editor's note: A preparation from cannabis.

**Editor's note: *Chelum* here refers to hashish.

powerful in exciting it. We may try and ascertain whether the word "lunacy" has any real claims to the derivation assigned to it. Anxious to test the reality or otherwise of lunar influence on the insane, I carried out during the year the following observations, adding to them notes of the pressure, temperature, and humidity of the atmosphere.

As they only extend over a year, they are perhaps not very valuable, but still the results are interesting; the more so, as they are, I believe, at variance with prevailing ideas. Thus, extremes of temperature are not necessarily accompanied by maniacal exacerbation, for the greatest heat, 110° F, was noted on June 4th and September 10th, and the greatest cold, 40°, on December 15th, and on neither day was any patient excited. Nor are extremes of pressure; for the Barometer was at its utmost height, 30–33, on November 23rd at its greatest depression, 29–31, on July 7th, without any cases of maniacal excitement.

Humidity apparently predisposes to excitement; for on the day of greatest rain, July 29th (when four inches were gauged), one patient was attacked; and in July, the month of greatest rain, (when _____ were gauged),* we had the maximum excitation; in the rainy months of June, July, August, September, and October we had 45.5 percent of all cases of excitement.

I should fancy that the mugginess of the rains has as much to say to these cases as the positive humidity. Now for lunar influence, or lunacy proper. The annexed Table will show that the lunations had but little influence on the patients attacked; the greatest number falling to the share of the new moon, and smallest but one to that of the full moon. And that the full moon has apparently but little influence will be seen from this Table (B), which shows that, while forty-nine cases of excitement occurred during the wax, eighty-nine occurred during the wane of the moon.

On the whole, I think the question is still an open one, to be decided by further experiment; and I believe that magnetic and electric observations will yield valuable results. These I hope to commence on the receipt of the instruments I have sent home for.

XI. I regret that I can only repeat the remarks in my Report for 1865 regarding the Asylum establishment. As a class, the keepers are of little

---

*Editor's note: The author left this blank.

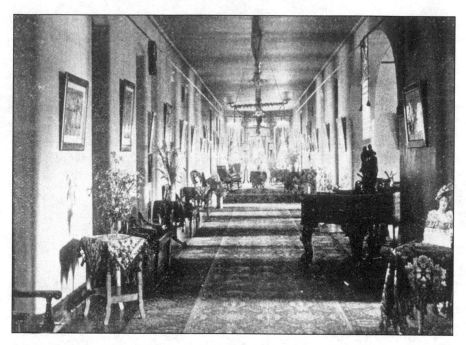

Interior view of a corridor in the asylum at Norristown, Pennsylvania, United States (1896). Courtesy of the National Library of Medicine, Bethesda, MD.

worth, and I have not received from Sergeant Frawley, the Overseer, the assistance I anticipated. He is greatly wanting in activity, and has not the confidence or respect of his subordinates.

XII. I append a list of the visits paid to the Asylum during the year by the Official Visitors:

Jan	None
Feb	Officiating Deputy Inspector General
Mar	Deputy Inspector General; Judge; Joint Magistrate
Apr	Deputy Inspector General
May	Ditto Ditto
June	Ditto Ditto
July	Ditto Ditto
Aug	Ditto Ditto
Sep	Ditto Ditto
Oct	Ditto Ditto Commissioner
Nov	Ditto Ditto
Dec	None

I have the honor to be, Sir,
Your most obedient Servant,
R. F. Hutchinson, M.D.
Superintendent, Lunatic Asylum

From W. A. Green (Inspector General of Hospitals, Lower Provinces, Office of Superintendent Government), *Annual Report of the Insane Asylums in Bengal for the Year 1867* (Calcutta: Office of Superintendent Government Printing, 1868), 71–75.

Elizabeth P. W. Packard
(1816–1897)

The Prisoners' Hidden Life, or Insane Asylums Unveiled
(1868)

Already in the eighteenth century, there were widely publicized reports about sane individuals being committed against their will as well as stories about the abuse of patients in asylums. By the second half of the nineteenth century, novels and short stories, such as Sheridan Le Fanu's *Uncle Silas* (1864) and Charlotte Perkins Gilman's *The Yellow Wallpaper* (1899), were replete with tales of madwomen kept in attics and of husbands or guardians attempting to drive their wards mad. Such horror stories were reinforced throughout the century by former patients who alleged they were mistreated in asylums. Their memoirs often had sensational titles, for example, Samuel Bruckshaw's *One More Proof of the Iniquitous Abuse of Private Madhouses* (1774) and Elizabeth Packard's *The Prisoners' Hidden Life, or Insane Asylums Unveiled* (1868). By the late nineteenth century, these reports helped lend credence to calls for a far-reaching reform of state hospitals.

The following is an excerpt from Elizabeth Packard's *The Prisoners' Hidden Life*. A champion for married women's rights, Packard accused her husband of committing her to the Jacksonville Insane Asylum in Illinois against her will. She claimed that her husband, in collusion with the asylum's director, kept her there for espousing Calvinist religious beliefs. Eventually gaining her freedom, she published a number of books in the years 1864–1868 about her experiences, going on to form one of the first antipsychiatry associations in the United States. Even in the absence of knowing the veracity of her claims, her account below shows how conventional ideals of femininity and family inflected early antipsychiatric sentiments.

Mrs. Cheneworth's Suicide—Medical Abuse

Mrs. Cheneworth hung herself in her own room, after retiring from the dancing party, last night. Her measure of grace was not sufficient to enable her to bear the accumulated burdens of her hard fate any longer, without driving her to desperation. I can not blame her for deliberately preferring death, to such a life as she has been experiencing in this Asylum. She has literally been driven to it by abuse.

She was entered in my ward, where she remained for several weeks, when she was removed to the lowest ward, where she has been murdered by slow tortures. If this Institution is not responsible for the life of Mrs. Cheneworth, then I don't know what murder is. She was evidently insane when she entered; she was not responsible, although her reason was not entirely dethroned. Her moral nature was keenly sensitive; her power of self-control was crushed by disease and medical maltreatment. She resisted until she evidently saw it was useless to expect justice, and was just crushed beneath this powerful despotism.

She was a lovely woman, fitted by nature and education to be an ornament to society and her family. Gentle and confiding, with a high sense of honor and self-respect, she despised all degrading associations. . . . She was a most accomplished dancer, having been trained in the school of the best French dancers in the country. Her complexion white and clear, with regular features, black, but mild and tender eyes, her hair was long, black, and beautiful. In short, she was a little, beautiful, fawn-like creature, when she came to this Institution. She had been here a short time once before, after the birth of her first child; and from her account I inferred that her restoration to reason was not then attended with the grim spectre of horrors which must have inevitably accompanied this.

She had left a young babe, this time, which her physician advised her to wean, since she was now in a delicate condition. Thus her overtasked physical nature, abused as it was by bad medical treatment, added to the double burden she was called to endure, could not sustain the balance of her mental faculties. Her nerves were unstrung, and lost their natural tone by the influence of opium, that most deadly foe of nature, which evidently caused her insanity. The opium was expected to operate as a quietus to her then excited nervous system; but instead of this, it only increased her nervous irritability. The amount was then increased, and this course persisted, until her system became drunk, as it were, by its influence. The effect produced was like that of excessive drinking, when it causes delirium tremens. Thus she became a victim to that absurd practice of the medical profession, which depends upon poisons instead of nature to cure disease.

What Mrs. Cheneworth wanted was, the nourishment of her exhausted physical nature, by rest, food, air, and exercise. She did not need to have the power of her system thrown into confusion by taxing them with poisons, which nature must either counteract and resist, or be overcome by them, and sink into death. Nature was importuning for help to bear her burdens, being already overtasked. But instead of listening to these demands, her blinded friends allowed her to be thus medically abused. After having suffered her to receive this treatment, and thus brought into a still worse condition—an insane state—when more than ever she needed help and the most tender, watchful care; then to be cast off in her helplessness upon strangers, who knew nothing of her character, her habits, her propensities, her cravings, her disposition, or her constitution; how could they reasonably expect her to thus receive the care necessary to her recovery? They probably did expect it, and on this false expectation placed her here for appropriate medical treatment.

What a delusion the world is laboring under, to expect such treatment here! Did they but know the truth, they would find that all the "medical treatment" they get here is to lock them up! and thus having hidden them from observation, and cut them off from all communication with their friends, they then inflict upon them what they consider condign punishment for being insane! Why can not their friends bestow upon them this "medical treatment" at home, without the expense of sending them to this

Asylum to get it? This is the sum and substance of all the "treatment" they get here, which they could not get at home—that is, they could not get *this treatment* from reasonable friends, any where, outside of these inquisitorial institutions. How doleful is this purgatory? thus legally upheld for the *punishment of the innocent!* Great God! Is this Institution located within the province of thy just government? or is this Satan's seat, that has not yet been subjected to thy omnipotent power? . . .

Alas! for poor Mrs. Cheneworth! her days for reasonable treatment expired when she was removed to the lowest ward, and consigned to the care of Elizabeth Bonner. This attendant was a perfect contrast to her former attendants in character, disposition, and habits. She was a large, coarse, stout, Irish woman, stronger than most men; of quick temper, very easily thrown off its balance, when, for the time being, she would be a perfect demon, lost to all traces of humanity. Her manners were very coarse and masculine, a loud and boisterous talker, and a great liar, with no education, and could neither read nor write.

To this vile ignorant woman was Mrs. Cheneworth entrusted, to treat her just as her own feelings dictated. Miss Bonner's first object was to "subdue her," that is, to break down her aspiring feelings, and bring her into a state of cringing submission to her dictation. Here was a contest between her naturally refined instincts, and Miss Bonner's unrefined and coarse nature. Any manifestation of the lady-like nature of Mrs. Cheneworth, was met by its opposite in Miss Bonner's servant-like nature and position, and she must lord it over this gentle lady. The position of the latter, as a boarder, must at her beck, be exchanged, by her being made to feel that she was nothing but a slave and menial. If she ventured to remonstrate against this wanton usurpation of authority over her, she could only expect to receive physical abuse, such as she was poorly able to bear. And O! the black tale of wrongs and cruel tortures this tender woman experienced at the hand of this giant like tyrant no tongue or pen can ever describe! She was choked, pounded, kicked, and plunged under water, and well nigh strangled to death. Mrs. Coe assured me this was only a specimen of the kind of treatment all were liable to receive at her hands, since she claimed that this was the way to cure them! and this insisted upon, was what she was put here to do. Being strong, she was peculiarly adapted to her place, since no woman or man could grapple with her successfully.

The last time I saw Mrs. Cheneworth was at the dance, after which she hung herself, being found suspended from the upper part of her window by the facing of her dress. I never saw a person so changed. I did not know her when Miss Bonner introduced me to her that evening. O, such a haggard look! such despair and wretchedness as her countenance reflected, I have never witnessed. My feelings were touched. I asked her to go with me, and putting my arm around her waist, she walked with me across the ward to the window looking South. Here we conversed confidentially, freely. She said, "O, Mrs. Packard, I have suffered everything but death since we were parted!"

"But how has your face become so disfigured by sores, and what causes your eyes to be so inflamed?"

"I fainted, and fell down stairs, and they poured camphor so profusely over my face, and into my eyes and ears, that I have, in consequence, been blind and deaf for some time."

I do not know whether her chin, which was red and raw, was thus caused or not. She said the fall had caused her to miscarry, and thus, thought I, you have had to bear this burden in addition to the load of sorrows already heaped upon your tender, weak person. Said I, "Have you any hope of getting out of this place—of ever being taken to your friends?"

"No! none at all! Hopeless, endless torment is all that is before me! O, if I could only get out of this place, I would walk to my father's house. It is only fourteen miles south here," pointing out the window, "but O, these iron bars! I can not escape through them." . . .

Here we leave Mrs. Cheneworth, and turn with sorrowing hearts, to the group of bereaved ones at home—those fondly loved ones, who have thus been called to lay upon the altar of sacrifice, this precious victim. O, could you have foreseen her sad fate, would you thus willingly have laid her upon such an altar? No, you would not. You could not, and lay claim to your humanity. You are not hard hearted and cruel towards this loved idol of your fondest affections. No, you would have cherished her with the tenderest care at home, had you thought it would have promoted her best good. Your hearts, I doubt not, wept the bitterest tears at the thought of being compelled to place her in an Insane Asylum. But these tears could not remove the necessity which you felt you had for so doing. Had you not reason in your own mind for believing that Insane Asylums were established for the benefit of the insane? Did you not suppose they had a competent medical faculty there, who knew better than yourselves how to treat such cases? Yes, so you thought, as you ought to have had reason to think.

But alas! for a blinded public! Alas! for man who is placed under an irresponsible human power. Such power, man is not fitted to be trusted with. Despotism too soon usurps the rule of reason and kindness, and might takes the place of right. Authority supplants kindness, truth, and honesty. After this love of domineering has once taken possession of the human soul, it can only be held by sinister, artful policy. Helplessness, weakness, and dependence are the virgin soil where tyranny and despotism hold their most resistless sway. But under the influence of our free government, power would probably cope with it successfully; therefore its policy consists in cutting off these victims from access to any power by which they would be exposed and dethroned. Therefore, they not only prevent communications with their friends while there, but forestall their confidence in their statements after they get out, assuring them they were so insane while there that they can not report correctly, and therefore their representations must be listened to as mere phantoms of a diseased imagination. Therefore, their friends hear as though they heard not.

But the hitherto blinded public can no longer plead ignorance as an excuse for not grappling successfully with this legalized despotism. No; the Legislature of the State are already informed, through their own Committee, of the imperative need of such enactments, as shall hereafter forever prevent such *abuse of power*, by any future Superintendent, as their present incumbent is found to be notoriously guilty of.

From Mrs. E.P.W. Packard, *The Prisoners' Hidden Life; or, Insane Asylums Unveiled* (Chicago: E.P.W. Packard and A. B. Case, 1868), 202–211.

Brain Science, Nerves, and Clinical Psychiatry

Nelson Sizer

(1812–1897)

*Forty Years in Phrenology:
Embracing Recollections of History,
Anecdote, and Experience*

(1891)

Although today it is often dismissed as little more than quackery, phrenology—the study of the shape and size of crania and how these relate to character attributes—was a serious discipline in the nineteenth century and a precursor to the field of neurology. Its founder, the Badenese anatomist and physician Franz Joseph Gall (1758–1828), observed brain-damaged patients and came to the conclusion that specific aptitudes, inclinations, and faculties were associated with certain parts of the brain, which, in turn, left peculiar traces on the skull.

Phrenologists, however, not only were involved in research. They practiced as itinerant lecturers, psychological examiners, and advisers. In the United States, one of the most successful group of phrenologists were the siblings Orson, Charlotte, and Lorenzo Fowler, who published a prominent journal on the subject and founded consulting firms in major cities throughout the Northeast. From 1838 until the turn of the century, they and their employees

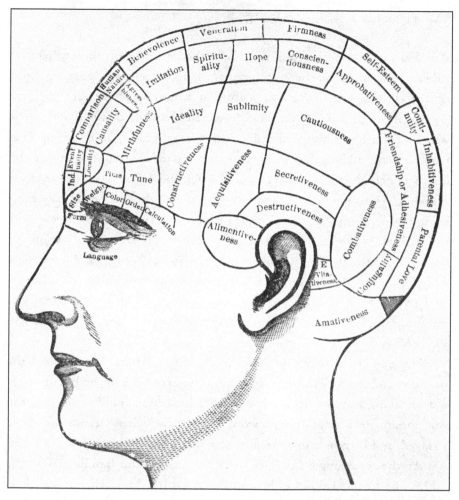

A model phrenological head. From Nelson Sizer and H. S. Drayton, *Heads and Faces, and How to Study Them: A Manual of Phrenology and Physiognomy for the People* (New York: Fowler & Wells, 1887), 195.

visited small towns, renting local churches or town halls and giving lectures on phrenology. Along the way, they were often asked to serve as counselors to parents, spouses, and business associates. The following excerpt from the memoirs of the practitioner Nelson Sizer, an employee of the Fowlers, gives us a sense of the ways in which phrenologists served as incipient psychotherapists.

Timid Child Managed—a Great Test

Another instance occurred in this town, the recital of which may serve to aid some mother or teacher in the management of an unduly cautious child. At the close of a lecture on the nature and training of the sentiments of Approbativeness and Cautiousness, in which I had said that half the trouble which people had with timid children was largely owing to their improper management; adding that however much afraid of strangers any bright, intelligent child, two or three years old, might be, I would undertake to get it willingly into my lap in twenty minutes. A bright and genial lady came up to the platform and said to me, "I have a boy two and a half years old, that I think is bright, but he has never been in the lap of any person not belonging to the family; even his grandpa, who has been in and out almost daily for the last year, can make no headway in overcoming the child's aversion to strangers. Now, if you will come into my house and get that boy into your lap, willingly, in twenty minutes or twenty hours, I will believe in Phrenology."

I found out where she lived and arranged to go there at one o'clock the next day and to enter the dining room in the extension of the house, without knocking and that neither she nor her husband should say any person was coming, or look at or say a word to "Charlie" when I came, nor while I stayed, and I was not to be treated as a stranger while there.

At the hour appointed I entered the house, the family was at the table. Charlie slipped out of his chair and left for the kitchen as quick as legs and "wings" could carry him. I instantly spoke in a tone of familiarity to the parents: "What made you eat up all the dinner so that I can have none? I will pick what I can get." I took a seat at the table and began to eat—and kept talking in a way that a child, which I felt certain was listening, would understand—then laying one hand on the father's head and the other on the mother's, kept on telling them what they were fond of and what they could do, and stealthily turning toward the open door into the kitchen, saw about half of the little head and one bright eye peeping around the door jamb, of course wondering who and what that stranger could be who seemed so much at home with the house, the dinner, and the parents. I went on examining the heads and talking, keeping my back toward the little spectator, who forgot that I saw him leave the room, and, perhaps supposed I did not know he had existence. He edged his way into the room, and as he was against the wall quite a distance from the door, I kept turning my back toward and my face directly from him so as to compel him to get very near me before he could see the face of the drollest man that ever he saw in his home. Of course the plan was to ignore the boy, yet to talk so that he could comprehend it. All at once I walked away from the boy to the opposite side of the room and looking up to a gaudy picture, representing Solomon's temple, with the Sanhedrin in session wearing their red robes, I said, "What a splendid picture Charlie has here!" and then I kept on describing the figures of the council and calling them men and ladies and boys, and I dropped my eye and he stood by my side eagerly looking to learn, for the first time, the mysteries of the great picture which, the stranger had said, was Charlie's. He had forgotten that I was a stranger in the sense of being dangerous. I had said nothing to him, had not looked at him, had not tried to have him come to me, but had let him alone, and talked steadily about what he could not understand, and he had got all the faculties of curiosity aroused, and his Cautiousness had gone to sleep.

I stooped and picked him up saying, "You can't half see it down there, I will show you all about it." And his finger on the picture with mine trying to tell me what he could of its new-found beauties. The fact that it was *his*, was a new thing to him, and I seemed to him to know more about his interests and possessions than his mother did.

I then set him down, for fear it would occur to him that I was a stranger, and walked right away from him and went where his father and mother sat, marked off a chart for the mother, and the boy was leaning against me, apparently very much at home, and trying to be interested in what I was doing. I opened my chart, which contained pictures, and told Charlie if he wanted to see the picture he might come now, and he climbed into my lap without assistance, while I kept the pictures of the book out of the reach of his eyes until he had got fairly into my lap. It was a struggle, and when he got fixed and gave a sigh of contentment, I turned toward the blazing and half tearful eyes of the mother interrogatively, and she burst out, "I give it up. Oh, how did you do it?"

I quietly replied, "I made no appeal to his Cautiousness, but did everything to allay that feeling, and to awaken curiosity and excite his judgment, imagination, and affection. Ignoring him was just what he needed, yet it was what others did not do, and you always tried to urge him to pay attention to the stranger, and make friends with him. That defeated its own purpose. I took a different course, and you see the result."

The boy talked of me for months afterward, and wanted me to "come some more." This method of curing timidity I always use when necessary, and it is wonderful how quickly other faculties can be awakened, and Cautiousness be allayed. A timid child is talked to and coaxed by every one that calls, and so grows worse. If left alone and unnoticed, it would soon get over its bashfulness.

"A Spoiled Child, and How It Was Done."

"Mistaken severity as well as mistaken kindness will equally, but very differently, spoil a child. As over-indulgence in every whim or imaginary want of a child leads to effeminacy, amiable selfishness, capricious exactions from friends and servants, and a general helplessness; so, on the other hand, too much strictness and severity in the training ruins the temper and makes a vixen to torture the next generation, or utterly crushes the spirit and makes life to the child a 'vale of tears.' We give a case in point:

"I examined in this place the head of a little girl four years old, and found Destructiveness and Combativeness very largely developed. Wondering why these organs should be so large, I referred to the heads of the father and mother and a younger child, and found that none of them had those organs in more than a medium degree. This, of course, excited my surprise, and I felt it necessary to account for the discrepancy, or ascertain the history of the case. Accordingly, I suggested to the parent that the child must have been very much annoyed and irritated by surrounding influences to induce at so early an age such extraordinary developments.

"The mother, with regretful earnestness, replied: 'That is true, and I will explain the reason. I have been a teacher and "boarded around," and seeing much slackness and imbecility in parental government, I firmly resolved if I ever had children, I would begin with them in season and make them go straight. Accordingly, this girl being my first child, I began early to make her toe the mark, and I used to train and whip her for every little offense or neglect. She has become fretful, peevish, and violent in temper, so that now, whipping only makes her worse. A few days ago I lost my temper and gave her a severe whipping, and the moment I got through with her she seized the fire-tongs, and with a severe blow she broke the back of her pet kitten that was sitting by the fire. When her anger had subsided she mourned piteously for the death of her pet, and she can not get over her loss. She is a very bad child when angry, and I do not know what I can do with her. I have, however, taken a very different course with my other one, and she is easily managed, though her natural disposition is no more amiable than that of the older one was at first. I fear I have spoiled my little girl by unnecessary strictness and severity.'"

This painful fact has doubtless since then helped me in hundreds of instances, to guide and aid other mothers in the adoption of better methods in the training of their precious pets, whose upgrowth to goodness and to God was the hope and the burden of their life. . . .

Insanity Cured by Phrenology

While here, I received a call from a friend residing twelve miles distant, at Suffield, Conn., where I married my wife and resided during 1843. He informed me that Henry Bissell, of Suffield, had recently received a blow upon the head in the region of the temple, and had become insane in consequence. He appeared somewhat strangely for a day or two, and then took the train for New York, and before arriving there, attracted attention by immoderate laughter at everybody and everything in the car. A gentleman who knew him happened to be on the train, and took him back to Hartford, left him in the asylum, and sent for his father. Here he had been for several weeks under treatment without any apparent benefit. On hearing these facts I wrote at once to the father, and sent it by my informant, stating the impression that the injury was upon the seat of Mirthfulness, hence his tendency to laugh and see absurdity in everything, and suggested that if the physician would apply leeches and ice to that part of the head which was injured, the symptoms of insanity would cease. The aged father, who was interested in our lectures on Phrenology at Suffield in 1841, recognizing the reasonableness of the views that I had taken of the cause and proper treatment of the case, on receiving my letter at eight o'clock that night he instantly harnessed his team for a dreary drive of seventeen miles to Hartford, and, reaching the asylum at eleven o'clock, after Dr. Butler had retired, he insisted upon seeing him at once. With my letter open in his hand, the anxious father met the doctor, who read it deliberately and said: "It looks reasonable, and we will try the treatment in the morning."

"No, doctor; we will try it to-night, if you please. I can not wait till morning."

"All right," said the doctor, "to-night, if you say so."

In half an hour the patient was under the treatment of leeches, in another half hour the injured part was under the influence of pounded ice, and he was fast asleep. The next morning he and his father took breakfast with the doctor; "he was clothed and in his right mind," and in a short time went home with his father, apparently cured.

The injury was directly over the organ of Mirthfulness, and the inflammation caused by the blow, produced the deranged action of that faculty. Thirty-seven years have now elapsed, since this injury was received and cured, and there has been no return of the symptoms of insanity. Had the inflammation been allowed to proceed, death, or mental derangement for life, might have been the consequence. The young man being my friend, I felt peculiar interest in the case.

Thus Phrenology throws a flood of light on the subject of insanity for those who wish to learn.

Trades Selected for Boys

"I am from Patterson, sir; you will remember I brought to you my three elder boys, and you selected for each of them the trade he was best fitted for, and they are thriving at them nicely, and say they could not and would not change trades on any account. They often talk about it, and each boasts over the other that he has the best trade of the lot. Now I have brought this one, and I shall put him to the trade you say he is best adapted to. I believe you know about it, for you have placed the other three so well, and the trades are so different; only think one is a jeweler, one is a butcher, and the other is a carpenter. I have one more besides this, and I shall bring him when he is old enough to put to business."

And this is not the only family who is doing a similar thing, and such work serves to keep us up to a sense of our responsibility.

From Nelson Sizer, *Forty Years in Phrenology: Embracing Recollections of History, Anecdote, and Experience* (New York: Fowler and Wells, 1891), 63–67, 73–74, 188–189, 295–296.

George Miller Beard

(1839–1883)

Cases of Hysteria, Neurasthenia, Spinal Irritation, or Allied Affections

(1874)

Similar to scholars in the eighteenth century, observers on both sides of the Atlantic during the last third of the nineteenth century came to believe that nerves played a pivotal role in human health. The brain was often compared to a battery producing electricity that passed its energy through nerve fibres in a manner akin to the way in which electrical wires function. Too much or too little nervous energy, it was believed, could lead to a disequilibrium that came to be known as a "nervous breakdown."

George Miller Beard became one of the most famous proponents of this view. Beard began his career as an electrotherapist, following a tradition, which went back to the eighteenth century, of administering electrical current to individuals suffering from any number of different ailments, including paralysis, rheumatism, indigestion, headaches, and impotence. In 1869, he published an article announcing a new diagnosis, neurasthenia, a disease he believed was caused by the hectic pace and demands of modern life.

Under this head I propose to detail a few cases of nervous disease—commonly called functional—that are at once exceedingly frequent and exceedingly annoying both to patients and physicians. I shall treat the subject mainly from the clinical and practical stand-point, reserving the discussion of its scientific and philosophic relations for another occasion.

By hysteria and allied affections I mean that large and increasingly numerous class of affections that pass among the people and among the profession by the vague and half-erroneous terms, spinal irritation, nervous exhaustion, general debility, general neuralgia, etc.

In a work in which I have long engaged, and which is now slowly progressing, I hope to be able to unify these diseases—to show that they have in general a common pathology, a common history, a common group of symptoms, and a common therapeutics. I shall seek to show that these diseases, or symptoms of diseases—or, as they might, perhaps, with better justice be called, results of disease—are expressions of a common nervous diathesis; that they are all liable to run into each other, and to act vicariously to each other; that they are part of the price we pay for civilization, being confined mostly to the enlightened peoples of modern times; and that they are, in all their dreary shapes, most abundant in the northern portions of the United States of America. . . .

General Principles of Treatment

I treat all these affections, by whatever name known, on the same general principles, varying and adapting the method according to individual need. Of the various methods of using electricity, I depend mainly on general faradization and central galvanization, using sometimes in alternation—in some cases finding the former, in others the latter, more beneficial.*

Internally, I use preparations of phosphorous and cod-liver oil, and sometimes arsenic. I make large use of the cod-liver oil emulsion. I have seen good results from the oxide and phosphide of zinc and chemical food.

Externally, I use ice and hot-water bags to the spine with studious caution, and mild and cautious counter-irritation to tenders points on the spine. My method of counter-irritating nervous patients is, to take one of Alcock's porous plasters and cut off a piece of about the size and shape of my little finger;[†] along the centre of this I place a little Spanish-fly ointment, and then apply over the tender spot, and let it stay there until it falls off. Counter-irritation thus used is not very annoying, and is quite effective. I use Alcock's porous plaster because it sticks better than anything I can find.

Except when I am experimenting, I use all these remedies, or several of them, simultaneously.

---

*Editor's note: Faradization involved applying alternating current, while galvanization referred to the application of continuous, direct current.

[†]Editor's note: Alcock's Porous Plasters were adhesives purported to have electrifying properties that could alter blood circulation.

Neurasthenia, Cerebrasthenia, Myelasthenia

The old and forgotten term, *neurasthenia*, I have for several years applied to the condition known in common language as *nervous exhaustion*; and I have recently subdivided this condition into *cerebrasthenia* and *myelasthenia*, according as the exhaustion is chiefly manifested in the brain or in the spinal cord. When the exhaustion shows itself chiefly in the brain, there are the symptoms of insomnia, headache, vertigo, flashes before the eyes, muscae volitantes, tinnitus, etc. When the exhaustion shows itself chiefly in the spinal cords, there are the symptoms of pain in the back, at any point below the first cervical and last dorsal vertebrae, and mostly between the shoulder and in the lumbar region; spinal tenderness (though not always); weakness of the lower limbs, and sometimes of the arms; flatulence; feeling of oppression on the chest; gastralgia, intercostal and abdominal; neuralgia of the bladder and sexual disturbance; numbness of the extremities, etc. While the term neurasthenia implies both cerebrasthenia and myelasthenia, yet in some cases the exhaustion seems to be almost exclusively confined to the brain alone, or to the spinal cord alone. . . . The meaning of these terms will be made more clear by the following cases:

Case I. Mr. L———,aged 86, was referred to me, June 25, 1873, by Dr. Geo. Baker. For several months, since January 1873, the patient had suffered from vertigo, feeling of tingling, pricking, and stinging over the surface of the body; pain in the back; dyspepsia; constipation, insomnia, and mental depression. The spinal irritation was quite variable in its seat, being sometimes in the lower, sometimes in the upper vertebrae. Sometimes there was tenderness of the cervical vertebrae, with stiffness of the neck.

The diagnosis was neurasthenia, including cerebrasthenia and myelasthenia; and the pretty evident cause was excess in sexual indulgence combined with over work in business.

I gave general faradization alternately with central galvanization, for one month; and, at the same time, used phosphide of zinc pills in doses of 1–10 of a grain, and chemical food. Counter-irritation was also employed over the tender vertebrae. July 5, he was much better. August 1, still better; and September 1 he resumed active business.

Case IV. Miss G———, a young lady of about 24 years of age, was first seen, with D.O.L. Mitchell, Nov. 23, 1871. The patient was of a very fine organization, and of slight, fragile build. Left an orphan at an early age, she had worked hard as a copyist in a telegraph office, where she toiled many hours a day to support herself and her younger brothers and sisters. For two years or more she had been in a condition of excessive debility, which her physician could control only imperfectly by medication.

She could not walk a single block, or even part of a block, and so remained constantly indoors. Her appetite was feeble and fickle; sleep was uncertain and disturbed; the circulation unequal. The pulse, though weak and nervous, was yet tolerably strong for a delicate lady, but was very susceptible to mental influence. Careful examinations had been able to detect no disease of the lungs or heart or of any organ; the uterus had not been examined.

Fainting spells, or spells resembling fainting, came over her after severe exertion; even the *shock* of *hearing* the door open fearfully agitated her, so that she suffered for a number of minutes. She dreaded the coming of a new doctor, and lived in a condition of painful apprehension when she learned that I was to be called in to see her.

To all medication she was extremely susceptible; even a few drops of dilute phosphoric acid seemed to do injury. Similarly tonics and stimulants were badly borne. Some mental depression accompanied all these symptoms; but the patient had considerable *force of will*, and when in good health was very energetic. There were no fits of laughing or crying.

After a careful and thorough trial of general faradization, central galvanization, and galvanization of the cervical sympathetic, I gave up the case. She bore electricity as she bore everything else—badly, and no amount of treatment succeeded in bringing her to that condition where she could tolerate an average dose of either treatment.

During the latter part of the treatment the uterus was carefully examined by Dr. Skene, who found a tendency to vaginismus and anteflexion; but these symptoms were regarded merely as accompanying or incidental phenomena, and were not treated.

After electrical treatment was abandoned time came slowly to the rescue, and, under the care of her physician, she so far improved as to be able to walk out, but she subsequently relapsed.

This case illustrates: First, that there are certain temperaments that will not bear electricity; secondly, that in nerve functional disturbances time, rest, and hygiene may cure or greatly relieve, after medication has failed. In all these cases special pains must be taken to avoid exertion, mental or muscular. A slight indiscretion may put back the patient for weeks or months. For the nervously exhausted to overdo, even for an hour, is a blunder that is almost a crime.

From George Miller Beard, *Cases of Hysteria, Neurasthenia, Spinal Irritation, or Allied Affections* (Chicago: Spalding, 1874), 1–4, 6-7.

Auguste Tamburini
(1848–1919)
"A Theory of Hallucinations"
(1881)

The Italian Auguste Tamburini was an academic psychiatrist who served as both director of one of Europe's oldest asylums (San Lazzaro) and as a professor of psychiatry and neurology. He eventually became director of the psychiatric institute in Rome in 1907. Tamburini's article on the theory of hallucinations, published in French in 1881, was among the most cited in late nineteenth-century neuropsychiatry. It quickly inspired countless researchers and clinicians to see hallucinations no longer as possessing some kind of semantic meaning, but instead as products of mechanical processes involving the brain and nervous system.

There has been much debate on the nature and brain localization of hallucinations. This is to be expected as these phenomena are not only important symptoms of insanity and a cause of delusions, but have also played a role in history. Four types of explanation are available for their origin: (1) peripheral; (2) intellectual; (3) psycho-sensorial; and (4) sensorial.

According to the peripheral view, as stated in the writings of Erasmus Darwin, Foville and Michéa, hallucinations are subjective sensations caused by the peripheral irritation of sensory organs. As evidence, the authors quote the development of unilateral hallucinations in association with morbid changes in peripheral sense organs or the distortion of image caused by manual pressure on the eye. This view fails to explain the presence of hallucination in cases when the peripheral sense organ has been completely destroyed.

The "intellectualistic" view of hallucinations attributes the origin to disturbances of imagination and memory and has been supported by Esquirol, Lauret, Lélut, Falret, Reil, Neumann, Parchappe, Brierre de Briesmont, Delasiauve, Maudsley, etc. According to these authors hallucinations are thoughts changed into sensations; they are projections, so to speak, of the sensorial aspects of ideas on to the external world. Hallucinations are sensory delusions. Against this view is the fact that hallucinations are often thematically unrelated to normal or pathological ideas. Likewise this hypothesis is unable to explain the clinical facts listed by those supporting the peripheral view.

The psycho-sensorial theory is a combination of the two views above, and explains more clinical observations than either of them alone. Both intellectual and peripheral centres would participate in the constitution of the hallucinatory phenomenon. The theory has been supported by Müller, Griesinger, Baillarger, Moreau de Tours, Marcé, Motet, and more recently by Ball. The problem with this view is that, because it describes hallucinations in a general way, it explains everything; even worse, it does not take into consideration recent advances in neurophysiology.

According to the fourth view, the one more in keeping with modern brain anatomy and physiology, hallucinations are the result of activity in the sensory centres of the brain. This view, therefore, postulates the existence of sensory centres in the central nervous system to which sensory information is conveyed by sensory nerves. Morbid changes in these brain sites would give rise to hallucinatory experiences. Already hinted at in the work of Baillarger and Schröder Van der Kolk, this view has recently been expressed with great clarity by Kahlbaum and Hagen, and adopted by Koppe, Jolly, Hoffmann, Luys and Ritti.

How is that sensations generated in these brain centres can give rise to images endowed with all features of reality? According to Hagen all peripheral stimuli arriving at the sensory centres are immediately diverted to two destinations: the ideational centres (where they will generate images in consciousness) and back to the periphery (by the principle of external projection). Stimuli generated in the brain sites themselves would suffer the same fate, thereby giving rise to apparent perceptions. This view explains all clinical facts but requires periodical updating according to the progress of brain anatomy and physiology.

The next question is, where are the brain centres for hallucinations? Krafft-Ebing, Hoffmann, Leidersdorf and others have not provided an answer and simply refer to them as the sites where sensory nerves terminate. Hagen and Kahlbaum, on the other hand, have suggested that these centres are, in fact, the basal ganglia or sensory brain (*Sinnhirn*). Bergmann, in turn, has claimed that the sensory nerves terminate in the walls of the cerebral ventricles where, by means of a resonance mechanism, perceptions are constituted. Hallucinations would result from an irritation in these areas: the third ventricle would be associated with visual hallucinations, the fourth ventricle with auditory ones. . . .

Recent work, however, seems to suggest that sensory fibres do terminate in the cortex itself. . . . Panizza's "Observations on the optic nerve" was originally published in the Journal of the Lombard Institute for August 1855 and reprinted a year later. It reports experiments carried out on mammals, birds and fish by two methods: (1) selective lesioning of cortical sites followed by evaluation of visual function, and (2) eyeball enuncleation followed by analysis of retrograde nerve atrophy. Panizza wrote that in the dog "removal of cortical substance under the parietal areas causes contralateral blindness." He also showed retrograde atrophy of the optic nerve in the rabbit, horse, dog, ox, and sheep. He mapped the atrophic changes in the geniculate bodies, thalamus and even in the fibres arriving in the striatal area.

Clinical data suggest that this also applies to the human. For example, a traumatic lesion of the left eye caused atrophy in a three-year-old; a post mortem after his early death at age 16 showed parietal-occipital atrophy involving the right thalamus and hemisphere. After a right stroke a second patient developed amaurosis of the right eye and post-mortem showed softening of the posterior hemisphere. Panizza concluded that in the mammal the optic nerve receives contributions from the geniculate bodies, thalamus, and occipital lobe. His work has been replicated by Hitzig and Ferrier. . . .

These findings may help to explain the genesis of hallucinations. If there are cortical centres where sensory impressions become perceptions (and where they are also stored as mnemonic images), then it would be surprising that they did not play a role in the production of hallucinations. In the same way that irritation of motor centres may cause disorganized (epileptic) movements, morbid changes in sensory ones would cause pathological sensations.

What, however, would the origin of the sensations be? They are likely to be mnemonic images, stored impressions, which after being revived by the morbid process would with varying vividness (according to the strength of the irritation) present themselves to consciousness. When accompanied by all sensory features they would be perceived as real and hence constitute hallucinations proper. When the irritation is unilateral or limited to a discrete cortical area, the hallucination will occur in one specific sense modality (e.g. visual or auditory) and be unilateral; if the morbid process is bilateral, diffuse and involving more than one sensory centre, a composite hallucination involving all sense modalities might be experienced.

Acceptance of this hypothesis should depend on its being (a) in keeping with what is known in brain physiology, (b) in agreement with the facts of clinical observation, and (c) able to explain the diverse clinical presentations of hallucinations as reported by those who postulate rival theories (peripheral, psychical or mixed).

With regards to (a) above it has already been stated that the sensory centre hypothesis is in keeping with current knowledge of cortical physiology. An inkling of this view, which would make sense even if no facts on cortical physiology were yet known (as it is presented in the work of Meynert, Wundt and Hughlings-Jackson), can be found in the work of Ferrier when he reported that eyeball and ear movements followed electrical stimulation of the sensory centres, and that these were likely to be related to the projection of experienced images on to the external world (which the experimental animal would perceive as real objects). Thus, whilst stimuli applied to the motor centres cause epileptic movements, stimuli applied to the sensory centres generate hallucinations.

But the hypothesis must also be in accord with clinico-pathological observations. The point here is to determine whether subjects presenting with clear cut hallucinations will also exhibit relevant cortical lesions on post-mortem. It must be remembered that hallucinations are a transient phenomenon which tends to occur during the early stages of psychoses and that the irritation that causes them in the first place is unlikely to persist until the patient comes to post-mortem. Hallucinations may also be replaced by the symptoms of mental degeneration. Furthermore, even if the subject died whilst experiencing hallucinations, lesions may not be visible because of their irritative nature, as it is indeed the case with regards to irritative lesions in motor areas. Therefore, it is easy to imagine how difficult it is to accumulate evidence to confirm the hypothesis. Very few cases meeting these requirements have been reported in the literature (such as those by Ferrier, Pooley, Atkins and Gowers). Their common feature is that visual hallucinations were experienced only during the early irritative stage, and that the destructive stage of the lesion was followed by loss of vision. . . .

The third condition dictates that the hypothesis provide adequate explanation for all clinical presentations of hallucinations. For example, how to explain the fact that hallucinations precede or follow delusions. Both situations can be accommodated by this theory on the basis that it is unlikely that lesions causing hallucinations always occur on their own. Often, in fact, they are accompanied by other brain lesions. So, if the first lesion is on a sensory centre, hallucinations will precede delusions; if it is on the ideational centre it will be the other way around. This explanation is valid provided that it is not assumed that ideation is but a complex form of activity taking place in the sensory centres themselves.

In favor of a separation between ideational and sensory centres is the fact that psychologically healthy subjects have no difficulty in recognizing interloping sensations as hallucinations. This capacity for insight, however, cannot be explained either by the peripheral or psychical theory of hallucinations. The peripheral theory is also rendered implausible by the fact that hallucinations tend to be cognitively complex; and the psychical theory by the fact that they are often sensorially vivid. Both objections are easily dealt with by the theory that hallucinations result from irritation of the cortical sensory centres. . . .

It can be concluded that many aspects of hallucinations not explained by other theories are accounted for by the view proposed in this paper. This is based on the most recent anatomical, physiological and clinical findings, and postulates that the fundamental mechanism for hallucinations is a state of morbid excitation of cortical sensory centres, of sites where sensory impression from the peripheral organs are collected and transformed into perceptions, and where their mnemonic images are stored.

From Auguste Tamburini, "A Theory of Hallucinations," *History of Psychiatry* 1 (1990): 151–156 (© History of Psychiatry, 1990), by permission of Sage Publications Ltd.

Richard von Krafft-Ebing
(1840–1902)

Psychopathia Sexualis
(1892)

Since ancient times, Western religions have inveighed against various forms of deviant sexual behavior. And while medicine often appeared to be less prudish about commending the benefits of an active sex life, physicians nonetheless often warned of the health dangers posed by venereal diseases and masturbation. Over the course of the nineteenth century, however, a new trend emerged, as researchers and practitioners began applying clinical notions of normality and abnormality to classify, diagnose, and treat sexual deviants.

Richard von Krafft-Ebing's *Psychopathia Sexualis* was the culmination of this trend. An older contemporary of Emil Kraepelin and Sigmund Freud, Krafft-Ebing practiced psychiatry in various German asylums and clinics, until eventually settling in Vienna. *Psychopathia Sexualis* detailed his work with patients complaining of "perversions," which at that time included homosexuality, sadism, masochism, and exhibitionism. First published in German in 1886, the book was a scholarly best seller, going through numerous reprints and new editions during Krafft-Ebing's lifetime. As these excerpts show, the book was readily available to the general public, leading many readers to see their sexual proclivities in a new light. In fact, many readers were so moved that they contacted Krafft-Ebing and shared their own stories with him. He, in turn, incorporated many of their tales into subsequent editions of his book (see cases 136 and 137, below). As a result, *Psychopathia Sexualis* gives us both a sense of how Krafft-Ebing operated—note his reliance on hypnosis, a very common form of treatment at this time—as well as insight into how self-identified "perverts" lived with their desires.

While up to this time contrary sexual instinct has had but an anthropological, clinical, and forensic interest for science, now, as a result of the latest investigations, there is some thought of therapy in this incurable condition, which so heavily burdens its victims, socially, morally, and mentally.

A preparatory step for the application of therapeutic measures is the exact differentiation of the acquired from the congenital cases; and among the latter, again, the assignment of the concrete case to its proper position in the categories that have been established empirically.

The diagnostic differentiation of the acquired from the congenital condition is made without difficulty in the early stages of the anomaly.

If sexual inversion has already taken place, then the history of the development of the case will throw light upon it.

The important decision, prognostically, as to whether the contrary sexual instinct is congenital or acquired, can only be made in such cases by means of the most minute details of the history.

The establishment of the fact that contrary sexual instinct existed before indulgence in masturbation is of great importance with reference to deciding whether the anomaly is congenital or not. In this, however, a difficulty arises, owing to the possibility of imperfect localization of past events (illusions of memory).

For the presumption of acquired contrary sexual instinct, it is important to prove the existence of hetero-sexual instinct before the beginning of solitary or mutual onanism.

In general, the acquired cases are characterized in that:—

1. The homo-sexual instinct appears secondarily, and always may be referred to influences (masturbatic neurasthenia, mental) which disturbed normal sexual satisfaction. It is, however, probable that here, in spite of the powerful sensual libido, the feeling and inclination for the opposite sex are weak *ab origine*, especially in a spiritual and aesthetic sense.

2. The homo-sexual instinct, as long as inversio sexualis has not taken place, is looked upon, by the individual affected, as vicious and abnormal, and yielded to only *faute de mieux*.

3. The hetero-sexual instinct long remains predominant, and the impossibility of its satisfaction gives pain. It weakens in proportion as the homo-sexual feeling gains in strength.

On the other hand, in congenital cases (a) the homo-sexual instinct is the one that occurs primarily, and becomes dominant in the vita sexualis. It appears as the natural manner of satisfaction, and also dominates the dream-life of the individual. (b) The hetero-sexual instinct fails completely, or, if it should make its appearance during the life of the individual (psycho-sexual hermaphroditism), it is still but an episodical phenomenon which has no root in the mental constitution of the individual and is essentially but a means of satisfaction of sexual desire. . . .

The prognosis of the cases of acquired contrary sexual instinct is, at all events, much more favorable than that of the congenital cases. In the former, the occurrence of effemination—the mental inversion of the individual, in the sense of perverse sexual feeling—is the limit beyond which there is no longer hope of benefit from therapy. In the congenital cases, the various categories established in this book form as many stages of psycho-sexual taint, and benefit is *probable* only within the category of the psychical hermaphrodites, though *possible* (*vide* the case of Schrenk-Notzing) in that of the urnings.*

The prophylaxis of these conditions becomes thus the more important,—for the congenital cases, prohibition of the reproduction of such unfortunates; for the acquired cases, protection from the injurious influences which experience teaches may lead to the fatal inversion of the sexual instinct.

Numerous predisposed individuals meet this sad fate, because parents and teachers have no suspicion of the danger which masturbation brings in its train to such children.

In many schools and academies masturbation and vice are actually cultivated. At present much too little attention is given to the mental and moral peculiarities of the pupils. If only the tasks are done, nothing more is asked. That many pupils are thus ruined in body and soul is never considered. In obedience to affected prudery, the vita sexualis is veiled from the developing youth, and the slightest attention given to the excitations of his sexual instinct. How few family physicians are ever called in, during the years of development of children, to give advice to their patients that are often so greatly predisposed!

---

*Editor's note: *Urning* was a nineteenth-century term for "homosexual."

It is thought that all must be left to Nature; in the meantime, Nature rises in her power, and leads the helpless, unprotected innocent into dangerous by-paths.

A more detailed treatment of this prophylactic side of the subject is impossible here.

To parents and teachers, the experiences detailed in this work, and numerous scientific works on masturbation, give suggestions.

The lines of treatment, when contrary sexual instinct exists, are the following:—

1. Prevention of onanism, and removal of other influences injurious to the vita sexualis.
2. Cure of the neurosis (neurasthenia sexualis and universalis) arising out of the unhygienic conditions of the vita sexualis.
3. Mental treatment, in the sense of combating homosexual, and encouraging hetero-sexual, feelings and impulses. . . .

Case 136. *Acquired Contrary Sexual Instinct.*— Mr. Z., aged 32, divorced. He comes of a hysteropathic mother. Maternal grandmother suffered with hysteria, and her brothers and sisters were neurotic. One brother is an urning. Z. was but poorly endowed mentally, and did not learn easily. No sickness besides scarlatina. When thirteen, he was taught to masturbate by companions in a school. Sexually, he was hyperaesthetic, and, at seventeen, began to indulge in coitus, with full pleasure and power. For reasons of position and money, he married at twenty-six. The marriage was very unhappy. After a year Mrs. Z. became incapable of coitus, by reason of uterine disease. Z. satisfied his inordinate desires with other women, *faute de mieux,* by masturbation. Besides, he gave himself up to play, led an absolutely dissolute life, became exceedingly neurasthenic, and sought to strengthen his weakened nerves by drinking great quantities of wine and brandy. To his essential cerebral asthenia were added peripheral alcoholic cramps and globus, and he became very emotional. His libido nimia continued unabated. On account of his disgust of prostitutes and fear of infection, satisfaction by coitus was exceptional. For the most part, the patient helped himself with onanism.

Four years ago he noticed weakening of erection and decrease of libido for women. He began to feel himself drawn toward men, and his lascivious dreams were no longer concerned with women, but with men.

Three years ago, while being rubbed by a bath-attendant, he became powerfully excited sexually (the attendant also had an erection, to patient's surprise). He could not keep from embracing and kissing the attendant, and allowing him to perform masturbation on him, the attendant doing it most willingly. From this time this mode of indulgence was all that he cared for. Women became a matter of entire indifference to him; he devoted himself exclusively to men. With them he practiced mutual masturbation, and had a longing to sleep with them. He abhorred pederasty. He was entirely satisfied until (August, 1890) an anonymous letter, warning him to be careful, brought him to his senses. He was much frightened, had hysterical attacks, and became much depressed. He was embarrassed before men, seemed like a pariah in society, contemplated suicide, and finally confessed to a priest, who comforted him. He now fell into a religious state (equivalent), and, out of remorse and to cure himself of his abnormal sexual inclinations, wished to go into a cloister. While in this state, my "Psychopathia Sexualis" fell into his hands. He was frightened and filled with shame, but found comfort in it, inasmuch as he concluded that he must have some malady. His first thought was to rehabilitate himself sexually in his own eyes. He overcame all disinclinations, and visited a brothel. At first he was not successful, on account of great excitement, but he finally succeeded.

Since, however, his contrary sexual inclinations were not overcome, in spite of all his efforts to put them down, he finally came to me, asking for assistance. He felt himself to be terribly unfortunate, and very near to despair and suicide. He saw destruction before him, and would be saved at any price.

His confession was interrupted by numerous hysterical attacks. Comforting and encouraging words about his future had a calming influence. . . .

Hip-baths, massage, ergot with antipyrin and pot. brom., ordered, with interdiction of onanism, intercourse with men, and lascivious thoughts of them.

After a few days the patient came complaining that he was not equal to the task. He said his will was too weak. In this precarious situation, it seemed that nothing but hypnotic treatment could bring improvement.

September 11, 1889. First Sitting. Bernheim's method [of hypnosis] used, in order to induce lethargy as quickly as possible.

Suggestions:—

1. I abhor onanism, and will not masturbate again.

2. I regard the inclinations for men disgusting,—horrible; and I shall never think men handsome and enticing.

3. Women alone I find enticing. Once a week I shall cohabit with pleasure and power.

The patient received these suggestions, and repeated them in a drawling tone.

The sittings took place every second day. After the fifteenth, it was possible to induce the somnambulistic stage of hypnosis with any post-hypnotic suggestions desired.

The patient improved morally and mentally, but symptoms of cerebral neurasthenia troubled him still, and, now and then, dreams of men occurred; and there were, also, in the waking state, inclinations towards men, which depressed him exceedingly. . . .

December 9, 1889, patient again came for treatment. Of late he had had lascivious dreams of men twice, but had experienced no inclination toward men in the waking state. He had also resisted the impulse to masturbate, though, while living alone in the country, he had had no opportunity for coitus. He had inclinations only for the opposite sex, and, as a rule, dreamed only of females. Returned to the city, he had indulged in coitus with pleasure. The patient felt himself morally rehabilitated, being almost free from neurasthenic symptoms; and, after three more hypnotic sittings, he declared himself perfectly well, and confident that he would not relapse. Such a relapse occurred, however, in September, 1890, when, after over-exertion on an excursion into the mountains, and emotional strain with want of opportunity for coitus, he again became neurasthenic.

Again he had dreams of men, and felt drawn toward attractive male forms; he masturbated many times, and, after returning to the city, found no real pleasure in coitus. By means of anti-neurasthenic treatment and hypnosis, it was possible to restore the previous condition.

In the course of the years 1890 and 1891 the patient now and then had contrary sexual feelings and dreams, but only when, as a result of emotional strain or excesses, his neurosis re-appeared. At such time satisfaction in coitus was wanting. He would then find it necessary to undergo a few hypnotic sittings, in order to restore his equilibrium—always with success.

At the end of 1891 the patient pointed with satisfaction to the fact that, since treatment, he had been able to avoid masturbation and male-intercourse, and had regained his self-confidence and self-respect.

Case 137. "I was born in 1858, out of wedlock. It was only late that I was able to trace my obscure origin, and obtain knowledge of my parents; and this knowledge is, unfortunately, very obscure and imperfect. My father and mother were cousins. My father died three years ago. He later married, and, as far as I know, had several healthy children.

"I do not think that my father had contrary sexual feelings. Without knowing him as my father, I often saw him when I was a child. He was a powerful, masculine man. As for the rest, it is said that, at the time of my birth, or before, he was sexually ill.

" . . . I think I may say that my vita sexualis was really first awakened after I had been seduced into mutual masturbation, in my thirteenth year, by a room-mate at the Institute. At that time ejaculation did not take place, but first about a year later. Nevertheless, I gave myself up to the vice of onanism passionately. At this time, however, the first signs of homo-sexual inclination were manifested. Youthful, powerful men, market-helpers, workmen, and soldiers took possession of my dreams and played an important role in my fancy while masturbating.

" . . . When, at the age of fourteen, I went to H., I lost sight of my lover and seducer. He was some years older than I, and was an official; and, in this capacity, when I was nineteen, I again met him once on the railway. We immediately cut the journey short, and lodged together, attempting mutual pederasty; but, on account of pain, immissio was not successful. We amused ourselves in mutual onanism. In H. I had sexual intercourse with two fellow-students, but this intercourse was confined to frequent mutual onanism, owing to the fact that they were not inclined to pederasty. . . .

"With my sojourn here, my vita sexualis has undergone a complete change. I have learned how easy it is to find persons who, partly for money and partly for desire, yield to our inclinations. I have also not been spared annoying experiences with cheats. Until the end of the last year (since then, owing to fear of venereal infection, I have not gone beyond mutual masturbation), I enjoyed male-love to the full extent, particularly in passive pederasty. I have never practiced active pederasty, because I have found no one able to endure the pain.

"Generally, I seek my lovers among cavalrymen and sailors, and eventually, among workmen, especially butchers and smiths. Robust forms, with healthy facial complexions, attract me especially. Leathern riding-trousers have a particular charm for me. I have no partiality for kissing and the like. I also love large, hard, and calloused hands.

"I do not wish to leave unmentioned that, under certain circumstances, I have great control of myself.

" . . . Until my thirty-eighth year I had not a clear understanding of my condition. I always thought that, by early and frequent masturbation, I had become averse to women, and hoped always that, when the right woman came, I should be able to abandon onanism and find pleasure in her. Here it was that I first came to fully understand my condition, after making the acquaintance of others suffering and feeling like myself. At first I was frightened; later I came to look upon my fate as something not dependent on myself. Too, I made no further effort to resist temptation.

"Two or three weeks ago 'Psychopathia Sexualis' fell into my hands. The work has made an unexpectedly deep impression on me. At first I read the work with an interest that was undoubtedly lascivious. The description of the cultivation of *mujerados*, for example, excited me uncommonly.* The thought of a young, powerful man being emasculated in this manner, in order, later, to be used for pederasty by a whole tribe of wild, powerful, and sensual Indians, so excited me that I masturbated five times during the next two days, fancying myself such a presumptive *mujerado*. The farther I read in the book, however, the more I saw its moral earnestness; the more I felt disgust with my condition; and the more I saw that I must do everything,

---

*Editor's note: George Miller Beard, for instance, describes *mujerados* as a group of men among the Pueblo Indians with "protuberant abdomens, well-developed mammary glands, rounded and soft limbs, shrunken genital organs, high, thin, cracked voices, and pubes devoid of hair. . . . In order to make a Mujerado a very strong man is selected; masturbation is performed upon him many times a day; he has to ride almost continuously on horseback without saddle. By this process the genital organs become much excited, and seminal losses are produced; the nutrition of the organs is interfered with; they grow smaller and weaker, and, in time, desire and power cease; then follow the changes in character, the desire to dress like a woman and to engage in feminine occupations, just as with the Scythians; courage and manhood are lost; wives and children, for those who have them, pass from their control." George M. Beard, *Sexual Neurasthenia (Nervous Exhaustion): Its Hygiene, Causes, Symptoms, and Treatment, with a Chapter on Diet for the Nervous* (New York: E. B. Treat, 1886), 100–101.

if it were possible, to bring about a change in my condition. When I had finished the book, I was determined to seek assistance from its author.

"The reading of this work had an undoubted effect. Since then I have masturbated only twice, and have practiced onanism with cavalrymen only twice. In every instance I have had really less pleasure and satisfaction than before, and I always have the feeling: 'Ah, if I could only be free from it!' Nevertheless, I confess that, even now, in the society of handsome soldiers, I immediately have erection.

"In conclusion, I may add that, in spite of, or, perhaps, on account of, onanism, I have never had pollutions. The ejaculation of semen, which usually consists of only a few drops, and it has always been so, takes place only after prolonged friction. If, for any reason, I have not masturbated for a long time, the ejaculation takes place quickly, and is more abundant. About twelve years ago Hansen tried in vain to hypnotize me." *

In the spring of 1891 the writer of the foregoing autobiography visited me, with the declaration that he could live no longer in his condition; that he looked to hypnotic treatment as the only hope of salvation, for he had not strength enough to resist his impulse to masturbation and satisfaction with persons of his own sex. He felt like a pariah; like an unnatural man; like one outside the laws of nature and society, and in danger of criminal prosecution. He felt moral repugnance when he performed the act with a man, but yet the sight of any handsome soldier actually electrified him. For years he had not had the slightest sympathy with women, not even mentally.

The patient looked to be exactly the person, physically and mentally, described by himself in his autobiography. His head was exquisitely hydrocephalic, and also plagiocephalic. At first attempts at hypnosis met with difficulties. Only by Braid's method, with the help of a little chloroform, was deep lethargy attained at the third sitting.[†] From that time simply looking at a shining object was sufficient. The suggestions consisted of the command to avoid masturbation, the removal of homosexual feelings, and the

---

*Editor's note: He is referring here to Carl Hansen (1833–1897), a Danish hypnotist who performed on stage in Vienna around this time.

†Editor's note: Braid's method refers to the method of hypnosis developed by James Braid (1795–1860), the Scottish surgeon who first coined the term *hypnosis*. Braid emphasized the importance of relaxation, directed attention, and suggestion in a successful hypnosis.

assurance that the patient would have inclination for women and be virile, and have pleasure only in hetero-sexual intercourse. Masturbation was indulged in but once; after the eighth sitting the patient dreamed of a woman.

When, after the fourteenth sitting, the patient had to return, on account of pressing business, he declared that he was quite free from any inclination to masturbate and to indulge in male-love, but that he was by no means absolutely free from his partiality for men. He felt returning interest in the female sex, and hoped to be freed finally from his unhappy condition by continuance of the treatment.

From Richard von Krafft-Ebing, *Psychopathia Sexualis* (Philadelphia: F. A. Davis, 1892), 319–321, 330–308.

Jean-Martin Charcot
(1825–1893)

"A Tuesday Lesson: Hysteroepilepsy"
(1888)

During the last quarter of the nineteenth century, the French neurologist Jean-Martin Charcot was among the most acclaimed experts in the world on hysteria. Conducting research and teaching at the famous Salpêtrière Hospital in Paris (1862–1893), Charcot used a novel combination of clinical observation, pathological anatomy, and photography to analyze hysterical episodes, breaking them down into discrete stages in order to enable more accurate diagnosis. By 1883, Charcot had turned the Salpêtrière into a hub for the study of hysteria: of the some five hundred women admitted to the hospital at that time, around 20 percent were diagnosed with hysterical symptoms. Charcot treated these mostly working-class patients with a regimen that included the use of ovarian compressor belts, hypnotism, and electrotherapy.

Charcot was a renowned self-promoter. His fame grew especially after he introduced a set of weekly public lectures, attended by students, physicians, researchers, artists, and writers from all over Europe. On Fridays, he gave carefully prepared presentations, employing diagrams, drawings, art, and even costumed patients to make his points. The Tuesday Lessons were reserved for more impromptu discussion of cases and for interviews with newly admitted patients. In both settings, Charcot typically illustrated his theses by using hypnotism to induce hysterical symptoms in his patients. The dramatic features of the lectures did not escape the notice of contemporaries, and, as the excerpt below shows, critics questioned whether Charcot's patients were merely getting caught up in the medical theater being staged.

(A female patient on a stretcher is brought into the amphitheater.)

CHARCOT: Here is a patient whom you saw last Friday. After a fall she developed a lower extremity contracture with a deformity of her right foot. Nothing is more frequent in hysterics than posttraumatic contractures. What could one make of such a case? I told you last time how important it is to treat and cure these contractures as soon as they appear. But now here we have an exception to this rule, and we have waited and watched this woman three or four days without interfering. I told you why we did this— with cases like this woman's, you may, in fact, be able to treat this through provoking a second sort of attack. Often with such attacks, a change occurs in the patient and a contracture that seemed permanently fixed before can completely disappear. You may say to me, "Isn't there something immoral about waiting and provoking such crises?" Surely not, if one can offer a treatment for a disorder that otherwise has no cure.

And I have shown you how there is a parallel relationship between transient hysteric attacks and the forms of hysteria like this one that last longer, five or six months. Often, those patients with contractures are not those who have fleeting hysteric attacks and vice versa. It is because of this doctrine, so soundly described by Dr. Pitres, that we can make use of hysterogenic points to provoke a transient attack as a form of therapy in the treatment of static hysteric signs. Now, this patient will be used for demonstration. I will tell you, however, that although I am practically certain of the outcome of this experiment, man is less predictable than machinery, and I will not be totally surprised if, in fact, we do not succeed. I have also

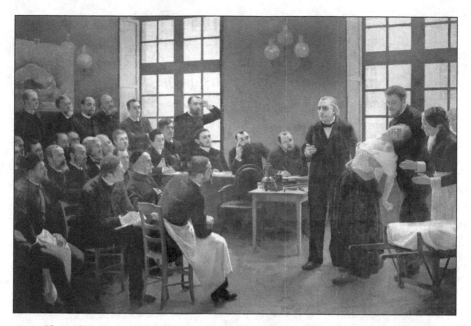

A Clinical Lesson with Charcot at the Salpêtrière 1887, by Andre Brouillet (1857–1914). This famous portrait depicts the neurologist Jean-Martin Charcot during one of his public lectures. Here he discusses the case of a patient (Blanche Wittmann), who has just been hypnotized by his assistant Joseph Babinski. Hopital Neurologique, Lyon, France. © Erich Lessing/Art Resource, NY.

heard that animal experiments performed before an audience often given different results from those seen in the laboratory. This may be the case here, since this is, in fact, a comparable clinical experiment. If we do not get the desired result, it still will be a significant lesson for you.

This patient has a hysterogenic point on her back, another under her left breast, and a third on her leg. We will focus on this latter one. If the attack proceeds as I believe it will, I will want you to focus on all its phases. This is not an easy task, and it took me many years to analyze the phenomena you will see. I first came to the Salpêtrière 15 or 20 years ago and inherited the well-run service of Dr. Delasiauve. From my first days I witnessed these hysteroepileptic attacks, and was very circumspect in making my early diagnoses. I said to myself, "How can it be that such events are not described in the textbooks? How should I go about describing these events from my first-hand experience?" I was befuddled as I looked at such patients, and this impotence greatly irritated me. Then one day, when reflecting over all these patients as a group, I was struck with a sort of intuition about them. I again said to myself, "Something about them makes them all the same." Indeed we have a particular disease before us—primary hysteria beginning with an epilepticlike attack that resembles so closely real epilepsy that it may be called hysteroepilepsy, even though it has nothing at all to do with true epilepsy. The epileptoid phase can be divided into a tonic and clonic portion. Then, after a brief respite, the phase of exotic movements begins, under one or two predominant forms, either vocalizations or extreme opisthotonus (*arc en cercle*). Then, the third phase supercedes, and suddenly the patient looks ahead at an imaginary image—indeed a hallucination, which will vary according to the setting. The patient may look with great fear or with joy, depending on what she sees. You saw this in a woman the other day when I touched her abdomen in the ovarian region. She rose from her bed, hurried into the corner, and said the most distressing things.

But I want you to appreciate especially the unfolding of an attack. I tell you all this beforehand so that you can mark each phase, since they are hard to appreciate without preparation. Importantly, the attack is not a series of individual small attacks, but a single event that unrolls sequentially. I use here the method of describing an archetype with the most complex and fully developed features described. This system is essential for all neurologic diagnosis; one must learn to identify the archetype. The epileptoid phase can be lacking and the attack begin with the movement phase, either vocalizations or back arching. Sometimes the movements never appear, and one only has hallucinations. There are as many as 20 variations, but if you have the key to the archetype, you immediately focus on the disease at hand and can say with confidence that in spite of the many possible variations, all these cases represent the same disorder. So, here we have this contracted foot that reportedly cannot be reduced either during the day or night. I have not specifically examined it at all times, but I surmise that this is in fact true. We are not dealing here with simulation, one of the greatest obstacles to neurology. (*The intern touches the hysterogenic point under the left breast. Immediately, the attack begins*).

CHARCOT: Now, here we have the epileptoid phase. Remember this sequence—epileptoid phase, arched back, then vocalizations. The arched back that you now see is rather pronounced. Now here comes the phase of emotional outbursts, which fuses with the back arching, and now there is a contracture phase. Such contractures can persist occasionally, and if this occurs in our patient, we will hardly have helped her. Now the epileptoid period starts again. Focus your attention this time on the two distinct epileptoid movement phases—first, the tonic, then the clonic. Note how this resembles true epilepsy. Now let us see if she is ovarian. *(The intern comes forwards and presses the ovarian region)*.

CHARCOT: Do this in a real epileptic and nothing will happen, showing you immediately the difference between epilepsy and hysteroepilepsy. In contrast to this situation, epilepsy has no direct link with the ovary. See how the attack is momentarily suspended by abdominal compression. Is it true that ovarian compression actually aborts the attack? This maneuver is contested in a number of textbooks, where the authors act as if they know what they are talking about. In both England and Germany there are some people who say they have never seen ovarian compression work, but these same people are those who are all too eager to generalize from their very limited experience. In that the phenomenon has been unequivocally demonstrated to occur in Paris, I find it only reasonable to believe it also occurs elsewhere.

Now we will release the compression, and you will see how the attack promptly recommences. Here comes the epileptoid phase again. Often outside of France, epileptoid behavior is still called epilepsy. I disagree with such terminology and distinctly calls this hysteroepilepsy or hysteria major. Here now comes the arched back. Note the consistent pattern, always predictable and regular. . . .

Let us press again on the hysterogenic point. Here we go again. Occasionally subjects even bite their tongues, but this would be rare. Look at the arched back, which is so well described in the textbooks.

PATIENT: Mother, I am frightened.

CHARCOT: Note the emotional outburst. If we let things go unabated, we will soon return to the epileptoid behavior. Now we have a bit of tranquility, or resolution, followed by a type of static contracted posture. I consider this latter deformity as an accessory phenomenon to the basic attack. *(The patient cries again: "Oh! Mother.")*

CHARCOT: Again, note these screams. You could say it is a lot of noise over nothing. True epilepsy is much more serious and also much more quiet.

I do not know what will be the final outcome for this woman's contractures, but I am glad to have been able to show you a rather typical attack. Let us review for emphasis: an epileptoid phase with two parts, tonic and iconic, followed by a phase of exotic movements, and then a phase of high emotional pitch, which, in this patient, is sad. All these are then followed by these strange contorted postures.

This patient was just a minute ago quite stiff, which is unusual. Most patients look quite natural and assume realistic poses during all of this. A final phase is quite rare and not seen in this patient—a period of delirium.

Here, after the phase of affective change, the cycle starts over and may continue for several days. Ovarian compression is effective only for some patients—these are called ovarian subjects. Clearly, all subjects are not ovarian. I can only emphasize again my stand on this, even though others have misquoted my opinions. From such misquotes, I have been said to advocate surgical operations in the form of ovarian ablation for hysteroepilepsy, such as are performed in America. What I have said is still true; there are certain patients who have ovarian tenderness and in such patients, ovarian compression can stop an individual attack, although not the disease. When I say stop an attack, I mean you can provide your patient with a respite. We will place around this patient's abdomen a compression belt, and she will temporarily be controlled. But some day she will have to remove it—she can't wear it forever, and she may well start her spells all over again. Ovarian compression is a preventative method and also a means to assure temporary peace. But I emphasize again, it is not a cure. Nor is ovarian resection. Do not be fooled, the ovary is not the only spot that can be compressed for effective control. . . .

It would seem by some accounts that hysteroepilepsy exists only in France; in fact, it has been said that it exists only at the Salpêtrière, as if I have created this condition by my own willpower. What a marvel this would be if I could, in fact, fabricate illnesses according to my whims or fantasies. But in fact all I am is a photographer. I describe what I see. And it is all too easy to show you that such phenomena have indeed occurred outside the walls of the Salpêtrière. First, the descriptions of possessed victims from the Middle Ages are full of similar descriptions. Dr. Richer,* in his monograph, showed how in the fifteenth century, the same syndrome

---

*Translator's note: Paul Richer was both artist and neurologist and always a close collaborator of Charcot. The reference is to Richer's *Clinical Studies on Hysteroepilepsy* (with 105 drawings and 9 engravings) (Paris: Delahaye et LeCrosnier, 1881).

occurred just as it does today. Furthermore, I have received numerous contemporary personal reports, primarily from North American sources, that have no inherent relationship to the Salpêtrière. These letters were inspired by my reports of hysteroepilepsy and demonstrate that elsewhere cases exist that are exactly comparable to our cases here.

In England there is a highly distinguished physician, Dr. Gowers, who does not believe my descriptions. He sees things quite differently. In his treatise on epilepsy he uses the term "hysteroid conditions" after epilepsy. He considers the first "epileptic phase" that we have seen today as true epilepsy and agrees that all the subsequent phenomena you have witnessed occur, but he calls them postictal. Why? Because the patient's crisis always starts with what appears to be epileptic. We are seeing the same things and calling it by different names. I maintain that the sequence of events is a single process and is fixed in stepwise relationship of each phase. It forms an entity called hysteroepilepsy, and I will not be convinced otherwise.

Prior to my becoming director of this service, my predecessors introduced terminology to distinguish patients with these mixed attacks (*attaques à crises mixtes*) of hysteroepilepsy from those with distinct attacks of alternating hysteria and true epilepsy (*attaques à crises séparées*). What does this latter term mean?

Let us take a look at another patient. (*Another woman comes in.*) From time to time, this woman has various attacks. She is hysterical but also truly epileptic. By this I mean she has two distinct and essentially different diseases, both belonging to the same general family as would be, for instance, gout and rheumatism occurring in the same patient. Now the two conditions are separate and remain so throughout the patient's life. They do not fuse or evolve one into the other. Let us not incorrectly create a Darwinism of such events. The pivotal feature in the doctrine of evolution is time, meaning multiple generations, and when I speak of two separate disorders, I speak of them in the context of one person's brief life.

In the case of separated crises, you have first an attack of hysteroepilepsy and then an attack of real epilepsy. In such a case, after a hysterical outburst, a patient may be found to have bitten her tongue. When the staff gets the patient back to bed and examines here, they will say, "No, she has had a real seizure" if she bit her tongue, and "Yes, it was a hysterical spell" if there was no tongue biting. The point here is that the two are entirely different types of events, although they may occur in the same patient. If one reports that a patient had a real seizure, this behavior is taken seriously. If the same patient is said to have a hysterical fit, even lasting six days, there would be no major concern. If she has a real seizure, she could progress to status epilepticus, so the physician is immediately notified. The temperature could rise. Life itself would be at stake. Therefore, the distinction between the two is paramount. In hysteroepileptic patients with a known hystero-genic point, you could compress it, not only experimentally, to induce hys-terical attacks, but more importantly, to stop them; whereas, if the attack is really a seizure, such compression will serve absolutely no purpose.

I will add that whereas potassium bromide has a palliative effect on true epilepsy, it will not help hysteroepileptic events. You can give tons of it without changing these patients. Primary hysteria is not epilepsy. Only in the patient's family tree will the two link together. By this I mean that a hysteroepileptic parent can have a child with true epilepsy and vice versa. But to be truthful, they could just as well give birth to manics or other chil-dren with forms of psychosis as well. I have told you before that the neu-rologic tree has many branches, and each one bears different fruits.

From Jean-Martin Charcot, *Charcot the Clinician: The Tuesday Lessons*, translated by Christopher G. Goetz (New York: Raven, 1987), 102–109. With permission of Christopher G. Goetz.

Emil Kraepelin
(1856–1926)

"About the Surveillance Ward at the Heidelberg Clinic for Lunatics"
(1895)

Emil Kraepelin's influence on modern psychiatry is difficult to over-estimate. His insistence that psychiatric disorders be understood in terms of their symptoms and course (not their etiology), his effort to identify statistical regularities in symptoms, his use of experimental techniques, and his development of a clinical picture for dementia praecox (schizophrenia) and cyclothymia (manic depression, or bipolar disorder) set in motion an agenda pursued by clinical psychiatry up to this very day. Assuming the position of director of the psychiatric clinic at the University of Heidelberg in 1891, he turned the facility into a site that combined teaching, research, and treatment.

The excerpt here describes his refinement of the surveillance ward at the Heidelberg clinic. Surveillance wards—large rooms that allowed staff to keep patients under "constant observation"—were first developed in Germany in the 1880s. These "scientific observatories," as one psychiatrist described them, constituted a new kind of institutional space, designed specifically to address the needs of a new urban, university-based psychiatry. Note the prevalence and use of psychoactive drugs on the ward.

I had been convinced of the need for a sufficiently large surveillance ward since my first year working at the Heidelberg clinic. Because of constant overcrowding in those rooms originally earmarked for the use of the surveillance ward, I had already considered it necessary to plan on a transfer from those wards to the adjoining and far more spacious ward for the semi-calm. With this revolution, I managed to completely get rid of the semi-calm ward during the day, in order to gain more space for scientific research rooms. Those rooms made available from the earlier surveillance ward were now only used as sleeping halls, whereas the small number of "semi-calm" patients were distributed among the three remaining wards—the surveillance ward and those for calm and agitated patients. . . .

At the outset, it must be granted that the described layout of the surveillance ward, as it once was, has certain significant disadvantages. It is certainly correct to insist that, above all else, a surveillance ward allow a clear view so that an unobstructed surveillance of all residents is possible. Admittedly in our clinic, rooms A–D are connected to one another via wide door openings, but it is not possible for a person to responsibly keep watch over more than at most two rooms at the same time. Fortunately such an awkward observation of each individual patient in the entire ward is not altogether necessary, as will become evident, so that practical operations have not been hindered in any noticeable way by the inadequate layout of the ward. In fact, it has proven to be an estimable advantage that, in some directions, the peculiar arrangement of rooms allows for a more effective segregation on the surveillance ward of individual patients with different classifications.

In order to get an exact picture of all relevant circumstances [on the ward], special questionnaires were filled out for 250 days—from 3 January to 9 September 1893 (in addition to the standard daily reports following the Munich model). These contained, first of all, a record of the names of all the patients who found themselves on the surveillance ward from day to day, followed by a brief report on the apparent reason for their stay. Attention was also paid to those patients transferred to the surveillance ward only at night. In addition, the names of all patients in beds in other wards (for whatever reason) were also included. Furthermore, all tranquilizer and sleeping medication doses were continuously recorded, along with the particular reasons and the level of success. The duration of and reasons for every individual isolation were also entered. Finally, a survey of the distribution of patients in different wards during the day and at night was conducted on a regular basis. The 250 questionnaires for men and women that were collected were each put into 5 consecutive groupings, each covering 50 days, in order to be able to track changes in ward operations during the entire period of observation.

The daily average occupancy of the clinic during the entire time was 109.34 patients, of which 62.54 were in the male and 46.80 in the female ward. Of this total number, an average of 46.65 patients (42.66 percent) found themselves in both wards, 23.08 (36.89 percent) of the men and 23.57 (50.37 percent) of the women. The surveillance ward for men accommodated, then, over one-third of the total number, while the one for women an average of one-half. The difference derives in part from the larger frequency of depressive and agitated conditions among the women. Among the daily residents of the surveillance ward, depressed and agitated patients made up 12.04—around 19 percent—of the total number of male occupants, while for women the number was 15.48, i.e., no less than 33 percent of all female patients. In addition, it should naturally be noted that the spatial expansion of the surveillance ward made increasing the number of beds for more than 25 additional patients very difficult and, thus, the impact of the changing number of total residents was felt more on the remaining wards than on the surveillance ward. During the entire observation period, the latter was filled almost to capacity on both sides of the clinic. The total amount of floor space in the patient rooms of the surveillance ward was around 231 square meters. Thus, on the basis of average occupancy, each patient had approximately 10 square meters of floor space or, since the height was 3.8 meters, 38 cubic meters of air space. . . .

The reasons why individual patients were placed in the surveillance ward, according to the survey report, were varied. In the case of the first group of patients, indications primarily involved somatic issues; the task of the surveillance ward was "care" for the patient in the stricter sense of the term. This includes those with genuine physical ailments of all kinds, namely those sick with fever. These are joined by the lame, paralytics in advanced stages, apoplectics, as well as those who are unhelpful and bedridden because of age, weakness, or other frailty or otherwise place greater demands on staff. Also the unhygienic should be counted here, especially those largely falling under the latter category of care. At any rate, there are also some feeble-minded, catatonics, and similar types who are not frail, but nevertheless, because of their lack of hygiene, require the better care provided by the surveillance ward. Finally, the physical condition of those who refuse food is a primary reason for accommodation on the surveillance ward. All patients who do not eat enough food are looked after in bed and are placed under constant supervision.

Those refusing food constitute the second main group of surveillance ward residents—those patients who suffer from severe depressive conditions. The primary task of the surveillance ward here consists of monitoring. It is well known that these patients provided the initial impetus for the construction of surveillance wards. All anxious and sad patients are part of this group, as long as there is concern about suicidal tendencies; also those patients who appear to be a danger to themselves for other reasons and, finally, those in a daze or stupor who do not fall under the first grouping, since one often has to reckon with sudden, unexpected, dangerous behavior on their part.

Besides monitoring, the surveillance ward offers these patients the possibility of lengthy bed rest, something that must be considered a form of therapy. This is perhaps the case to a greater extent for another group of patients whom we primarily try to treat on the surveillance ward: the frenetic. The majority of these are manic patients, especially periodic and circular forms, as well as some paralytics and hebephrenics. These patients, like those who are anxiously agitated and demanding, can be supported most easily in bed on the surveillance ward and, in this manner, be satisfactorily influenced.

Alongside the three main groups of patients discussed so far, there is a small number of persons on the surveillance ward who are best accommodated here for a variety of reasons. The common goal is generally a more precise observation of the patients. Here it would be worth mentioning the new admissions about whom there are questions as to which of the above groups they might belong, prisoners under investigation, morphine and cocaine addicts, epileptics requiring special and on-going examinations (body weight, urine samples, digestion tests, etc), and, finally, some patients requiring a certain measure of segregation while being monitored because of particular sensitivities, deformities, or infectious or disgusting ailments. . . .

To get a full picture of operations on the surveillance ward, it is necessary to know the extent to which narcotics and sleeping medications have been given. If we count all those medications for which we methodically distribute a daily dose of an opium or bromine treatment, a daily average of 7.16 men and 7.36 women received tranquilizers or sleeping medications. Due to the varying occupancy levels on both wards, the percentage for men would be 11.45 percent and 15.74 percent for the women. The higher figure for women can be explained easily, being due to the fact that disproportionately more agitated patients were registered among their ranks. On average, among the men, 8.5 percent of day shift and 6.1 percent of night shift patients were counted as agitated; for the women, the figures were 24.4 percent for the day shift and 8.3 percent for the night shift. The large discrepancy during the day shift moved toward parity during the night shift, something that perhaps speaks to the fact that the agitation of women is determined to a greater degree by external influences than is the case with the men. Also the greater frequency of periodic manic and circular forms of milder agitation among the women vis a vis the more severe paralytic, epileptic, and alcoholic frenetic conditions found among the men plays a certain role here.

Considering the significantly higher number of agitated patients among the women, the amount of sleep medications and tranquilizers administered on the male side appears disproportionately too large. The cause of this most probably lies in the exceptionally high number of patients. The male ward can normally accommodate around 55 patients; nevertheless, on average there were 62.5 patients here, and, one day, the number reached 70. Thus, it appeared impossible to adequately separate the disruptive patients from the others, so we had to rely more frequently on sleeping medications than would have been necessary under better circumstances, in order to establish some quiet during the night. Most often, sleeping medications were naturally administered on the surveillance ward, since it was here that those patients resided who most needed sedation both for themselves and for their surrounding environment. This situation is made very clear in the following summary, which cites the percentage of patients in the entire clinic and the percentage of patients on the surveillance ward who, on average, received daily sleeping medication. Opium treatment for anxious patients is not included here.

| | Time Periods (I–V) | | | | |
	I	II	III	IV	V
Men					
Sleeping Medication Total (pct)	7.42	8.50	10.60	12.39	9.85
On the Surveillance Ward	12.71	14.48	18.52	23.08	15.56
Percentage of Agitated Patients	6.24	7.08	10.16	9.43	9.59
Women					
Sleeping Medication Total (pct)	12.12	9.15	11.56	10.82	14.05
On the Surveillance Ward	14.59	11.63	13.06	12.11	15.20
Percentage of Agitated Patients	22.15	20.09	21.26	24.15	34.70

Without question, the proportion of patients who received sleeping medication is greater on the surveillance ward than throughout the entire clinic, but this difference is everywhere more pronounced on the male side. From this, we can conclude that the administration of sleeping medication to men was essentially rooted in the effort to be able to care for disruptive patients with the least amount of injury to their neighbors on the surveillance ward; whereas for the women, the need for sleeping medication appears hardly lower in the other wards and accords with the large number of agitated elements in general. . . .

The following table provides information about the types of medication administered, in which, though, a number of medications (duboisin, chloral hydrate, chloral morphine) are not cited. Alcohol that is used more frequently as a sleep aid in cases of mild anxiety and fatigue psychosis is also not taken into account, while habitual consumption without medical justification was completely eliminated. The figures refer to daily doses; when it comes to bromine and opium, the unit is generally the sum of a number of separate doses during the day.

	Trional	Sulfate	Hyoscine	Morphine	Opium	Bromine
Men	347	721	20	—	420	279
Women	228	511	206	74	509	312

Among men, actual sleeping medications, trional and sulfate, predominate, which can be explained by the need to establish quiet during the night in over-crowded wards. By contrast, among the women, the experimental administration of the quick-acting and powerful narcotics hyoscine and morphine was noticeably common. In these cases, then, it involved combating sudden bouts of agitation as effectively as possible. The correspondence of this result with our earlier table is self-evident, though it should not be overlooked that in the selection of medication, the personal inclinations and experiences of the ward physician naturally plays a very important role. The more substantial use of (almost always) methodically administered opium and bromine on women is obviously tied to the previously established greater frequency of depressive conditions among the female sex.

From Emil Kraepelin, "Über die Wachabteilung der Heidelberger Irrenklinik," *Allgemeine Zeitschrift für Psychiatrie und psychisch-gerichtliche Medizin* 51 (1895): 1–21. Translated by Greg Eghigian.

Sigmund Freud

(1856–1939)

"The Origin and Development of Psychoanalysis"

(1910)

Sigmund Freud studied neurology at the University of Vienna. Soon after receiving his medical degree, in 1885, he went to Paris to observe the famous Jean-Martin Charcot. Leaving Paris in 1886, Freud returned to Vienna with an interest in the psychological origins of hysteria. He soon established his own private practice and a partnership with his colleague Josef Breuer (1842–1925). Together the two men developed the outlines of a new approach to psychiatric disorders, stressing the roles of memory, trauma, and therapeutic talk. Freud and Breuer soon parted ways, and Freud went on to elaborate his own school of thought—psychoanalysis.

In 1909, Freud came to the United States—his only visit—at the invitation of the president of Clark University, the psychologist G. Stanley Hall. There, Freud gave a series of lectures intended to introduce Americans to the new field. The warm reception he received was a harbinger of things to come, as the United States proved to be far more receptive to psychoanalytic thinking than did his home continent of Europe.

First Lecture

Ladies and Gentlemen: It is a new and somewhat embarrassing experience for me to appear as lecturer before students of the New World. I assume that I owe this honor to the association of my name with the theme of psychoanalysis, and consequently it is of psychoanalysis that I shall aim to speak. I shall attempt to give you in very brief form an historical survey of the origin and further development of this new method of research and cure.

Granted that it is a merit to have created psychoanalysis, it is not my merit. I was a student, busy with the passing of my last examinations, when another physician of Vienna, Dr. Joseph Breuer, made the first application of this method to the case of an hysterical girl (1880–82). We must now examine the history of this case and its treatment, which can be found in detail in *Studien über Hysterie*, later published by Dr. Breuer and myself.

But first one word. I have noticed, with considerable satisfaction, that the majority of my hearers do not belong to the medical profession. Now do not fear that a medical education is necessary to follow what I shall have to say. We shall now accompany the doctors a little way, but soon we shall take leave of them and follow Dr. Breuer on a way which is quite his own.

Dr. Breuer's patient was a girl of twenty-one, of a high degree of intelligence. She had developed in the course of her two years' illness a series of physical and mental disturbances which well deserved to be taken seriously. She had a severe paralysis of both right extremities, with anasthesia, and at times the same affection of the members of the left side of the body; disturbance of eye-movements, and much impairment of vision; difficulty in maintaining the position of the head; an intense Tussis nervosa; nausea when she attempted to take nourishment; and at one time for several weeks a loss of the power to drink, in spite of tormenting thirst. Her power of speech was also diminished, and this progressed so far that she could neither speak nor understand her mother tongue; and, finally, she was subject to states of "absence," of confusion, delirium, alteration of her whole personality. These states will later claim our attention.

When one hears of such a case, one does not need to be a physician to incline to the opinion that we are concerned here with a serious injury, probably of the brain, for which there is little hope of cure and which will probably lead to the early death of the patient. The doctors will tell us, however, that in one type of cases with just as unfavorable symptoms, another, far more favorable, opinion is justified. When one finds such a series of symptoms in the case of a young girl, whose vital organs (heart, kidneys) are shown by objective tests to be normal, but who has suffered from strong emotional disturbances, and when the symptoms differ in certain finer characteristics from what one might logically expect, in a case like this the doctors are not too much disturbed. They consider that there is present no organic lesion of the brain, but that enigmatical state, known since the time of the Greek physicians as hysteria, which can simulate a whole series of symptoms of various diseases. They consider in such a case that the life of the patient is not in danger and that a restoration to health will probably come about of itself. The differentiation of such an hysteria from a severe organic lesion is not always very easy. But we do not need to know how a differential diagnosis of this kind is made; you may be sure that the case of Breuer's patient was such that no skillful physician could fail to diagnose an hysteria. We may also add a word here from the history of the case. The illness first appeared while the patient was caring for her father, whom she tenderly loved, during the severe illness which led to his death, a task which she was compelled to abandon because she herself fell ill.

So far it has seemed I best to go with the doctors, but we shall soon part company with them. You must not think that the outlook of a patient with regard to medical aid is essentially bettered when the diagnosis points to hysteria rather than to organic disease of the brain. Against the serious brain diseases medical skill is in most cases powerless, but also in the case of hysterical affections the doctor can do nothing. He must leave it to benign nature, when and how his hopeful prognosis will be realized. Accordingly, with the recognition of the disease as hysteria, little is changed in the situation of the patient, but there is a great change in the attitude of the doctor. We can observe that he acts quite differently toward hystericals than toward patients suffering from organic diseases. He will not bring the same interest to the former as to the latter, since their suffering is much less serious and yet seems to set up the claim to be valued just as seriously.

But there is another motive in this action. The physician, who through his studies has learned so much that is hidden from the laity, can realize in his thought the causes and alterations of the brain disorders in patients suffering from apoplexy or dementia, a representation which must be right up to a certain point, for by it he is enabled to understand the nature of each symptom. But before the details of hysterical symptoms, all his knowledge, his anatomical-physiological and pathological education, desert him. He cannot understand hysteria. He is in the same position before it as the layman. And that is not agreeable to any one, who is in the habit of setting such a high valuation upon his knowledge. Hystericals, accordingly, tend to lose his sympathy; he considers them persons who overstep the laws of his science, as the orthodox regard heretics; he ascribes to them all possible evils, blames them for exaggeration and intentional deceit, "simulation," and he punishes them by withdrawing his interest.

Now Dr. Breuer did not deserve this reproach in this case; he gave his patient sympathy and interest, although at first he did not understand how to help her. Probably this was easier for him on account of those superior qualities of the patient's mind and character, to which he bears witness in his account of the case.

His sympathetic observation soon found the means which made the first help possible. It had been noticed that the patient, in her states of "absence," of psychic alteration, usually mumbled over several words to herself. These seemed to spring from associations with which her thoughts were busy. The doctor, who was able to get these words, put her in a sort of hypnosis and repeated them to her over and over, in order to bring up any associations that they might have. The patient yielded to his suggestion and reproduced for him those psychic creations which controlled her thoughts during her "absences," and which betrayed themselves in these single spoken words. These were fancies, deeply sad, often poetically beautiful, day dreams, we might call them, which commonly took as their starting point the situation of a girl beside the sick-bed of her father. Whenever she had related a number of such fancies, she was, as it were, freed and restored to her normal mental life. This state of health would last for several hours, and then give place on the next day to a new "absence," which was removed in the same way by relating the newly-created fancies. It was impossible not to get the impression that the psychic alteration which was expressed in the "absence" was a consequence of the excitations originating from these intensely emotional fancy-images. The patient herself, who at this time of her illness strangely enough understood and spoke only English, gave this new kind of treatment the name "talking cure," or jokingly designated it as "chimney sweeping."

The doctor soon hit upon the fact that through such cleansing of the soul more could be accomplished than a temporary removal of the constantly recurring mental "clouds." Symptoms of the disease would disappear when in hypnosis the patient could be made to remember the situation and the associative connections under which they first appeared, provided free vent was given to the emotions which they aroused. "There was in the summer a time of intense heat, and the patient had suffered very much from thirst; for, without any apparent reason, she had suddenly become unable to drink. She would take a glass of water in her hand, but as soon as it touched her lips she would push it away as though suffering from hydrophobia. Obviously for these few seconds she was in her absent state. She ate only fruit, melons and the like, in order to relieve this tormenting thirst. When this had been going on about six weeks, she was talking one day in hypnosis about her English governess, whom she disliked, and finally told, with every sign of disgust, how she had come into the room of the governess, and how that lady's little dog, that she abhorred, had drunk out of a glass. Out of respect for the conventions the patient had remained silent. Now, after she had given energetic expression to her restrained anger, she asked for a drink, drank a large quantity of water without trouble, and woke from hypnosis with the glass at her lips. The symptom thereupon vanished permanently."

Permit me to dwell for a moment on this experience. No one had ever cured an hysterical symptom by such means before, or had come so near understanding its cause. This would be a pregnant discovery if the expectation could be confirmed that still other, perhaps the majority of symptoms, originated in this way and could be removed by the same method. Breuer spared no pains to convince himself of this and investigated the pathogenesis of the other more serious symptoms in a more orderly way. Such was indeed the case; almost all the symptoms originated in exactly this way, as remnants, as precipitates, if you like, of affectively-toned experiences, which for that reason we later called "psychic traumata." The nature of the symptoms became clear through their relation to the scene which caused them. They were, to use the technical term, "determined" (determiniert) by the scene whose memory traces they embodied, and so could no longer be described as arbitrary or enigmatical functions of the neurosis.

Only one variation from what might be expected must be mentioned. It was not always a single experience which occasioned the symptom, but usually several, perhaps many similar, repeated traumata cooperated in this effect. It was necessary to repeat the whole series of pathogenic memories in chronological sequence, and of course in reverse order, the last first and the first last. It was quite impossible to reach the first and often most essential trauma directly, without first clearing away those coming later.

You will of course want to hear me speak of other examples of the causation of hysterical symptoms beside this of inability to drink on account of the disgust caused by the dog drinking from the glass. I must, however, if I hold to my programme, limit myself to very few examples. Breuer relates, for instance, that his patient's visual disturbances could be traced back to external causes, in the following way. "The patient, with tears in her eyes, was sitting by the sick-bed when her father suddenly asked her what time it was. She could not see distinctly, strained her eyes to see, brought the watch near her eyes so that the dial seemed very large (macropia and strabismus conv.), or else she tried hard to suppress her tears, so that the sick man might not see them."

All the pathogenic impressions sprang from the time when she shared in the care of her sick father. "Once she was watching at night in the greatest anxiety for the patient, who was in a high fever, and in suspense, for a surgeon was expected from Vienna, to operate on the patient. Her mother had gone out for a little while, and Anna sat by the sick-bed, her right arm hanging over the back of her chair. She fell into a revery [sic] and saw a black snake emerge, as it were, from the wall and approach the sick man as though to bite him. (It is very probable that several snakes had actually been seen in the meadow behind the house, that she had already been frightened by them, and that these former experiences furnished the material for the hallucination). She tried to drive off the creature, but was as though paralyzed. Her right arm, which was hanging over the back of the chair, had 'gone to sleep,' become anasthetic [sic] and paretic, and as she was looking at it, the fingers changed into little snakes with deaths-heads. (The nails). Probably she attempted to drive away the snake with her paralyzed right hand, and so the anasthesia [sic] and paralysis of this member formed associations with the snake hallucination. When this had vanished, she tried in her anguish to speak, but could not. She could not express herself in any language, until finally she thought of the words of an English nursery song, and thereafter she could think and speak only in this language." When the memory of this scene was revived in hypnosis the paralysis of the right arm, which had existed since the beginning of the illness, was cured and the treatment ended.

When, a number of years later, I began to use Breuer's researches and treatment on my own patients, my experiences completely coincided with his. In the case of a woman of about forty, there was a tic, a peculiar smacking noise which manifested itself whenever she was laboring under any excitement, without any obvious cause. It had its origin in two experiences which had this common element, that she attempted to make no noise, but that by a sort of counter-will this noise broke the stillness. On the first occasion, she had finally after much trouble put her sick child to sleep, and she tried to be very quiet so as not to awaken it. On the second occasion, during a ride with both her children in a thunderstorm the horses took fright, and she carefully avoided any noise for fear of frightening them still more. I give this example instead of many others which are cited in the "*Studien über Hysterie.*"

Ladies and gentlemen, if you will permit me to generalize, as is indispensable in so brief a presentation, we may express our results up to this point in the formula: Our hysterical patients suffer from reminiscences. Their symptoms are the remnants and the memory symbols of certain (traumatic) experiences.

A comparison with other memory symbols from other sources will perhaps enable us better to understand this symbolism. The memorials and monuments with which we adorn our great cities, are also such memory symbols. If you walk through London you will find before one of the greatest railway stations of the city a richly decorated Gothic pillar"—"Charing Cross." One of the old Plantagenet kings, in the thirteenth century, caused the body of his beloved queen Eleanor to be borne to Westminster, and had Gothic crosses erected at each of the stations where the coffin was set down. Charing Cross is the last of these monuments, which preserve the memory of this sad journey. In another part of the city, you will see a high pillar of more modern construction, which is merely called "the monument." This is in memory of the great fire which broke out in the neighborhood in the year 1666, and destroyed a great part of the city. These monuments are memory symbols like the hysterical symptoms; so far the comparison seems justified. But what would you say to a Londoner who today stood sadly before the monument to the funeral of Queen Eleanor, instead of going about his business with the haste engendered by modern industrial conditions, or rejoicing with the young queen of his own heart? Or to another, who before the "Monument" bemoaned the burning of his loved native city, which long since has arisen again so much more splendid than before?

Now hystericals and all neurotics behave like these two unpractical Londoners, not only in that they remember the painful experiences of the distant past, but because they are still strongly affected by them. They cannot escape from the past and neglect present reality in its favor. This fixation of the mental life on the pathogenic traumata is an essential, and practically a most significant characteristic of the neurosis. I will willingly concede the objection which you are probably formulating, as you think over the history of Breuer's patient. All her traumata originated at the time when she was caring for her sick father, and her symptoms could only be regarded as memory symbols of his sickness and death. They corresponded to mourning, and a fixation on thoughts of the dead so short a time after death is certainly not pathological, but rather corresponds to normal emotional behavior. I concede this: there is nothing abnormal in the fixation of feeling on the trauma shown by Breuer's patient. But in other cases, like that of the tic that I have mentioned, the occasions for which lay ten and fifteen years back, the characteristic of this abnormal clinging to the past is very clear, and Breuer's patient would probably have developed it, if she had not come under the "cathartic treatment" such a short time after the traumatic experiences and the beginning of the disease.

We have so far only explained the relation of the hysterical symptoms to the life history of the patient; now by considering two further moments which Breuer observed, we may get a hint as to the processes of the beginning of the illness and those of the cure. With regard to the first, it is especially to be noted that Breuer's patient in almost all pathogenic situations had to suppress a strong excitement, instead of giving vent to it by appropriate words and deeds. In the little experience with her governess' dog, she suppressed, through regard for the conventions, all manifestations of her very intense disgust. While she was seated by her father's sick bed, she was careful to betray nothing of her anxiety and her painful depression to the patient. When, later, she reproduced the same scene before the physician, the emotion which she had suppressed on the occurrence of the scene burst out with especial strength, as though it had been pent up all along. The symptom which had been caused by that scene reached its greatest intensity while the doctor was striving to revive the memory of the scene, and vanished after it had been fully laid bare. On the other hand, experience shows that if the patient is reproducing the traumatic scene to the physician, the process has no curative effect if, by some peculiar chance, there is no development of emotion. It is apparently these emotional processes upon which the illness of the patient and the restoration to health are dependent. We feel justified in regarding "emotion" as a quantity which may become increased, derived and displaced. So we are forced to the conclusion that the patient fell ill because the emotion developed in the pathogenic situation was prevented from escaping normally, and that the essence of the sickness lies in the fact that these "imprisoned" (*dingeklemmt*) emotions undergo a series of abnormal changes. In part they are preserved as a lasting charge and as a source of constant disturbance in psychical life; in part they undergo a change into unusual bodily innervations and inhibitions, which present themselves as the physical symptoms of the case. We have coined the name "hysterical conversion" for the latter process. Part of our mental energy is, under normal conditions, conducted off by way of physical innervation and gives what we call "the expression of emotions." Hysterical conversion exaggerates this part of the course of a mental process which is emotionally colored; it corresponds to a far more intense emotional expression, which finds outlet by new paths. If a stream flows in two channels, an overflow of one will take place as soon as the current in the other meets with an obstacle.

You see that we are in a fair way to arrive at a purely psychological theory of hysteria, in which we assign the first rank to the affective processes. A second observation of Breuer compels us to ascribe to the altered condition of consciousness a great part in determining the characteristics of the disease. His patient showed many sorts of mental states, conditions of "absence," confusion and alteration of character, besides her normal state. In her normal state she was entirely ignorant of the pathogenic scenes and of their connection with her symptoms. She had forgotten those scenes, or at any rate had dissociated them from their pathogenic connection. When the patient was hypnotized, it was possible, after considerable difficulty, to recall those scenes to her memory, and by this means of recall the symptoms were removed. It would have been extremely perplexing to know how to interpret this fact, if hypnotic practice and experiments had not pointed out the way. Through the study of hypnotic phenomena, the conception, strange though it was at first, has become familiar, that in one and the same individual several mental groupings are possible, which may remain relatively independent of each other, "know nothing" of each other, and which may cause a splitting of consciousness along lines which they lay down. Cases of such a sort, known as "double personality" ("double conscience"), occasionally appear spontaneously. If in such a division of personality consciousness remains constantly bound up with one of the two states, this is called the conscious mental state, and the other the unconscious. In the well-known phenomena of so-called post hypnotic suggestion, in which a command given in hypnosis is later executed in the normal state as though by an imperative suggestion, we have an excellent basis for understanding how the unconscious state can influence the conscious, although the latter is ignorant of the existence of the former. In the same way it is quite possible to explain the facts in hysterical cases. Breuer came to the conclusion that the hysterical symptoms originated in such peculiar mental states, which he called "hypnoidal states" (*hypnoide Zustände*). Experiences of an emotional nature, which occur during such hypnoidal states easily become pathogenic, since such states do not present the conditions for a normal draining off of the emotion of the exciting processes. And as a result there arises a peculiar product of this exciting process, that is, the symptom, and this is projected like a foreign body into the normal state. The latter has, then, no conception of the significance of the hypnoidal pathogenic situation. Where a symptom arises, we also find an amnesia, a memory gap, and the filling of this gap includes the removal of the conditions under which the symptom originated.

I am afraid that this portion of my treatment will not seem very clear, but you must remember that we are dealing here with new and difficult views, which perhaps could not be made much clearer. This all goes to show that our knowledge in this field is not yet very far advanced. Breuer's idea of the hypnoidal states has, moreover, been shown to be superfluous and a hindrance to further investigation, and has been dropped from present conceptions of psychoanalysis. Later I shall at least suggest what other influences and processes have been disclosed besides that of the hypnoidal states, to which Breuer limited the causal moment.

You have probably also felt, and rightly, that Breuer's investigations gave you only a very incomplete theory and insufficient explanation of the phenomena which we have observed. But complete theories do not fall from Heaven, and you would have had still greater reason to be distrustful, had any one offered you at the beginning of his observations a well-rounded theory, without any gaps; such a theory could only be the child of his speculations and not the fruit of an unprejudiced investigation of the facts.

Second Lecture

Ladies and Gentlemen: At about the same time that Breuer was using the "talking-cure" with his patient, M. Charcot began in Paris, with the hystericals of the Salpêtrière, those researches which were to lead to a new understanding of the disease. These results were, however, not yet known in Vienna. But when about ten years later Breuer and I published our preliminary communication on the psychic mechanism of hysterical phenomena, which grew out of the cathartic treatment of Breuer's first patient, we were both of us under the spell of Charcot's investigations. We made the pathogenic experiences of our patients, which acted as psychic traumata, equivalent to those physical traumata whose influence on hysterical paralyses Charcot had determined; and Breuer's hypothesis of hypnoidal states is itself only an echo of the fact that Charcot had artificially reproduced those traumatic paralyses in hypnosis.

The great French observer, whose student I was during the years 1885–86, had no natural bent for creating psychological theories. His student, P. Janet, was the first to attempt to penetrate more deeply into the psychic processes of hysteria, and we followed his example, when we made the mental splitting and the dissociation of personality the central points of our theory.* Janet propounds a theory of hysteria which draws upon the principal theories of heredity and degeneration which are current in France. According to his view hysteria is a form of degenerative alteration of the nervous system, manifesting itself in a congenital "weakness" of the function of psychic synthesis. The hysterical patient is from the start incapable of correlating and unifying the manifold of his mental processes, and so there arises the tendency to mental dissociation. If you will permit me to use a banal but clear illustration, Janet's hysterical reminds one of a weak woman who has been shopping, and is now on her way home, laden with packages and bundles of every description. She cannot manage the whole lot with her two arms and her ten fingers, and soon she drops one. When she stoops to pick this up, another breaks loose, and so it goes on.

Now it does not agree very well, with this assumed mental weakness of hystericals, that there can be observed in hysterical cases, besides the phenomena of lessened functioning, examples of a partial increase of functional capacity, as a sort of compensation. At the time when Breuer's patient had forgotten her mother-tongue and all other languages save English, her control of English attained such a level that if a German book was put before

---

*Editor's note: Freud here refers to Pierre Janet (1859–1947), a French neurologist and psychologist who wrote on hysteria and hypnosis.

her she could give a fluent, perfect translation of its contents at sight. When later I undertook to continue on my own account the investigations begun by Breuer, I soon came to another view of the origin of hysterical dissociation (or splitting of consciousness). It was inevitable that my views should diverge widely and radically, for my point of departure was not, like that of Janet, laboratory researches, but attempts at therapy. Above everything else, it was practical needs that urged me on. The cathartic treatment, as Breuer had made use of it, presupposed that the patient should be put in deep hypnosis, for only in hypnosis was available the knowledge of his pathogenic associations, which were unknown to him in his normal state. Now hypnosis, as a fanciful, and so to speak, mystical, aid, I soon came to dislike; and when I discovered that, in spite of all my efforts, I could not hypnotize by any means all of my patients, I resolved to give up hypnotism and to make the cathartic method independent of it.

Since I could not alter the psychic state of most of my patients at my wish, I directed my efforts to working with them in their normal state. This seems at first sight to be a particularly senseless and aimless undertaking. The problem was this: to find out something from the patient that the doctor did not know and the patient himself did not know. How could one hope to make such a method succeed? The memory of a very noteworthy and instructive proceeding came to my aid, which I had seen in Bernheim's clinic at Nancy. Bernheim showed us that persons put in a condition of hypnotic somnambulism, and subjected to all sorts of experiences, had only apparently lost the memory of those somnambulic experiences, and that their memory of them could be awakened even in the normal state.* If he asked them about their experiences during somnambulism, they said at first that they did not remember, but if he persisted, urged, assured them that they did know, then every time the forgotten memory came back.

Accordingly I did this with my patients. When I had reached in my procedure with them a point at which they declared that they knew nothing more, I would assure them that they did know, that they must just tell it out, and I would venture the assertion that the memory which would emerge at the moment that I laid my hand on the patient's forehead would be the right one. In this way I succeeded, without hypnosis, in learning

---

*Editor's note: Hippolyte Bernheim (1840–1919) was known for his contention that hypnosis was little more than a form of ritualized suggestion.

from the patient all that was necessary for a construction of the connection between the forgotten pathogenic scenes and the symptoms which they had left behind. This was a troublesome and in its length an exhausting proceeding, and did not lend itself to a finished technique. But I did not give it up without drawing definite conclusions from the data which I had gained. I had substantiated the fact that the forgotten memories were not lost. They were in the possession of the patient, ready to emerge and form associations with his other mental content, but hindered from becoming conscious, and forced to remain in the unconscious by some sort of a force. The existence of this force could be assumed with certainty, for in attempting to drag up the unconscious memories into the consciousness of the patient, in opposition to this force, one got the sensation of his own personal effort striving to overcome it. One could get an idea of this force, which maintained the pathological situation, from the resistance of the patient.

It is on this idea of resistance that I based my theory of the psychic processes of hystericals. It had been found that in order to cure the patient it was necessary that this force should be overcome. Now with the mechanism of the cure as a starting point, quite a definite theory could be constructed. These same forces, which in the present situation as resistances opposed the emergence of the forgotten ideas into consciousness, must themselves have caused the forgetting, and repressed from consciousness the pathogenic experiences. I called this hypothetical process "repression" (*Verdrängung*), and considered that it was proved by the undeniable existence of resistance.

But now the question arose: what were those forces, and what were the conditions of this repression, in which we were now able to recognize the pathogenic mechanism of hysteria? A comparative study of the pathogenic situations, which the cathartic treatment has made possible, allows us to answer this question. In all those experiences, it had happened that a wish had been aroused, which was in sharp opposition to the other desires of the individual, and was not capable of being reconciled with the ethical, aesthetic and personal pretensions of the patient's personality. There had been a short conflict, and the end of this inner struggle was the repression of the idea which presented itself to consciousness as the bearer of this irreconcilable wish. This was, then, repressed from consciousness and forgotten. The incompatibility of the idea in question with the "ego" of the patient was the motive of the repression, the ethical and other pretensions of the individual were the repressing forces. The presence of the incompatible wish, or the duration of the conflict, had given rise to a high degree of mental pain; this pain was avoided by the repression. This latter process is evidently in such a case a device for the protection of the personality.

I will not multiply examples, but will give you the history of a single one of my cases, in which the conditions and the utility of the repression process stand out clearly enough. Of course for my purpose I must abridge the history of the case and omit many valuable theoretical considerations. It is that of a young girl, who was deeply attached to her father, who had died a short time before, and in whose care she had shared—a situation analogous to that of Breuer's patient. When her older sister married, the girl grew to feel a peculiar sympathy for her new brother-in-law, which easily passed with her for family tenderness. This sister soon fell ill and died, while the patient and her mother were away. The absent ones were hastily recalled, without being told fully of the painful situation. As the girl stood by the bedside of her dead sister, for one short moment there surged up in her mind an idea, which might be framed in these words: "Now he is free and can marry me." We may be sure that this idea, which betrayed to her consciousness her intense love for her brother-in-law, of which she had not been conscious, was the next moment consigned to repression by her revolted feelings. The girl fell ill with severe hysterical symptoms, and, when I came to treat the case, it appeared that she had entirely forgotten that scene at her sister's bedside and the unnatural, egoistic desire which had arisen in her. She remembered it during the treatment, reproduced the pathogenic moment with every sign of intense emotional excitement, and was cured by this treatment.

Perhaps I can make the process of repression and its necessary relation to the resistance of the patient, more concrete by a rough illustration, which I will derive from our present situation.

Suppose that here in this hall and in this audience, whose exemplary stillness and attention I cannot sufficiently commend, there is an individual who is creating a disturbance, and, by his ill-bred laughing, talking, by scraping his feet, distracts my attention from my task. I explain that I cannot go on with my lecture under these conditions, and thereupon several strong men among you get up, and, after a short struggle, eject the disturber of the peace from the hall. He is now "repressed," and I can continue my lecture. But in order that the disturbance may not be repeated, in case the man who has just been thrown out attempts to force his way back into the room, the gentlemen who have executed my suggestion take their chairs to the door and establish themselves there as a "resistance," to keep up the repression. Now, if you transfer both locations to the psyche, calling this "consciousness," and the outside the "unconscious," you have a tolerably good illustration of the process of repression.

We can see now the difference between our theory and that of Janet. We do not derive the psychic fission from a congenital lack of capacity on the part of the mental apparatus to synthesize its experiences, but we explain it dynamically by the conflict of opposing mental forces, we recognize in it the result of an active striving of each mental complex against the other.

New questions at once arise in great number from our theory. The situation of psychic conflict is a very frequent one; an attempt of the ego to defend itself from painful memories can be observed everywhere, and yet the result is not a mental fission. We cannot avoid the assumption that still other conditions are necessary, if the conflict is to result in dissociation. I willingly concede that with the assumption of "repression" we stand, not at the end, but at the very beginning of a psychological theory. But we can advance only one step at a time, and the completion of our knowledge must await further and more thorough work.

Now do not attempt to bring the case of Breuer's patient under the point of view of repression. This history cannot be subjected to such an attempt, for it was gained with the help of hypnotic influence. Only when hypnosis is excluded can you see the resistances and repressions and get a correct idea of the pathogenic process. Hypnosis conceals the resistances and so makes a certain part of the mental field freely accessible. By this same process the resistances on the borders of this field are heaped up into a rampart, which makes all beyond inaccessible.

The most valuable things that we have learned from Breuer's observations were his conclusions as to the connection of the symptoms with the pathogenic experiences or psychic traumata, and we must not neglect to evaluate this result properly from the standpoint of the repression-theory. It is not at first evident how we can get from the repression to the creation of the symptoms. Instead of giving a complicated theoretical derivation, I will return at this point to the illustration which I used to typify repression.

Remember that with the ejection of the rowdy and the establishment of the watchers before the door, the affair is not necessarily ended. It may very well happen that the ejected man, now embittered and quite careless of consequences, gives us more to do. He is no longer among us, we are free from his presence, his scornful laugh, his half-audible remarks, but in a certain sense the repression has miscarried, for he makes a terrible uproar outside, and by his outcries and by hammering on the door with his fists interferes with my lecture more than before. Under these circumstances it would be hailed with delight if possibly our honored president, Dr. Stanley Hall, should take upon himself the role of peacemaker and mediator. He would speak with the rowdy on the outside, and then turn to us with the recommendation that we let him in again, provided he would guarantee to behave himself better. On Dr. Hall's authority we decide to stop the repression, and now quiet and peace reign again. This is in fact a fairly good presentation of the task devolving upon the physician in the psychoanalytic therapy of neuroses. To say the same thing more directly: we come to the conclusion, from working with hysterical patients and other neurotics, that they have not fully succeeded in repressing the idea to which the incompatible wish is attached. They have, indeed, driven it out of consciousness and out of memory, and apparently saved themselves a great amount of psychic pain, but in the unconscious the suppressed wish still exists, only waiting for its chance to become active, and finally succeeds in sending into consciousness, instead of the repressed idea, a disguised and unrecognizable surrogate-creation (*Ersatzbildung*), to which the same painful sensations associate themselves that the patient thought he was rid of through his repression. This surrogate of the suppressed idea—the symptom—is secure against further attacks from the defences of the ego, and instead of a short conflict there originates now a permanent suffering. We can observe in the symptom, besides the tokens of its disguise, a remnant of traceable similarity with the originally repressed idea; the way in which the surrogate is built up can be discovered during the psychoanalytic treatment of the patient, and for his cure the symptom must be traced back over the same route to the repressed idea. If this repressed material is once more made part of the conscious mental functions—a process which supposes the overcoming of considerable resistance—the psychic conflict which then arises, the same which the patient wished to avoid, is made capable of a happier termination, under the guidance of the physician, than is offered by repression. There are several possible suitable decisions which can bring conflict and neurosis to a happy end; in particular cases the attempt may be made to combine several of these. Either the personality of the patient may be convinced that he has been wrong in rejecting the pathogenic wish, and he may be made to accept it either wholly or in part; or this wish may itself be directed to a higher goal which is free from objection, by what is called sublimation (*Sublimierung*); or the rejection may be recognized as rightly motivated, and the automatic and therefore insufficient mechanism of repression be reinforced by the higher, more characteristically human mental faculties: one succeeds in mastering his wishes by conscious thought.

Forgive me if I have not been able to present more clearly these main points of the treatment which is to-day known as "psychoanalysis." The difficulties do not lie merely in the newness of the subject.

Regarding the nature of the unacceptable wishes, which succeed in making their influence felt out of the unconscious, in spite of repression; and regarding the question of what subjective and constitutional factors must be present for such a failure of repression and such a surrogate or symptom creation to take place, we will speak in later remarks.

From Sigmund Freud, "The Origin and Development of Psychoanalysis," translated by Henry W. Chase, *American Journal of Psychology* 21 (1910): 181–218.

Vincent

"Confessions of an Agoraphobic Victim"

(1919)

Since ancient times, observers have been aware that some individuals are plagued by delusional fears. During the second half of the nineteenth century, clinicians began to apply the term *phobia* to a variety of these extremes forms of anxiety. One of the earliest phobias to draw attention was the fear of certain, typically public, spaces. In 1871, the Berlin psychiatrist Carl Westphal (1833–1890), having encountered patients complaining of an inability to cross or go down particular streets, dubbed this condition *agoraphobia*. Like neurasthenia, agoraphobia appeared to many to be a peculiarly urban phenomenon, and up until World War I, it was diagnosed primarily in men. The following autobiographical description of agoraphobia gives a sense of how the malady was experienced as a form of nervousness around the turn of the century.

For some time I have been planning to commit to writing personal observations of my condition, sensations and experiences during a long period of suffering from a malady which, for lack of a better name, medical men have termed "Agora-phobia"—fear of an open place.

As I am unacquainted with medical literature I do not know how much has been written on this subject. Only one case of "confessions" has come to my notice. Some time ago I read several pamphlets on "Religion and Medicine"—Emmanuel Church publications—one of which discussed various "nervous" disorders, among them the "phobias." In the course of the discussion there was introduced testimony of a man who had been grievously afflicted with agoraphobia. I devoured these "confessions" with the greatest avidity. It was the first and only time I had read any testimony of an individual thus afflicted.

This same pamphlet stated that the man had since become almost cured. Encouraged by these good tidings I tried to practice mental poise and tranquility for several weeks. During those few weeks I saw wonderful improvement in my condition. However, I lapsed gradually into my old habit of self-neglect, and with this neglect improvement in my health ceased.

The testimony taken from the above mentioned pamphlet leads one to infer that the affliction came upon the victim rather suddenly, and that the symptoms of the malady were present only occasionally: namely, when the man was on certain streets and at definite places on these streets.

If the above inference is correct I have to testify that my case is quite different. In the first place, my malady came upon me gradually and went through definite stages of development. Second, I am conscious of my affliction every minute that I am awake.

I am now in mid-life and I have not seen a well day since I was about twelve years of age. Before I experienced any of the symptoms of agoraphobia I recall that a strange affliction came over me, an affliction that seemed to baffle the country doctors who were consulted. I was taken suddenly with "spells" which lasted about thirty minutes. During these attacks I was entirely conscious and rational. As I remember the affliction, a sort of chill came over me—not like an ordinary chill, but a sort of "coldness" that produced a very unusual sensation, or perhaps, a lack of sensation would describe it more accurately. I have an impression that the physicians suggested that it might possibly have been due to a temporary stoppage of circulation. At any rate the remedy applied was vigorous rubbing of my body with rough towels, or with the bare hands by those attending me; sometimes, when it was convenient, a hot bath was resorted to; stimulants were also administered. I was more liable to these attacks during times of excitement. For instance, I recall that one of the worst attacks I ever had came over me while I was attending the funeral of a relative. When there seemed to be no outward cause that brought on the attacks, it was noted by my parents that they recurred periodically; I believe it was every fourteen days or was it eleven days?

My own belief now is that the illness referred to was due to some disorder of the nervous system. At any rate, after a few months I outgrew the tendency. However, I was not a well boy. I was abnormally timid and more or less melancholy, and was given to worry and brooding.

In this connection I would remark that I was born with an active, nervous temperament, and was always, as a boy, more or less timid. I was abnormally alert when there was possibility of danger. I remember how I used to run and leap like a fawn when passing through tall grass and weeds in the summer time, fearing lest I should encounter snakes, which were rather common.

When my strange illness came upon me I worried over it, fearing that I should die in one of the attacks. During this overwrought state of mind I was much affected by a terrible tragedy which took place in our community. One of my playmates, a boy about eleven years of age, disappeared one day. The supposition was that he had fallen into the river and had been drowned. On this theory, the river was dragged day after day for more than a week, but no body was discovered. Then the theory was advanced that he had been kidnapped, or perhaps, he being a venturesome lad, had started out to "see the world" and had met with foul play. I recall very well how the entire community was stirred and what effect it had on the boys and girls of the village and neighborhood. Finally, one morning in late autumn, the body of my playmate was found on the bank of the river, at a bend in the stream just below the village. But he had not been drowned—his throat was cut from ear to ear. The murder had been committed in a cellar in the village by a half-crazed woman who had later carried the body, by night, and placed it on the bank of the river.

This whole affair had a most depressing effect upon me. After that I almost feared to be alone, was afraid to go to the barn in the day time, and suffered when put to bed in the dark. Perhaps the worry over my illness, together with the depressing effect of the tragedy, brought on a severe attack of nervous dyspepsia. This resulted in malnutrition for my oversensitive nervous system which, perhaps, laid the foundation for the "phobias."

It was during the months which followed that I remember having experienced the first symptoms of agoraphobia. There was a high hill not far from my home in the country where we boys used to coast in the winter time. One evening while coasting, in company with other boys of the neighborhood, I experienced an uncomfortable feeling each time we returned to the top of the hill. It was not a well defined symptom of this horrible (I use the term deliberately) malady, but later experiences have taught me that it possessed the unmistakable earmarks. As the months went by the symptoms developed, with the result that I avoided hill-tops, so far as possible.

Later, perhaps a year or so, I commenced having a dread of wide fields, especially when the fields consisted of pasture land and were level, with the grass cropped short like the grass on a well-kept lawn. I likewise commenced to dread high things, and especially to ascend anything high. I even had a fear of crowds of people, and later of wide streets and parks.

I have outgrown the fear of crowds largely, but an immense building or a high rocky bluff fills me with dread. However the architecture of the building has much to do with the sort of sensation produced. Ugly architecture greatly intensifies the fear.

In this connection I would remark that I have come to wonder if there is real art in many of the so-called "improvements" in some of our cities, for, judging from the effect they produce on me, they constitute bad art.

But the one thing that I would make plain is that the malady is always present. As I write in my study I am painfully conscious of it—in fact, I am conscious of it during every hour that I am awake. The fear, intensified, that comes over me while crossing a wide street is, it seems to me, an outcropping of a permanent condition.

It is not pain that I feel, but it seems to me that it is more than a dread. I am not nervous, as some people whom I know—I mean in the same way, but it certainly is a case of "nerves." Let me illustrate:—I enter a home and sit in an arm-chair chatting with my friend; I soon find myself gripping the arm of the chair with each hand. My toes curl in my shoes, and there is a sort of tenseness all over my muscles.

At times my phobias are much more pronounced than at other times. Sometimes, after a strenuous day, on the following morning, I find myself almost dreading to walk across a room; at other times I can cross a street without any pronounced discomfort. Manual labor improves my condition. Walking and riding horseback are beneficial.

Usually I feel better in the evening than in the morning, partly because the darkness seems to have a quieting effect upon me. I love a snow storm a regular blizzard, and feel much less discomfort in going about the town or riding on a train on such days, probably because one's view is obstructed. In fact I welcome stormy days, strange to say, with a zest that is hard to appreciate; in short, some of the most stormy days of the hard winters of this region stand out as bright spots in my life. On such days I make it a point to be out and about the town.

I dread going out on water in a boat, especially if the surface is smooth; I much prefer to have the waves rolling high. The most restful place in all the world for me is in a wood, where there is much variety in the trees and plenty of underbrush, with here and there low hills and little valleys, and especially along a winding brook. I love "the quiet places by the woods." Also the little lakes with their narrow bays and wooded shoreline. I love quiet, restful landscape. It seems to rest my eyes and soothe my spirit. On the other hand, let the landscape be bold and rugged and bleak and it strikes terror to my soul.

I lived in New Haven during four years, while a student at Yale, and never climbed to the top of East Rock. And the big Green near the university always made me very uncomfortable when I looked at it.

I ride a bicycle along streets with comparative comfort where I should suffer agony were I to walk. In walking I feel less uncomfortable in passing along the street if I carry a suit-case or traveling-bag—something to grip.

When I think of the agony which I have experienced for many years I am astounded at the endurance of the human spirit. Let me illustrate:—I have such a dread of crossing a long bridge on foot that it would require more courage for me to walk to the part of my town situated across the river than it would to face a nest of Boche machine guns. And yet day after day, month after month, and year after year I have carried in my soul the dread of such an eventuality.

No one knows the truth about my condition. It is one of the characteristics of the victim of the disease to conceal it most cunningly. I think I am an honest man in all essential things. My credit is good at the banks. But I have deliberately told lies to avoid embarrassing situations and have even changed my plans to have my lies "come true."

I have never mentioned my condition to a physician. I have passed several examinations for life-insurance policies—in fact, have never been refused a policy by any life insurance company. I eat and sleep well, am rather strong and wiry physically. My occupation makes heavy demands on the vitality and entails considerable mental exercise, but I am seldom unable to take up my duties on account of indisposition. However, in my own mind I am a nervous wreck, weak, worthless, and unworthy of the high respect which the community accords me.

In spite of all this I seem to exercise marked power of leadership in my town, and am known as a public speaker of ability.

Of course, the paramount question with me is: Is there hope of a cure? Can I ever take my place in the world unhandicapped as other men are, and enjoy a single day undepressed by dark dread? If I could be as other men, it seems to me that my usefulness should be increased a hundredfold. Those who have not been thus afflicted cannot understand just what I mean.

I see a man hobbling past my house on crutches, a cripple for life, and I actually envy him. At times I would gladly exchange places with the humblest day-laborer who walks unafraid across the public square or saunters tranquilly over the viaduct on his way home after the day's work.

From Vincent, "Confessions of an Agoraphobic Victim," *American Journal of Psychology* 30 (1919): 295–299.

PART III

The Militant Age

By the turn of the twentieth century, many were questioning the optimistic outlook that had been voiced in the nineteenth century. The precipitous increase in the asylum population, the apparent emergence of new nervous disorders, and the often disappointing results of therapies led some to fear that, instead of progressing, public health was on the decline. This perception of decline encouraged countless public figures to express the view that Western civilization itself was in a state of degeneration, caught up in a process of atavistic devolution. The carnage of World War I (1914–1918), which brought about unprecedented loss of life and a mass outbreak of neurotic disorders, reinforced the conclusion that aggressive scientific, medical, and political intervention was needed in order to avoid catastrophe. Between 1914 and 1950, Western publics adjusted themselves to radically new attitudes toward life and death, health and illness, pain and suffering.

One of the most popular innovations predated the war. Eugenics, a field whose name was coined by Francis Galton (1822–1911), held that various physical and mental attributes were inherited and that it was incumbent upon society to regulate reproduction toward the goal of a healthier population. Eugenics grew to enjoy broad public support across the political spectrum, and in the years 1910–1940, the movement inspired legislation restricting marriage and compelling the sterilization of those deemed mentally ill or disabled.

It was the Great War, however, that provided the impetus for more comprehensive change. The conflict proved to be an economic, political, demographic, and public health disaster for most every country involved. Around 9 million men were killed in action, twice that number were wounded, and perhaps another 9–10 million civilians died of famine or disease brought on by the war. Military hospitals were flooded by soldiers with brain injuries and neurotic symptoms. Back home, public health officials reported a rise in nervous complaints among women and children. With scarce resources being directed primarily at the war effort, asylum patients proved especially vulnerable. In Germany, around 140,000 of them died between 1914 and 1918, most from hunger and malnutrition.

There is compelling evidence to indicate that the wartime emphasis on triage—giving treatment priority to those patients most likely to survive—moved physicians and policymakers in central Europe after the war to entertain more radical ideas about handling mental disorders and disabilities. In 1920, jurist Karl Binding and psychiatrist Alfred Hoche published *Permission for the Destruction of Life Unworthy of Life*, a tract justifying the killing of what Hoche referred to as "the mentally dead." To be sure, this was an extreme and mostly unpopular position, but it reflected how far some mainstream experts were willing to go in combating mental disorders.

Many more psychiatrists and neurologists pinned their hopes for successful cures on biomedical research. One of the great success stories took place during the first decade of the twentieth century, when scientists discovered that general paresis—an illness marked by progressive dementia and paralysis and constituting perhaps 15 percent of the cases in psychiatric hospitals at the time—was, in fact, the result of syphilis infection earlier in life. The successful treatment of syphilis with the chemical compound arsphenamine (developed in 1910) seemed to offer the promise of a bold new future for psychiatric research.

In general, between 1920 and 1950, psychiatry showed steady interest in finding bodily cures for ostensibly mental disorders. In addition to refinements of earlier regimens, such as sedatives, hydrotherapy, and electrotherapy, there were new, involved treatments designed to provoke fevers, seizures, or coma in patients: malaria fever therapy, insulin therapy, and metrazol therapy. And, of course, there was the lobotomy, a surgical procedure first developed in 1935 in which brain tissue was deliberately destroyed in order to effect personality changes. In time, many physicians and the public came to view these treatments as reckless and unethical. But it needs to be remembered that they were all the products of mainstream scientific and medical research. After all, the developers of malaria fever therapy and the lobotomy both received Nobel Prizes for their work.

That said, the two world wars were bookends for a period of heroic and, at times, risky medicine. The same was true of public policy. Mass death, radical political movements, civil wars, inflation, unemployment, and austerity led voters and states to entertain more drastic solutions. Unsurprisingly, perhaps, the 1930s and 1940s were the heyday for eugenic legislation. In Germany, where Adolf Hitler (1889–1945) and the Nazi Party assumed power in 1933, the government instituted a set of lethal "racial hygiene" policies. By the end of World War II, the country had sterilized some three hundred thousand "morally feeble-minded" individuals and killed around two hundred thousand "incurable" psychiatric patients, all for the espoused benefit of the "Aryan race."

One might term the Nazi episode a politicization of madness and psychiatry, but this would ignore the fact that insanity and its treatment have always had political dimensions. Perhaps, instead, it makes more sense to consider how, in the twentieth century, policymakers, clinicians, and the lay public became more self-reflexive, more deliberate in their use of psychiatry and psychotherapy as political tools. This was certainly true in the Soviet Union, where, beginning in the 1960s, the regime began diagnosing political dissidents with mental disorders and committing them to psychiatric facilities. The international public outcry prompted clinicians to formulate a universal ethical code of professional conduct.

Western Europe and the United States also faced criticism after World War II. The rise of human rights, consumer rights, disability rights, feminist, and anticolonialism movements sparked often acerbic debates about psychiatry's past, present, and future. This crystallized in the form of the antipsychiatry movement, an international array of professionals and patients who questioned medicine's and the state's authority to manage those deemed mentally ill. While some categorically rejected psychiatry's prerogatives, others sought to reform mental health care by orienting it around social reintegration. Both "social psychiatry" and "community mental health care" grew out of this latter impulse. Their goals and methods, reinforced by the development of effective new drugs in the 1950s and fiscal concerns in the 1970s, helped bring about the large-scale emptying of asylums known as deinstitutionalization.

War and Neurosis

Fritz Kaufmann
(1875–1941)

"The Systematic Cure of Complicated Psychogenic Motor Disorders among Soldiers in One Session"
(1916)

Although hysteria was long associated with girls and young women, French and German clinicians during the last third of the nineteenth century began recognizing the increasing prevalence of the illness in men. In particular, industrial workers of all kinds complained of a variety of nervous ailments for which there was no apparent organic lesion. In Germany, these functional illnesses earned the name "traumatic neuroses" and were generally believed to be caused by jarring shocks to the nervous system. The fact that large numbers of workmen used this diagnosis to claim social insurance benefits, however, made many policymakers, companies, and physicians wonder whether these men were simply malingering. By the early twentieth century, a very lively debate raged not only about whether the traumatic neuroses were somatic or psychological in origin, but also about whether they were the manifestation of genuine disease or of simply a weak character.

The issue of male hysteria came to a head during World War I. In Germany, more than six hundred thousand servicemen were treated in military hospitals for nervous diseases in the years 1914–1918. By the last year of the war, 5 percent of all hospital beds in the country were reserved for hysteria cases. The need to get men treated and returned to service as quickly as possible led clinicians to tinker with traditional treatments. One such treatment was developed by Fritz Kaufmann, staff physician at the Nervous Illness Station of the Reserve Infirmary at Ludwigshafen. Before the war, Kaufmann had experimented on a twenty-year-old hysterical girl, applying strong electric currents for as long as ten minutes, combined with verbal suggestion. Her rapid recovery, he claimed, inspired him to conceive a wartime version he called "the surprise attack."

The psychogenic disorders that are coming to our attention among combat soldiers differ in no significant way from the clinical picture that peacetime practice offers. One particular type has struck me in the evidence I have encountered, namely, the large number of patients presenting manifestations of complicated motor hyperstimulation and breakdown. The strong tremor is the symptom that virtually all patients with hyperstimulation have in common. One encounters the symptoms isolated in extremities and linked to contractions on the ends of extremities or throughout the entire extremity, soon thereafter becoming a general tremor, complicated by ticklike twitches, stutters, pseudospastic paresis, saltatory reflex spasms, etc.

With my patients, it has appeared irrelevant to the particulars of the individual case whether it develops acutely after a grenade explosion, or whether the psyche flees into neurosis after chronic, severe attacks, or under certain circumstances, following an intermediary influenza or intestinal catarrh, or, finally, whether the psychogenic disorder grafts on to an organic disorder as an hysterical component and then develops further.

In contrast to many, I consider it necessary to conduct a symptomatic treatment of the patient with psychogenic stimulations and stoppages as promptly as possible, as soon as the acute fatigue symptoms—which are almost never absent among patients in the field—remit. For if it is true that hysteria is not "cured" as soon as the discrete symptoms disappear, it is also true that there are many patients for whom motor symptoms constitute the only verifiable pathological disturbance, even while there is no sign of hysterical character or other hysterical stigmata. In such monosymptomatic cases, one heals the illness by removing the symptoms, even if a certain "illness inclination" remains. . . .

As far as my own overview of the situation, once they become ill, psychogenic patients, especially those afflicted with the above-cited complicated disorder, are most often sent to standard way stations in a reserve infirmary on the home front. Depending on the individual treating physician, they are treated more or less with suggestion. There can be no doubt that any path to treatment can reach its goal if only it is paved with correct suggestion. Individuals such as [Max] Nonne in Hamburg achieve noteworthy success with hypnosis: for the most part, however, their slogan is "convalescence" and "exercise." I do not fear encountering any resistance when I contend that a large portion of those patients treated with convalescence and exercise are eventually released as unfit for service, many with high pensions, some who still "require outside attention and care."

This leads to unhappy consequences for the families; it also leads to the loss of human labor power for the state; another, not insignificant, consequence is the considerable burden on the military budget. . . .

Since I was unsatisfied with the success of the standard form of suggestive therapy in older cases—and almost all the cases in my unit were of this kind—I went back to a kind of treatment that I first used in 1903 as an assistant at the Erbs Clinic. It was common practice in the Erbs Clinic, as was the case elsewhere, to treat hysterical paralyses with energetic faradic brushing, often with good success.

On the basis of my successful experience with the *surprise attack*—based on and reinforced by Nonne's announcement that various forms of psychogenic motor disorders were cured through one hypnotic session—from the end of 1915, I turned to the surprise attack method that I will describe in the following.

From everyday experience, we know that innervation that has derailed because of a mental shock quite frequently is put back on the right track by a new mental shock. We are now in the position to artificially give patients, similar to the case I described earlier, just such a shock by using a strong electric current and accompanying this with appropriate verbal suggestion in the form of orders, all in an effort to cure them.

Our method brings together four components:

1. suggestive preparation
2. application of strong alternating currents with the aid of ample word suggestion
3. strict conformity to military forms of subordination and the giving of word suggestions in the form of orders
4. insistent demand for a cure in one session

Re: 1. Suggestive preparation, as I was able to convince myself repeatedly (in the case of the psychogenic deaf and dumb), is not essential, but very desirable. . . . One must emphasize to the patient already during the days in preparation that the treatment is painful, that, however, he will be safe and cured by the current in one session.

Re: 2. A mental shock can only be achieved only if severe pain is triggered by the current. At times, especially with those patients who have never been electrified, one gets by with moderately strong currents, since, in these cases, the novelty of the sensation is uncommonly suggestive enough to have its effect. Frequently, however, especially with older cases, it is necessary to apply strong currents. I mostly use the sinusoidal current of the Erlanger Pantostat, which was less uncomfortable than the faradic current, and I eventually combine this with galvanic current, especially in cases where simultaneous hysterical anasthesia needed to be removed.* Naturally, one may indiscriminately choose body parts for application. If these body parts (not to be injured by the current) are the site of the primary symptom—for instance, the legs in the case of pseudospastic walking disorders with tremors—these are, of course, electrified. By contrast, for example, in cases of treating hysterical aphonia, I place the large electrode plate on the lower spinal column, while the arm is worked on with the Erbs normal electrode or perhaps the electric brushes, but the larynx is left untouched. Everything else is left to word suggestion and other suggestive methods. I let the electric current work for about 2–5 minutes, then exercises are done, followed by more electrification, etc.

---

*Editor's note: The Erlanger Pantostat was a portable electrical device commonly used at the time for this purpose. By 1926, around fifteen thousand had been sold worldwide.

Re: 3. An extraordinarily important aid in this kind of suggestive treatment are the disciplinary qualities of the treating officer: military discipline demands the most absolute, blind subordination to the orders of the superior, and this successfully creates the fertile ground for a suggestive procedure. *With patients who have psychogenic disorders from intake on, it is necessary to conform strictly to military protocol,* as far that is possible; and then, during the surprise attack treatment, harshly grab people without appearing brutal, giving *instructions in the form of short orders* using military commands. After an electrification, I let those with shakes in the legs or with pseudocerebral ataxia do marching exercises under tough military orders (exactly like the barrack yard). Those with head tremors have to practice "eyes right" and "eyes left" orders, etc.

Re: 4. *Success can only be achieved with unrelenting persistence in carrying out the treatment.* One cannot let up, even if the cure does not happen after the first few minutes; one cannot tire of constantly emphasizing that this goal will be reached; one must seek to convince the patient in every way possible that you are in the position to force your own strong will upon him. One cannot be afraid of exercising at a slow pace with spastics, those with tremors, and ataxics. One cannot stop constantly ordering the aphonic patient after strong electrification to pronounce "A," using the aid of energetic gestures (like an orchestra conductor prompting the fortissimi). In short, you must participate in the treatment with your entire personality. Success is not inevitable, however, *even if on many occasions it emerges after a half hour, an hour, or several hours of constant effort. . . .*

It has proved to be expedient with hard-to-influence patients to take occasional breaks of a few minutes during the session and to leave the patients alone for awhile. It is essential to avoid letting those present talk during the break about things that could distract the patient; rather, it is advised that you use the break to make comments directed at colleagues and assistants who are present in order to suggestively influence the patient. Everything must be employed to have a suggestive impact. Very often I have encountered the first signs of the return of normal function right after the breaks. It is well worth emphasizing that, during the treatment, the contact between doctor and patient may not be disturbed by attempts on the part of those present to rush to the aid of the physician by word or deed. . . .

An additional word about the continued treatment of such patients is necessary. It appears advisable not to release them immediately during the first days after the cure, but rather to keep them on hand for several weeks, in order to be able to offer every possibility of counteracting a potential relapse. Since the paths for pathological innervation in our patients have already become established, a relapse is a particular concern when mala voluntas plays a role. Thankfully, this is seldom the case. But even patients with the best intent to be healthy easily relapse, if one does not allow sufficient time for the normal innervation to again generally solidify itself. This can best take place under the watchful eyes of the physician who achieved the symptomatic cure. It is likely not necessary to mention that convalescence in the infirmary must be undertaken in the proper manner.

These people are no longer suited for combat. After several weeks of convalescence, for the most part, we have released the patients as fit for nonactive duty or as infirmary assistants. Unfortunately, we are not yet mandating catamneses. On the basis of numerous experiences that have been reported to us by authorities, I have doubts about whether releasing [these men] as fit for nonactive duty was appropriate; nonactive duty offers numerous possibilities that can have an adverse effect on the delicate balance of nerves and cause a relapse. Perhaps it is best to release these people as fit for work at their former trade.

From Fritz Kaufmann, "Die planmäßige Heilung komplizierter psychogener Bewegungsstörungen bei Soldaten in einer Sitzung," *Münchener medizinische Wochenschrift, Feldärztliche Beilage* 63 (1916): 802–804. Translated by Greg Eghigian.

W.H.R. Rivers
(1864–1922)
"War Neurosis and Military Training"
(1918)

Like Germany, Great Britain was surprised by the number of men developing war neurosis or "shell shock," as it came to be known in the English-speaking world. During the war, eighty thousand British cases of war neurosis were diagnosed, while after the war, some two hundred thousand veterans were awarded pensions for war-related nervous diseases. The physician and anthropologist William Rivers was among those called on to treat these men during the war. Influenced by evolutionary biology, Rivers had become interested in nervous illnesses before the war. After the war started, he was introduced to Freud's ideas and soon after began applying psychoanalytic concepts and methods at Craiglockhart War Hospital, near Edinburgh. There, Rivers treated shell-shocked officers, the most famous being the war poets Siegfried Sassoon and Wilfred Owen, by encouraging them to talk about their traumatic memories.

Excluding from the category of neurosis cases of simple exhaustion or concussion and disorders of circulation or digestion due to infection, and excluding also definite psychoses, cases of war neurosis fall into three main groups, though intermediate and mixed examples are of frequent occurrence.

The first group comprises cases in which the disorder finds expression in some definite physical form, such as paralysis, mutism, contracture, blindness, deafness, or other anaesthesia, or in some convulsive seizure. The characteristic common to all these symptoms is that they are such as can be readily produced in hypnotism or other state in which suggestion is especially potent. . . . In the meantime I shall be content to speak of this group as hysteria, the term by which it was generally known before the war and one which, in spite of its unsatisfactory character, is still widely used.

The second group consists of cases in which the disorder shows itself especially in the lack of physical and mental energy, in disorders of sleep and of the circulatory, digestive, and urogenital systems. On the mental side there is usually depression, restlessness, irritability and enfeeblement of memory, and on the physical side tremors, tics, or disorders of speech. This group is usually know as neurasthenia in this country, but in this case I shall anticipate the results of my later discussion and speak of it by the term anxiety neurosis.

The third group, with which I shall have little to do in this report, is characterized by the definitely psychical form of its manifestations. This groups comprises a number of different varieties. In some case the most obvious symptom is mental instability and restlessness with alternations of depression and excitement or exaltation, similar to those of manic-depressive insanity. In other cases there are morbid impulses of various kinds, including those towards suicide or homicide. In others the chief symptoms are obsessions or phobias, while others suffer from hallucinations or delusions. The special feature of all these cases is that the symptoms resemble in kind those of the definite psychoses, but have neither the severity nor the fixity which makes the seclusion of the patient or any legal restriction in the management of his affairs necessary. . . .

[A] brief sketch of the aims and methods of military training has led me to distinguish three main processes—suggestion, repression, and sublimation, while others of less importance in relation to neurosis are habituation and sidetracking. I can now consider how these different factors will affect officers and men respectively. The heightening of suggestibility, though probably an inevitable result of any kind of military training, is preeminently one which affects the private soldier. It is the private soldier especially who is submitted to the commands of others, while the officer is not only less fully drilled, but the periods in which he is subject to the commands of others are relieved by other periods in which he is the dispenser of commands and orders.

Sublimation, on the other hand, has more effect on the officer. It is doubtful how far the honor and welfare of the regiment or other unit appeals to the private soldier in general, though it is perhaps almost if not quite as definite among the non-commissioned as among the commissioned officers of the old army. In the new army, it probably means little or nothing to the ordinary soldier, in whose case any sublimation due to military training has its source in comradeship or in his feelings of respect and duty towards his officers, and especially towards either his platoon- or company-commander. It is because the aggregate with which he acts is composed of men with whom he has become comrade and friend, that this aggregate comes to have an influence upon him, while in other cases the relation towards his officer is more important. In each case, however, the result is the production of a state of dependence which works in the same direction as the factor of suggestibility already considered. The point of especial importance in relation to the incidence of neurosis is that the fact of comradeship to some extent, and far more the state of dependence on his officer, diminish the sentiment of responsibility and thus tend to enhance suggestibility or, perhaps more correctly, work in the same direction as suggestibility. In the case of the officer, on the other hand, the relation towards his men brings with it responsibilities which are perhaps more potent than any other element of his experience in determining the form taken by his nervous disorder, if he should break down. It is these responsibilities and other conditions associated with them which lead to his being so especially prone to suffer from the state of anxiety neurosis.

The third main factor, repression, is very important in relation to the incidence of different forms of neurosis in officers and men. The officer is driven by his position to repress the expression of emotion far more persistently than the private soldier. It is the special duty of the junior officer to set an example in this respect to his men, to encourage those who show signs of giving way. In the proper performance of this duty, it is essential that the officer shall appear calm and unconcerned in the midst of danger. The difficulty of keeping up this appearance after long continued strain or after some shock of warfare has lessened the power of control produces a state of persistent anxiety which is the most frequent and potent factor in the production of neurosis, and is especially important in determining the special form it takes. The private soldier has to think only or chiefly of himself; he has not to bear with him continually the thought that the lives of forty or fifty men are immediately, and of many more remotely, dependent on his success in controlling any expression of fear or apprehension.

A factor of minor importance, but one which is nevertheless worth mentioning here, is that the officer is less free to employ the picturesque or sulphurous language which is one of the instruments by which the Tommy finds a safety valve for repressed emotion.

The preceding argument has led us to the conclusions that of the three main agencies upon which the success of military training depends one, suggestion, is especially potent and prominent in the case of the private, while the other two, sublimation and repression, have by far the greatest effect in the case of the officer. One of the chief results of military training is to increase the suggestibility of the private, and this increased tendency in one direction is but little counteracted by sublimation or complicated by the necessity for vigorous repression. The factor of sublimation may even tend to enhance his dependence and suggestibility. In the case of the officer, any increase in suggestibility produced by his training is largely compensated by the necessity for individual and spontaneous action, while the *esprit de corps* and other means of sublimation only tend in many cases to heighten his sense of responsibility and thus add still another cause for his anxieties. There are many officers, both commissioned and non-commissioned, to whom the honor of the regiment or battalion is quite as potent as responsibility for the lives of others in producing the state of anxiety which forms the essential element in the production of their neurosis.

I have now considered how far the different forms of war neurosis can be traced to the influence of military training and the nature of military duties. It is gradually becoming apparent, however, that the conditions of military training and active service are very far from exhausting the factors by which war neurosis is produced. A large part, perhaps even a majority of the prolonged cases of functional nervous disorders which fill our hospitals, can be traced directly to circumstances which have come into being after some shock illness, or perhaps only the ordinary process of leave, has removed the soldier from the actual scene of warfare. I have now to inquire how far the influence of military training and the nature of military duties assist in producing the neurosis of the hospital and the home.

Histories of cases of war neurosis show that officers after some shock or illness suffer for a time from those symptoms which I have ascribed to suggestion, but whether owing to treatment or spontaneous change, these symptoms soon disappear. It may be that the failure to be content with a simple but crude solution of a conflict which satisfies the private soldier is due to superior education, but the nature of his training and duties also contribute to this result. If the disability were the unwitting outcome of a conflict between the instinct of self-preservation and a simple conception of military duty, it might suffice to be paralyzed or mute, but if the morbid state depends primarily upon sentiments of responsibility towards his military unit or his comrades, such a solution is not likely to satisfy his nature long. His conflict differs from that of the private soldier in that it is founded largely upon acquired experience rather than upon instinctive trends. It is more actively conscious than the process which has produced a paralysis or mutism. These disabilities fail altogether to touch the special anxieties which have taken the foremost place in the production of his illness.

In the state of weakened volition produced by shock or exhaustion it seems to the officer that he will never again be able to exert the vigor of control and initiative which alone enabled him to maintain the upper hand in the conflict of the trenches, and with this realization, the former conflict is replaced by one still more painful and enervating, in which sentiments of duty struggle ineffectually against a conviction of unfitness.

In this conflict military training and duty take a most important place. There are many officers whose conflict would be solved or would have never existed, if it were merely a matter of personal safety. It is the knowledge, born of long experience, that the honor of their military unit and the safety of their comrades depend on their efficiency which forms in many cases by far the most potent factor in the production and maintenance of anxiety states. To the private soldier, devoid of such responsibilities, the mere solicitude about his safety forms a less potent motive for conflict, and one which is more easily solved. Once the disability due to suggestion has disappeared spontaneously or by treatment, there may be no obvious conflict left. The instinct of self-preservation, to which his disability has been essentially due, will of course still be there, ready to reassert itself if the occasion arise, but any conscious conflict is so readily solved in accordance with obvious standards of social conduct that there is no opening for the occurrence of any state of anxiety sufficiently profound to act as the basis of neurosis.

The conclusion reached in the preceding pages is that the private soldier is especially apt to succumb to that form of neurosis which closely resembles the effects produced by hypnotism or other form of suggestion, because his military training has been of a kind to enhance his suggestibility. The officer, on the other hand, is less prone to this form of neurosis and falls a victim to it only when there is some organic injury which acts as a continuous source of suggestion. On the other hand the officer is especially liable to anxiety neurosis, because the nature of his duties especially puts him into positions of responsibility which produce or accentuate mental conflicts set up by repression, thus producing states of anxiety, the form taken by his nervous disorder. . . .

Treatment

If the argument of this report is sound, that the cases of functional nervous disorder hitherto labeled hysteria are produced by suggestion and depend on the enhanced suggestibility of the private soldier, it might seem at first sight the obvious course to make use of this heightened suggestibility in the treatment, and to use suggestion, either with or without the production of hypnotic state. If, however, suggestion be used in the ordinary crude way to remove symptoms, this line of treatment will only tend still further to heighten the suggestibility of the patient and to increase the tendency to similar disorders whenever he returns to the field. If at the time that the symptoms are removed suggestions are given against the occurrence of similar disabilities in the future, more could be said for this line of treatment, but this of course would not affect the heightened suggestibility which is the root of the evil.

The argument of this report points rather to a course in which treatment should be directed to lessen the suggestibility by a process of reeducation. This process should be so designed as to make the soldier understand the nature of the disorder which has afflicted him. He should be made to realize the essentially mental basis of his trouble and be thus put into a position in which, even if the disability recurs, he will not long be satisfied with it as a solution of the situation. This line of treatment has the disadvantage that it sometimes succeeds in doing away with the paralysis or other symptoms only to replace the physical disability by a state of anxiety; but a soldier in whom the conflict between the instinct of selfpreservation and duty is so pronounced as to lead to this result is very unlikely to show any more real success if treated by suggestion. Here, however, as in so many other departments of psychotherapy in connection with the war, we are hampered by our almost total ignorance concerning the after-history of soldiers who have been subjected to different modes of treatment. It is possible that there are sufferers from suggestion neurosis who are capable of long and valuable service if the symptoms due to suggestion are treated by means similar to those by which they have been produced.

In cases of anxiety neurosis the lines of causation considered in this report offer less help in treatment than in prevention. The knowledge of the process by which this state has been produced often greatly helps a patient, especially in removing and diminishing depression, or even shame, consequent upon failure. If he can be brought to see that his illness is the outcome of definite agencies over which he has had no control, or has been due to excess rather than defect in certain good qualities, the symptoms may be greatly relieved and the patient set upon a path which, if the exigencies of military service allow, may enable him again to perform his military duties. The knowledge of causation set forth in this report is useful in thus providing a groundwork for the process of reeducation.

From: W.H.R. Rivers, "War Neurosis and Military Training," *Mental Hygiene* 2 (1918): 513–533.

The New Focus
on the Body

Anonymous
"Autopsychology of the
Manic-Depressive"
(1910)

Hydrotherapy—the use of water to treat ailments—dates back to ancient times. By the end of the nineteenth century, it was enjoying something of renaissance and had become a staple in the psychiatric treatment of disorders. Among the most prominent applications of hydrotherapy at the time were two regimens. The first was the continuous bath, by which the patient was fastened in a hammock, placed in a tub, then covered with a canvas sheet that allowed his or her head to remain exposed. The tub was then filled with water of varying temperatures, with the treatment lasting hours or even days. The second regimen—the wet sheet pack—involved firmly wrapping patients in sheets dipped in water of varying temperatures (40–100°F, or 5–38°C). The treatments were often justified on the basis that they relieved cerebral congestion and removed bodily toxins.

The following excerpt is an autobiographical report by a woman who underwent hydrotherapy at the Government Hospital for the Insane in Washington, DC, around the turn of the twentieth century. It is interesting not only because the patient—a trained nurse by profession—discusses her attitude toward the treatment, but also because she provides a firsthand account of the experience of manic depression (now known as bipolar disorder). Her physician Eva Reid published this account, remarking that, at the time of writing this, the woman was in a "state of hypomania." Upon later coming to her senses, she was allowed to reread her statement, and "while she confirmed the truth of all her statements, she affirmed that she had forgotten many of her strange experiences at that time, and the recalling of them to her was painful in the extreme."

Early in January, 1908, I was seized with an unspeakable physical weariness. There was a tired feeling in the muscles unlike anything I had ever experienced. A peculiar sensation appeared to travel up my spine to my brain. I had an indescribable nervous feeling. My nerves seemed like live wires charged with electricity. My nights were sleepless. I lay with dry, staring eyes gazing into space. I had a fear that some terrible calamity was about to happen. I grew afraid to be left alone. The most trivial duty became a formidable task. Finally mental and physical exercise became impossible; the tired muscles refused to respond, my "thinking apparatus" refused to work, ambition was gone. My general feeling might be summed up in the familiar saying "What's the use." I had tried so hard to make something of myself, but the struggle seemed useless. Life seemed utterly futile.

One day it seemed to my disordered mind that one of the vertebrae in the dorsal region was pressed into position. The blood seemed to be carried to my brain in such quantities that the skull was too small to contain the brain enclosed therein. The feeling of emptiness gave way to a sensation of fullness and pressure. It seemed as though the condition of cerebral anemia had given place to one of congestion. By beating my head against the floor and walls I believed that I had loosened up the sutures and gave the brain a chance to expand. It certainly gave me relief. On two occasions a slight epistaxis seemed to relieve the pressure and clear my thinking processes. This confirmed my theory of cerebral congestion. I had a feeling that cranial nerves on the left side were adhering to the skull as ivy clings to a stone wall. Beating my head against the wall appeared to tear them loose from their support and relieve the tension. The muscles which heretofore had refused to respond to stimuli now refused to remain at rest. To keep physically quiet was an utter impossibility. The strain of trying to keep still was fast wearing me out. I would lie in bed and jump up and down on the springs; I would make numerous excuses to go for a drink and to the toilet, simply to be doing something. My thought processes which hitherto had been retarded, and their expression difficult, now began to flow with lightning rapidity. Thoughts crowded into my mind too rapidly for expression. Talking was the greatest relief imaginable. Formerly I was afraid to be left alone, now the one thing for which I longed was solitude. This was denied me. I was at this time a patient in a general hospital, of which I was formerly assistant superintendent of nurses, and it was considered necessary to "special" me night and day. Constant observation was maddening. There was an ever-present fear that in my constant talking, which I was unable to control, I would reveal professional secrets that had been entrusted to my care. In my official capacity as assistant superintendent I had been the receptacle of many confidences by the doctors, superintendent, nurses, and patients. These confidences—many of them too sacred to be bared for common curiosity—weighed on me constantly, and I dreaded lest in my delirium I would reveal them. Over-anxiety to retain mastery of my mind caused an extreme tension of the nerves all over my body. The presence of a nurse, always at my bedside, drove me frantic. Restraint was irritating and almost fatal. The fact that I was being watched and observed rendered sleep impossible. Drugs had no effect. I begged to be sent to the Government Hospital for the Insane. My one desire was to get away from over-anxious and over-curious friends and acquaintances. On March 1, 1909, I was removed at my own request to the Government Hospital, to recover, to go permanently insane, or to die. I confidently expected the last would be my fate.

Words fail to describe the feeling of relief I experienced when I was at last placed in a strong room at my own request. To be alone, to be shut off from the observation of the anxious and the curious, to be free to act and talk in any way my distorted fancy dictated was relief unspeakable. Here I was among strangers who cared nothing for the secrets I disclosed. They did not even stop to listen to them. They did not appear to be surprised or shocked at my wildest words or actions. I was not told a hundred times a day that I *must* keep quiet. I talked, laughed, cried, sang, shouted, and danced to my heart's content. The giving up of all attempt at self-control brought the needed rest and sleep.

The condition of my mind for many months is beyond all description. My thoughts ran with lightning-like rapidity from one subject to another.

I had an exaggerated feeling of self importance. All the problems of the universe came crowding into my mind, demanding instant discussion and solution—mental telepathy, hypnotism, wireless telegraphy, Christian Science, women's rights, and all the problems of medical science, religion, and politics. I even devised means of discovering the weight of the human soul, and had an apparatus constructed in my room for the purpose of weighing my own soul the minute it departed from my body. At one time I was elected to Congress by my own district. I was teacher, preacher, reformer, lawyer, judge, physician, actress, artist, poet, and writer, all within a wonderfully short space of time. Probably my most important delusion was that I was at the Government Hospital for the purpose of thorough investigation, supervision, and reformation. Each article of clothing and bedding given me was tested by pulling on it with all my might. If it tore, I immediately condemned it as being unfit for use, and tore it into shreds. I decided it was manufactured by convict labor, and utterly unfit to be used by an august person like myself. The crockery I tested by throwing it against the walls and ceiling. If it broke it proved to me conclusively that it was unfit for use in a government institution. I felt it my duty to train and instruct the nurses. My efforts in this direction seemed unappreciated. The valuable instruction so freely tendered was set at naught, spurned and trampled underfoot. In fact, I do not think they even stopped to digest it. Although my egotism was unbounded, yet I never for one moment was happy. Always being accustomed to bear responsibility, the exalted role I played served only to increase the burden of care. The propagation of all reforms for the betterment of the human race devolved upon me. I arranged programs and entertainments for Decoration Day, Fourth of July, Labor Day, Thanksgiving, and Christmas. I staged "Tillie the Mennonite Maid," managed a circus, conducted revival meetings for the benefit of the colored men who worked on the lawn. I made countless speeches, watching the facial expression of the other patients to see the effects of my oratory. This was usually far from encouraging. I designed cartoons, composed newspaper articles, diagnosed cases, prescribed treatment, planned kindergarten games. I sang by the hour, with an idea of chest expansion and voice culture. I tried cases in court, weighed the evidence pro and con, and rendered my valuable (?) decisions. I "bossed" the carpenters who repaired the porch where I sat. I gave advice to the painters. I never failed to obey the biblical injunction to "entertain strangers." For the benefit of the visitors who came in the ward, I performed athletic "stunts," improvising apparatus. This often necessitated the removal of the bolts from the beds. The bowls in which the soup was served made excellent missels [sic] with which to practice for a baseball pitcher. The pieces were even more useful. They made more noise, and could be used to make deep indentures in the walls of my room. The doors were of pine, and by scratching them deeply with pieces of broken dishes I could smell the odor of the pine tree, which was very agreeable. My inability to throw straight was all that saved the electric light in my room. The hair from the inside of my pillow and mattress was just what I needed to make a wig in which to impersonate an old lady in my plays. The ticking from the pillow was converted into a sunbonnet to represent the girl whose picture is on the back of the music of "School Days." The blankets torn into strips made excellent bandages, and were just what I needed for teaching purposes. I tore the sheets into strips and arranged designs for kindergarten games on the floor. In all this I had a feeling of resourcefulness, and many times called to mind the saying of the superintendent of our hospital: "If there's one think [sic] I admire it's a woman of resources." Thoughts chased one another through my mind with lightning rapidity. I felt like a person driving a wild horse with a weak rein, who dares not use force, but lets him run his course, following the line of least resistance. Mad impulses would rush through my brain, carrying me first in one direction then in another. To destroy myself or to escape often occurred to me, but my mind could not hold one subject long enough to formulate any definite plan. My reasoning was weak and fallacious, and I knew it.

My sleep was so fraught with dreams that I derived little benefit therefrom—dreams, delusions, and reality were so closely interwoven that even now I cannot tell one person from another. Hallucinations of sight were probably present. From the lower ventilator of my room came many animals nightly. These had been rescued from an untimely death by the antivivisectionists. The most formidable of these was a young alligator which gave me quite a shock when he first appeared. The sparrows and cats seen from my window acted "dopey." I concluded they had been fed arsenic as an experiment. The nurses and physicians were recognized as persons I had known, or of whom I had heard. One nurse was Ida Tarbell, in the hospital for the purpose of investigation; another was Ellen Terry, another Sis Hopkins, another a lion tamer from the circus. One of the patients was

Hetty Green, also investigating.* The nervous mechanism of the eye seemed to be affected. A distinct myopia was present. On only a few occasions did hallucinations of smell appear. Once I smelled burning rubber very distinctly, and on two occasions my room was filled with the perfume of flowers. One patient I imagined had been drinking embalming fluid, and each time she came near me I was nauseated by the odor. My sense of taste was impaired. Food and drink were obnoxious to me. I realized the importance of proper nourishment, however, and forced myself to eat and drink everything that was brought to me. I had fleeting delusions that the food was poisoned, but I still persisted in eating.

The sensation of physical pain which I endured is beyond my powers of description. Every afternoon I was seized by the most violent paroxysm of pain which racked every nerve in my body. The alimentary system throughout felt as though it were one rotten mass. With more or less regularity a convulsion would attack the intestines at about the sigmoid flexure, work its way up the descending colon, across the transverse, down the ascending colon, up through the coils of the small intestines; lessening in force it would attack the stomach, wriggle through the esophagus and disappear. My head would be drawn back and I would rest on my head and heels. By carefully massaging up and down on either side of the spinous process of the vertebrae the tension would gradually be relieved. One night the circulation in my lower extremities seemed to stop. My limbs were paralyzed. This was accompanied by an indescribable feeling at the base of the spine, and a tingling of the nerve trunks. After much pinching, massaging, and manipulation the circulation was again restored. From two until four in the afternoon during the hottest months, it seemed impossible to derive any oxygen from the air. Respiration was labored and painful. From time to time I suffered all the symptoms and complications of every disease known to medical science from exophthalmic goiter to scarlet fever. Carcinoma of the lungs was my favorite malady.

Hydrotherapy worked wonders. What I enjoyed most was the shower and spray. It was invigorating and refreshing, and seemed to give me a new

---

*Editor's note: Ida Tarbell (1857–1944) was a writer famous for her exposé of John D. Rockefeller and the Standard Oil Company. Ellen Terry (1847–1928) was an acclaimed stage actress. *Sis Hopkins* was a beloved stage play that chronicled the exploits of an awkward, rural girl. Hetty Green (1834–1916) was an eccentric heiress, famous for her stinginess.

lease of life. The packs I disliked at first. The restraint of the blankets around me was maddening, it seemed like a dare, and on several occasions I wriggled myself loose and escaped. However, after I became accustomed to them they were soothing and I frequently slept while being treated in this manner. The continuous bath was restful and quieting. My circulation was poor, and I suffered from cold even in the warmest weather. The continuous bath appeared to restore the circulation, and the warmth in the tub was grateful and soothing. The sheet thrown over me in the tub was irritating and worried me constantly. I wanted to be free to splash around as I pleased.

The two things I could not endure were restraint and observation. Had my lot fallen in a hospital where restraint was used I tremble to think what the outcome would have been. Sitting on the porch under the eye of a nurse seemed an unnecessary curtailment of my liberties. Several times I escaped, but was always followed and returned. To have someone watching me was unendurable, inasmuch as I realized in a way how foolish my words and actions were. One night one of the supervisors came in my room and stood for a minute watching me eat my supper. This maddened me so that I threw the tray and all its contents at her head.

The first symptom of recovery was a gradually increasing power to direct my thoughts into desired channels. I discovered that what seemed to be fact were in many cases delusions. Suddenly one day a feeling of self-control returned. The rapidity of thought seemed greatly lessened, and I was once more able to concentrate my mind on one subject for more than a few minutes at a time. Then came the feeling that I was well and must go home. Previous to this I realized my abnormal mental condition, and had no desire to see or be seen by my friends. Now I was seized with an eager longing to see my relatives and friends. It was like coming back from the dead. I overcame my restlessness by cleaning, scrubbing, mending, and writing. My brain seemed unusually active and clear. I wrote for hours at a time; essays, poems, aphorisms, etc., flowed from my pen with great rapidity. I again began to take an interest in my personal appearance, and gradually returned to my normal mental state.

From Eva Charlotte Reid, "Autopsychology of the Manic-Depressive," *Journal of Nervous and Mental Diseases* 37 (1910): 606–620.

Herman Lundborg
(1868–1943)
"The Danger of Degeneracy"
(1922)

In the wake of the popularity of Charles Darwin's (1809–1882) theory of the evolution of species by natural selection, a number of writers, policymakers, and researchers during the last third of the nineteenth century became concerned that Western civilization, instead of progressively evolving, was devolving or degenerating. Among the signs they believed that pointed to this degeneration were increasing crime rates and the growing number of those institutionalized as mentally ill and "feeble-minded." Over the course of the first decades of the twentieth century, local, national, and international organizations formed to press governments and individuals to more aggressively combat degeneracy. These impulses crystallized in the form of eugenics—a scientific and social movement demanding that society could and should be deliberately improved by encouraging those with the most desirable physical and mental attributes to reproduce and discouraging all others.

One of the regions where eugenics enjoyed strong support was Scandinavia. There, beginning in the 1930s and continuing after World War II, states passed a series of laws instituting the sometimes voluntary, sometimes mandatory, sterilization of the mentally ill and mentally disabled. Hundreds of thousands were sterilized under these laws: eleven thousand in Denmark between 1929 and 1960, fifty-eight thousand in Finland between 1935 and 1970, and forty thousand in Norway between 1934 and 1977. In Sweden, where sixty-three thousand were sterilized in the years 1934–1975, 90 percent were women. The following outline of eugenic principles and policies is the work of Swedish psychiatrist and neurologist Herman Lundborg. Lundborg was the head of the Institute for Race Biology (founded in 1922) in Uppsala, Sweden, and an advocate for strong eugenic legislation to protect what he termed a "Western world in danger."

Eugenic Theses and Guide-Lines

A.

1. A good *national-material* is the greatest riches a country can possess. The material of the people depends in the highest degree upon the quality of the hereditary mass. This is different in different nations.

2. *Heredity and selection* are the chief influences which govern life in this world. *Environment* is certainly also of significance, although it cannot develop new qualities but can only modify those already present, in the one or the other direction.

3. *Families and nations are governed by strict laws* in the same way as the private individual. One of the first tasks laid upon every civilized nation is the careful investigation of these biological laws of nature, and afterwards the regulation and arrangement of the conditions of society to suit these laws. If we break them we must ourselves bear the consequences: we degenerate and go under. These laws, however, are not altogether and only stern avengers. Rightly understood and obeyed they form a richly yielding source of improvement and progress.

4. *A glaring waste of the national-material* is to be found at present among many of the civilized nations and even with us. Material of great, and to a large extent irreplaceable, value is being lost with alarming rapidity. And it cannot be recovered in the same hasty manner as it is being thrown away.

5. *Many reasons co-operate* in bringing this about. The principal seem to be: (a) the sinking birthrate among the middle classes (among the peasant population) who possess stronger race energy than the other strata of society; (b) great industrial activity; (c) hasty race-mixture between nations, who from a race-biological point of view, stand too far apart; (e) [*sic*] luxury and the worship of mammon with the destruction of moral worth, which accompanies it, etc.

6. *The system of having none, one or two children* practiced by the more valuable strata of the people, while at the same time the lower and inferior strata increase relatively quickly, must lead to the deterioration of the race and the degeneration of the nation. The better off classes, especially the women of these classes, without any valid reason, show an increasing disposition to withdraw from parenthood. By so doing they shirk their duty and betray their own people. The decided individualism of our time, the

great claims made on life, together with the decided over-estimation of the power of environment and education, are important reasons leading in this direction. The public opinion in a country and the authorities of the State have also a heavy burden of guilt to bear in this respect.

7. *Industrial and agricultural occupations* demand, at least at times, increased and new energy. Partly for this reason and partly to defend the country from outward foes, owing to a low birth-rate in a country, foreigners belonging to an inferior race must be called in. In ancient Rome during its decline and fall the circumstances were exactly the same. Race-mixtures arise in such cases causing a mixed nation of inferior quality. This must sooner or later overthrow the ancient civilisation of the country. Chaos and anarchy become the ruling powers. Other nations force their way in and gradually the older civilisation is obliterated.

8. *It certainly lies within the boundaries of possibility to take up seriously the struggle against these threatening and destructive factors.* Such a course implies, however, that all good citizens within a country, irrespective of their social, political, and religious views, should unite their forces and work together for a common goal, rich in promise, the defence of their own national against internal revolutionary and race-degenerative tendencies.

For this is demanded: *good will and combination, financial self-sacrifice, greater morality and real love of humanity.*

3.

1. An energetic *work of enlightenment* on the subject ought to be carried on. Beginning with Universities, High Schools and Training Colleges as the starting point, public opinion ought to be worked upon by means of both lectures and writing. Medical men and teachers out to be specifically educated in the science of heredity and race-culture. The feeling of responsibility towards the coming generations must be aroused. No full-grown person ought to be ignorant concerning the great significance of parenthood, and all must learn to understand the meaning of *well-born from a biological point of view.*

2. *Race-biological institutes for investigation* with the object of studying hereditary questions and eugenic problems on all sides ought to be established in every civilized country as soon as possible. This had already been done in Sweden. The institute ought to be guided by genealogical, medical-biological, and social-economical principles. The instinct of self-preservation

ought now, after the world war, to drive the civilized nations towards starting this work without delay.

3. *Severe diseases among the people* such as alcoholism, sex diseases and
tuberculosis must be fought against strenuously.

4. *A simple and industrious manner of life* must be inculcated among all
classes of the population, at the same time that due exercise of the body and
sound sport are striven after. Luxury and an unchecked desire for pleasure
do not bring honour to any nation; they counteract the development of race
in a favourable direction.

5. *Social "swamps"* ought to be drained by means of wise reforms and
far-sighted law-making. The necessary supervision and care is not yet
given to individuals who are really degenerate—and such are to be found
in large numbers, both in our own land and in other civilized countries—
but they are allowed to influence the race in an obstructive and dangerous
manner. We ought to pay the greatest attention to political questions
regarding the population and allow the eugenic point of view always to
have full consideration.

6. The State and private persons ought to unite in building pattern
homes out in the country as a counter-balance to the *industrialism* which so
often proves an enemy to the race and to the health of the people. A sound
agricultural population with a high birth-rate is a necessary condition of life
for a nation that does not wish to degenerate. An independent peasant class
makes the groundwork, "backbone" of a nation. This class ought therefore
to be helped and cherished as much as possible. The de-population of the
countryside must be sternly opposed, but not by the introduction of industrialism there also. Home colonization ought to be encouraged.

7. *Emigration*, which has caused considerable drain on the life-blood of
the nation, ought, if possible, to be regulated and kept within proper
bounds.

8. We must also pay attention to *immigration* so that inferior individuals belonging to foreign races cannot enter the country and settle without
any hindrance. A mixture between nations who, from a race-biological
point of view, stand high and others containing lower race-elements, such
as gipsies [sic], Galicians, certain Russian tribes, etc., is certainly to be condemned.

9. The science of eugenics, which is a real *patriotic movement* according
to the true meaning of the words, has for its object the strengthening and

improvement of our people both bodily and mentally, and ought therefore to be able to reckon on having the support of all classes of society.

10. Widely spread *national societies* ought to be formed in all the civilized countries with the object of working for *race-culture, the health of the people and the improvement of morality.*

Rich citizens within the country could hasten the spread of eugenic ideas in a high degree by means of financial and moral support. These ideas ought not to remain in the long run only futile desires.

From Herman Lundborg, "The Danger of Degeneracy," *Eugenics Review* 14 (1922): 41–43.

The Decision in *Buck v. Bell*
(1927)

In the United States, Indiana passed the first eugenic sterilization law in 1907. Other states soon followed suit, including Virginia in 1924 (The Racial Integrity Act). Carrie Buck (1906–1983) and her mother, Emma, were both committed involuntarily to the Virginia Colony for Epileptics and Feeble Minded in Lynchburg, Virginia. The superintendent of the facility, Albert Priddy, judged both women, as well as Carrie's seven-month-old daughter, Vivian, to be feeble-minded, later testifying in court that the women "belong to the shiftless, ignorant, and worthless class of anti-social whites of the South." Priddy chose Carrie Buck to be the first person to be sterilized under the new law.

The case went to court, where expert testimony was solicited from a teacher, a field worker, and the eugenicist Harry Laughlin. Their testimony painted a picture of Emma and Carrie Buck as sexually promiscuous and morally degenerate. The case was eventually appealed to the U.S. Supreme Court—in the meantime, Priddy had died and his position was taken by J. H. Bell—which upheld the law with only one dissenting vote. Carrie Buck was sterilized on 19

October 1927. Virginia's sterilization law was repealed in 1974. In 2001 the Virginia State Assembly expressed its "profound regrets" for the state's involvement in eugenics, and in May 2002, Governor Mark Warner formally apologized on behalf of Virginia, calling the eugenics movement "a shameful effort in which state government never should have been involved." All told, some thirty U.S. states had similar laws, under which around sixty-five thousand individuals were sterilized.

U.S. Supreme Court
Buck v. Bell,
Superintendent of State Colony for Epileptics and Feeble Minded
Argued April 22, 1927. Decided May 2, 1927.
Mr. Justice Holmes delivered the opinion of the Court.

This is a writ of error to review a judgment of the Supreme Court of Appeals of the State of Virginia, affirming a judgment of the Circuit Court of Amherst County, by which the defendant in error, the superintendent of the State Colony for Epileptics and Feeble Minded, was ordered to perform the operation of salpingectomy upon Carrie Buck, the plaintiff in error, for the purpose of making her sterile. 143 Va. 310, 130 S. E. 516. The case comes here upon the contention that the statute authorizing the judgment is void under the Fourteenth Amendment as denying to the plaintiff in error due process of law and the equal protection of the laws.

Carrie Buck is a feeble-minded white woman who was committed to the State Colony above mentioned in due form. She is the daughter of a feeble-minded mother in the same institution, and the mother of an illegitimate feeble-minded child. She was eighteen years old at the time of the trial of her case in the Circuit Court in the latter part of 1924. An Act of Virginia approved March 20, 1924 (Laws 1924, c. 394) recites that the health of the patient and the welfare of society may be promoted in certain cases by the sterilization of mental defectives, under careful safeguard, etc.; that the sterilization may be effected in males by vasectomy and in females by salpingectomy, without serious pain or substantial danger to life; that the Commonwealth is supporting in various institutions many defective persons who if now discharged would become [274 U.S. 200, 206] a menace, but if incapable of procreating might be discharged with safety and become self-supporting with benefit to themselves and to society; and that experience has shown that heredity plays an important part in the transmission of insanity, imbecility, etc. The statute then enacts that whenever the superintendent of certain institutions including the abovenamed State Colony shall be of opinion that it is for the best interest of the patients and of society that an inmate under his care should be sexually sterilized, he may have the operation performed upon any patient afflicted with hereditary forms of insanity, imbecility, etc., on complying with the very careful provisions by which the act protects the patients from possible abuse.

The superintendent first presents a petition to the special board of directors of his hospital or colony, stating the facts and the grounds for his opinion, verified by affidavit. Notice of the petition and of the time and place of the hearing in the institution is to be served upon the inmate, and also upon his guardian, and if there is no guardian the superintendent is to apply to the Circuit Court of the County to appoint one. If the inmate is a minor notice also is to be given to his parents, if any, with a copy of the petition. The board is to see to it that the inmate may attend the hearings if desired by him or his guardian. The evidence is all to be reduced to writing, and after the board has made its order for or against the operation, the superintendent, or the inmate, or his guardian, may appeal to the Circuit Court of the County. The Circuit Court may consider the record of the board and the evidence before it and such other admissible evidence as may be offered, and may affirm, revise, or reverse the order of the board and enter such order as it deems just. Finally any party may apply to the Supreme Court of Appeals, which, if it grants the appeal, is to hear the case upon the record of the trial [274 U.S. 200, 207] in the Circuit Court and may enter such order as it thinks the Circuit Court should have entered. There can be no doubt that so far as procedure is concerned the rights of the patient are most carefully considered, and as every step in this case was taken in scrupulous compliance with the statute and after months of observation, there is no doubt that in that respect the plaintiff in error has had due process at law.

The attack is not upon the procedure but upon the substantive law. It seems to be contended that in no circumstances could such an order be justified. It certainly is contended that the order cannot be justified upon the existing grounds. The judgment finds the facts that have been recited and that Carrie Buck "is the probable potential parent of socially inadequate offspring, likewise afflicted, that she may be sexually sterilized without detriment to her general health and that her welfare and that of society will be promoted by her sterilization," and thereupon makes the order. In view of the general declarations of the Legislature and the specific findings of the Court obviously we cannot say as matter of law that the grounds do not exist, and if they exist they justify the result. We have seen more than once that the public welfare may call upon the best citizens for their lives. It would be strange if it could not call upon those who already sap the strength of the State for these lesser sacrifices, often not felt to be such by those concerned, in order to prevent our being swamped with incompetence. It is better for all the world, if instead of waiting to execute degenerate offspring for crime, or to let them starve for their imbecility, society can prevent those who are manifestly unfit from continuing their kind. The principle that sustains compulsory vaccination is broad enough to cover cutting the Fallopian tubes. Jacobson v. Massachusetts, 197 U.S. 11 , 25 S. Ct. 358, 3 Ann. Cas. 765. Three generations of imbeciles are enough. [274 U.S. 200, 208] But, it is said, however it might be if this reasoning were applied generally, it fails when it is confined to the small number who are in the institutions named and is not applied to the multitudes outside. It is the usual last resort of constitutional arguments to point out shortcomings of this sort. But the answer is that the law does all that is needed when it does all that it can, indicates a policy, applies it to all within the lines, and seeks to bring within the lines all similarly situated so far and so fast as its means allow. Of course so far as the operations enable those who otherwise must be kept confined to be returned to the world, and thus open the asylum to others, the equality aimed at will be more nearly reached.

Judgment affirmed.

Mr. Justice Butler dissents.

From U.S. Supreme Court, Buck v. Bell, 274 U.S. 200 (1927), FindLaw, http://laws.findlaw.com/us/274/200.html.

Julius Wagner-Jauregg
(1857–1940)
"The Treatment of Dementia Paralytica by Malaria Inoculation"
(1927)

The Viennese psychiatrist Julius Wagner-Jauregg did his studies at an experimental pathology institute, where he first became acquainted with using laboratory animals in experiments. He then became a professional psychiatrist, in 1883, with virtually no experience in treating patients. His interests soon led him to investigate the possible therapeutic benefits of induced fevers for psychiatric disorders, and in 1917, Wagner-Jauregg began inoculating patients with malaria-infected blood in order to produce these fevers.

Malaria inoculation grew to be a widely accepted treatment, particularly for general paresis (progressive paralysis), during the years 1920–1950. Physicians generally infected patients by injection or mosquito bites or by rubbing infected blood on open cuts. After about a week, the patient experienced chills and nausea, followed by a series of alternating spells of fever and chills. Fevers reached as high as 106°F (41°C). Quinine sulfate was then administered to treat the malaria. In 1927, Wagner-Jauregg was awarded the Nobel Prize for Physiology or Medicine. The following excerpt comes from the lecture he gave that year.

Nobel Lecture, December 13, 1927

Two paths could lead to a cure for progressive paralysis: the rational and the empirical. The rational path appeared to be practical, as since Esmarch and Jessen, in 1858, attention had been drawn to a connection between progressive paralysis and syphilis. If incontestable proof that progressive paralysis was a syphilitic brain disease was first given much later (I mention in this connection the names Wassermann and Noguchi), therapeutic attempts to apply anti-syphilitic treatments were nevertheless instituted much earlier.

Established psychiatry, it is true, soon turned away from the specific therapy. In all the textbooks it was stated that the mercury cure was of no use against paralysis and was usually harmful. . . .

The discovery of arsphenamine (Salvarsan) by Ehrlich brought new hope. The disappointment which soon followed was due to quite insufficient dosages. As one reads the reports of writers who have given arsphenamine in large doses and in rapidly repeated courses of treatment, and when one hears of the remissions obtained, in number and in duration far superior to the number of remissions observable in untreated paralysis, it cannot confidently be maintained that arsphenamine is ineffective against progressive paralysis. Yet it seems indeed, disregarding rare exceptions, that sooner or later a point is reached where arsphenamine treatment is unable to halt the fatal progression. The augmentation of the treatment by the employment of bismuth preparations could not change this.

There are, however, still always writers who expect the cure of paralytics from specific treatment alone.

But the question is not one of prestige between specific and non-specific treatment, but of what is the most far-reaching therapeutic effect on the disease obtainable.

And thus we have arrived at the empirical method.

Progressive paralysis has always been regarded as an incurable disease leading within a few years to insanity and death.

Nevertheless there were records of cured cases of progressive paralysis; cases in which there was such a complete retrogression of all the symptoms of the disease that it was possible for the person concerned to go about his life and business independently for many years. And even though such cases were extraordinarily rare, there were still relatively frequent remissions of a considerable duration in which the symptoms of the disease already developed retrogressed to a greater or less extent. Thus, in principle at least, progressive paralysis was necessarily a curable disease. And Francis Bacon, Lord Verulam, had already pronounced that it must be of the greatest interest for the physician to study healed cases of incurable diseases.

Now, the observation has been made that, in the rare cases of cure and in the frequent remissions of progressive paralysis, a febrile infectious disease or protracted suppuration had often preceded the improvement in the state of the disease. In that lay a pointer. These cures following febrile infectious diseases, of which I had experienced striking instances myself, led me to propose as early as 1887 that this natural experiment should be imitated by a deliberate introduction of infectious diseases, and I suggested at that time malaria and erysipelas as suitable diseases. I singled out as a particular advantage of malaria that there is the possibility of interrupting the disease at will by the use of quinine, but I did not then anticipate to what degree these expectations from induced malaria would be fulfilled.

At that time I did not proceed to the direct application of these proposals, apart from an unfortunate experiment with erysipelas, and I also hardly had the authority then to carry on with them.

On the other hand I attempted to imitate the action of a febrile infectious disease by the use since 1890 of tuberculin which Koch had just introduced. At first this was used not only in progressive paralysis, but also in other mental disturbances, not infrequently with beneficial consequences. (This was to some extent a forerunner of the use of protein therapy, which later attained a great advance.) As there were among these, some cases of progressive paralysis, my interest soon concentrated on this disease because a favourable result cannot be so easily regarded as fortuitous as in other psychoses.

It was ascertained by means of a preliminary experiment of a large number of paralytics that those treated with tuberculin (with a maximum dose at that time of 0.1) showed more and longer-lasting remissions and a longer duration of life than an equal number of untreated paralytics. Afterwards, this treatment was carried out systematically and with an increasing dose of tuberculin (up to 1.0), and simultaneously a vigorous iodine-and-mercury treatment, later accompanied by arsphenamine injections, was also introduced.

In 1909, at the International Medical Congress in Budapest I gave some information on these methods of treatment, which were thus the first combined treatment—i.e. specific and non-specific—of a syphilitic disease.

Qualitatively the remissions which were obtained by means of the mercury- tuberculin treatment did not differ from those to be attained through induced malaria. The complete disappearance of the mental disturbances and the resumption of business activity, even in professions which make greater intellectual demands—such as civil servant, officer, barrister, solicitor, teacher, industrialist, actor, etc.—and the duration of the remissions was in individual cases quite remarkable; amounting to up to fifteen years.

But the number of relapses was great, the lasting remissions were in the minority. I attempted to increase the effectiveness of the non-specific treatment by the utilization of various vaccines—staphylo-streptococcal vaccine, typhus vaccine—without altering the frequency of discouraging relapses in the slightest.

In the course of this experimentation with treatments I was able to observe repeatedly that particularly complete and long-lasting remissions presented themselves precisely in those cases in which an unintentional infectious disease, such as pneumonia or an abscess, appeared during the course of the treatment.

In 1917, therefore, I commenced to put into practice my proposal made in the year 1887, and I injected nine cases of progressive paralysis with tertian malaria. The result was gratifying beyond expectation: six of these nine cases showed an extensive remission, and in three of these cases the remission proved enduring, so that I was able to present these cases of cured patients who have without interruption taken up again their former occupations, to this year's annual meeting of the German Psychiatric Society as having been able to follow them for ten years. After the result of this first experiment was pursued for two years, I went on, in the autumn of 1919, to continue this experimental treatment on a large scale, and I made a report on it in 1920 to the annual meeting of the German Psychiatric Society in Hamburg.

Whereas the earlier non-specific methods of treatment of progressive paralysis had met with little approval, it was otherwise with the malaria treatment. After Weygandt and Nonne, stimulated by Mühlens in Hamburg, had first tested the method of treatment on a large number of patients, it found quick acceptance in many psychiatric clinics and insane asylums, and is currently used, as far as I am informed, in all the countries of Europe, in North and South America, in South Africa, in the Dutch East Indies, and in Japan.

The overwhelming majority of writers agree that with this method remissions can be obtained which are on a scale far exceeding those attained by any other method.

Nevertheless, the malaria treatment should not simply replace specific treatment but should be used in conjunction with it. Some writers believed at first that they could dispense with the specific treatment, in that they obtained brilliant remissions by malaria alone. But the question is how to obtain the maximum therapeutic effect from the treatment. So, I undertook comparative investigations in which paralytics admitted to the clinic were treated alternately, the one with malaria only, the other with malaria followed by neoarsphenamine. The superiority of the combined specific-nonspecific treatment was clearly shown.

The cases which had been subsequently treated with neoarsphenamine had 48.5% full remissions, those with no subsequent treatment only 25%. On the other hand, the number of deaths in the latter group was higher—18.7% against 12%—and likewise the number of rapidly deteriorating cases was 22% against 6.7%.

The malaria treatment is thus to be associated with a specific treatment. Insofar as neoarsphenamine is concerned, the drug should be given first after the fever has subsided, as otherwise the malaria is cut short. In my clinic now 5.00 grams of neoarsphenamine are given over six weeks after each malaria treatment.

Malaria treatment is the more effective the earlier in the course of the paralysis it is carried out. Therefore it is impossible to get a correct picture of its potential effectiveness by simply calculating that out of such and such a number of paralytics treated with malaria so many per cent obtained complete remission. It depends very much on how many among the material in question were in the initial stages of paralysis and how many were in the advanced stages.

We have therefore for some time singled out from the first, those cases of paralysis on their very first arrival at my clinic which from the degree and duration of their illness promised a favourable outcome and followed their progress separately. It was shown, that of these cases 84.8% obtained a full remission and 12.1% a partial remission, and that out of the total number of this series only one in thirty-eight had to be committed to the asylum.

Hence it was shown that progressive paralysis is, in principle, curable and that the practical success of the malaria treatment will be the greater the earlier the diagnosis of the illness is established—the more, that is, that the early stages of paralysis are recognized by physicians. It has become apparent that it is unwise to employ other methods of treatment against paralysis before the malaria treatment, as this means time wasted.

As the malaria treatment is the more effective the earlier it is employed, it would thus be best if it were carried out immediately on those luetics who are threatened with progressive paralysis. Which luetics are these? We know that they are those luetics in whom the cerebrospinal fluid in the advanced period of latency gives a positive reaction.

It is due to the late Kyrle of Vienna that the malaria treatment was extended to these luetics in that in these cases, which are not yet immediately threatened, he prescribed a course of arsphenamine to precede the malaria, and a second course to follow it. The results in respect of the readjustment of the cerebrospinal fluid, which in such cases with other methods of treatment is on the contrary frequently very refractory, were so gratifying that already a large number of syphilologists have become acquainted with these methods. And it is to be hoped that once these methods become public property, psychiatrists will have very much fewer paralytics to treat.

That the malaria treatment attained so great a dissemination is due to some favourable results, only apparent during its application, which could therefore not been expected from the beginning.

It would have been difficult in many places to continue the malaria treatment if it had not been possible to maintain for an unlimited period a malaria strain by continual passage through human beings—that is in the asexual cycle. This was at first doubted, or at least the feat was stated, that such a strain would, in the course of its passage, change its properties, i.e. might become either no longer infectious or too virulent. These fears have proved groundless. In my clinic there is a malaria strain in use that since September 1919 has made about two hundred passages through human beings, without its infectiousness, its virulence, and its therapeutic properties having been altered. Similar experiences have been had in many places.

The uninterrupted breeding of such a strain is, however, only possible where there is access to a sufficiently large number of paralytics needing treatment and possibly also of luetics in the advanced latency.

In places with little patient material, however, such a strain of induced malaria will always die out again, and it would involve great and often insurmountable difficulties to always procure a new case of natural malaria again to start a treatment, for the malaria virus will not breed in cultures.

Fortunately, however, the malaria parasites in human blood remain infectious for some time outside the human body, and this capacity can, by special methods of preservation be maintained for up to three days and in rare exceptions even longer, so that it is possible to send the virus over considerable distances by various means of transport.

It is therefore possible to supply with malaria virus an area of a very large radius from a centre, especially if use is made of the most modern form of transport, air mail. In this way we once successfully supplied malaria blood to Constantinople from Vienna.

It was finally a fortunate circumstance, which was not expected from the first, that tertian malaria brought on by injection proved to be so extraordinarily sensitive to quinine that a few grams of quinine suffice to cure the malaria completely and permanently, so that there is no fear of a relapse. It was through this that the great expansion which induced malaria has gained was first made possible.

When tertian malaria is acquired naturally the attacks of fever may also be cut short very effectively with quinine, but the patients remain carriers of the plasmodium and frequently relapse sooner or later. How would it have been possible to release so many paralytics and advanced syphilitics from the hospitals when outside they first of all ran the continual risk of a relapse and secondly, particularly where there were anopheles, were a danger to their environment?

The patient inoculated with malaria who has been adequately treated with quinine neither endangers himself further (in the sense of a malaria relapse), nor can he endanger his environment. However, he can from the moment of infection up to the elimination of the malaria present a danger to his environment, as malaria can be transferred from him to other persons through the sting of the anopheles, and that is then not induced malaria, but natural malaria, with its resistance to quinine.

This danger, which was assumed with the presence of anopheles in places of treatment, can be excluded with a fair degree of safety, if the patients are kept under mosquito-proof netting during the whole duration of the treatment. This has been done in several countries, such as England and Sweden.

The question is whether it is not possible to meet this danger in yet another way. An experiment was made in my clinic in 1924 with a large number of patients and mosquitoes to see if induced malaria could be transferred to other patients through anopheles; the experiment was without results. Such transfers have, however, been obtained by other writers[;]

notably Shute and James, and also Warrington Yorke, in England, have carried out numerous successful transfers of induced malaria by means of anopheles. The Vienna strain has, however, been proved at that time to be free of gametes by an experiment of the Italian malariologist D. Vivaldi. The strains which were transferable through anopheles have all proved to be gamete producers; and the English writers mentioned in particular state that the transference by anopheles is the easier, the richer in gametes the donor's blood is.

Plehn and Schulze of Berlin, and Vonkenel of Munich, also reported on such gamete-free strains.

I have therefore in the preceding year made the demand that everyone who practices malaria therapy, should procure a gamete-free strain and thus eliminate the danger of a transfer by means of anopheles.

More recent investigations carried out in my clinic this year have, however, shown that this demand cannot be realized, as gamete-free malaria strains cannot be obtained by transferring preserved blood unaltered from one place to another. That is to say that it has been shown that from the moment malaria blood leaves the human body, the malaria parasites deviate from the normal course of development; they leave the red blood corpuscles and assume gametic forms.

We thus have in the preserved blood, not a gamete-free strain, but predominantly gamete-containing injection blood.

Thus the propagation of a gamete-free strain would not be possible with preserved blood but only by direct transfer from one patient to another. It would not be possible to effect this by transferring the blood but only by transferring the patients.

Induced malaria is, however, of itself a dangerous disease. The attacks of fever usually reach 40°C by the third attack. The temperature often remains above 40°C for many hours in the later attacks. It frequently reaches 41°C. The highest temperature that I have observed was 42°C. In addition, the attacks frequently assume the quotidian type or take that course right from the beginning. It appears, incidentally, that paralysis plays a role in the appearance of the quotidian type, as in luetics of advanced latency the malaria usually remains tertian. Perhaps in this respect, however, different strains of malaria behave differently, since Bravetta in Novara has at his disposal a strain of which he reports that it causes without exception attacks of the tertian type.

The high temperatures on the one hand and the brief pauses in the quotidian type on the other, make on the usually already weakened organism of the paralytic, especially on his heart, often too great demands; and thus we and others also have seen not by any means infrequent cases of death during the fever period or immediately afterwards.

However, by various measures, this danger has been decreased to such an extent that fatal cases are now almost never seen. We use several methods to this end. Something can frequently be effected by the mode of inoculation. That is to say that, if one inoculates intracutaneously with a small quantity of blood, about 0.1 cm^3, the fever usually develops into the tertian type, especially when the blood groups of the donor and recipient correspond, and the avoidance of the quotidian type is already an alleviation.

In other cases we mitigate the fever with small doses of quinine (0.2–0.3) which must not, however, be given two days in succession, otherwise the fever ceases entirely. After a single administration of such a dose, the fever disappears for some days, during which the patient recovers; and when the fever sets in again it runs a milder course, as a rule. Alternatively one gives 0.1 quinine every two or three days from immediately after the injection, and in this way obtains a general alleviation of the course of the fever.

Finally, in cases which on account of their physical constitution or on account of their age—somewhere between 55 and 70—appear particularly endangered, a division of the course into two parts has been proved particularly successful. In such patients the fever will be interrupted by quinine after two to at the most four attacks. This is followed by a six weeks' pause taken up with injections of neoarsphenamine, after which the patient will be infected a second time. He has meanwhile recovered, and now endures the continuation of the cure very well.

In this connection the question also arises, how many attacks of fever are necessary for a successful malaria cure? This can only be decided by experience, as we have no biological evidence as to when the optimum activity occurs. In my clinic the fever is, as a rule, terminated after eight attacks. English writers, by comparing therapeutic results after a shorter or longer duration of the fever period have likewise come to the conclusion that the optimum therapeutic effect lies at around eight attacks.

Some writers have let their patients have very much longer fevers. However, I believe that it is much better to give to a patient in whom a course of some eight attacks of fever has had an unsatisfactory result, a second course soon afterwards, than to endanger the reconstruction which should follow each malaria injection by weakening the patient too severely by continuing the course too long.

This reconstruction as an aftereffect of induced malaria, and the long duration of its aftereffect in general, is something that must be taken into account by every explanation of the mode of action of induced malaria.

The improvement in the physical and mental health of the patients is not as a rule demonstrable immediately after the last attack of fever and never to the full extent. On the contrary, it often happens that a paralytic who on completion of the treatment has been committed to the asylum as uncured, presents himself again after six or twelve months and states that he has taken up his occupation again.

The most convincing, because numerically demonstrable, expression of this delayed action of induced malaria is in the reactions of the serum and of the cerebrospinal fluid. The immediate effect of the malaria treatment on these reactions is negligible, and the changes do not run parallel with the clinical symptoms. It does change however, if these reactions are repeatedly investigated at intervals.

Kyrle has already noticed that in the malaria treatment of advanced syphilitics distinguished by a positive cerebrospinal fluid, the immediate effect of the treatment was relatively small. However, after the space of a year the cerebrospinal fluid was negative, although since the malaria, no further treatment had taken place, and in spite of the fact that before the malaria treatment the most vigorous specific therapy had been applied without any result.

The same thing happens with paralytics, only at an even slower tempo. In them the negativity of the cerebrospinal fluid reactions often first appears two, three, and even four years after the malaria treatment and still without any specific or non-specific treatment being introduced after the latter.

My assistant D. Dattner reported three years ago on the results of treatment from a particular aspect on a series of 129 paralytics treated with malaria in the period between the beginning of 1922 and the beginning of 1924; 66 of them underwent cerebrospinal fluid examinations at more frequent intervals up to the present day. They were thus cases in whom the malaria treatment lay about three to five years behind. Of these cases, repeated examinations of the cerebrospinal fluid in 1927 showed completely negative findings in 36, and nearly negative findings in 23. This favourable result, however, had first appeared in many of them two or more years after the cessation of the malaria treatment and without any further treatment having been administered in the meantime.

It has been shown by these investigations that the serum reaction is more refractory than the cerebrospinal fluid reaction.

The regularly repeated examination of the serum and cerebrospinal fluid also provides good evidence to establish a prognosis for the remissions achieved. Relapses, that is, do occur, but they form by far the minority beside cases which have attained a full remission. However, the cases in which this progressive improvement in the cerebrospinal fluid appears, do not relapse; but the contrary does not hold good. Curiously enough, this progressive improvement of the cerebrospinal fluid appears also in a number of the cases which do not improve clinically. It is thus of prognostic value only in conjunction with the clinical findings.

How is the action of induced malaria on the paralytic process to be explained? It is certain that it is not the high temperature alone that is effective. The spirochaetes, it is true, disappear from the brain during the fever. When, however, the fever has passed, they are immediately to be found again in the brain, at least in cases where the course is not successful, as Forster has shown. Where are they in the meantime? Does malaria act against syphilis in general or predominantly against progressive paralysis? We know that syphilitic processes in the secondary period are also influenced by malaria, yet this action appears to be less permanent than the action on progressive paralysis. Vascular syphilis appears to be less favourably affected than progressive paralysis. Further, it has been experienced that soon after the malaria treatment gummata appear, even in cases in which the paralytic process has been favourably affected.

It appears then, that malaria besides a non-specific action against the syphilitic infection, also exerts a specific elective action on the cerebral process of progressive paralysis, including advanced infection of the cerebrospinal fluid.

It is also very likely that malaria creates favourable conditions for all reparatory processes because of its cyclic course, and because ultimately a rapid transition takes place from a serious state of illness to a full recovery. The superiority of induced malaria over the different types of stimulation therapy, e.g. by the injection of vaccines and proteins, has been shown by

Schilling and his colleagues on the cytological blood-picture, and by Donath and Heilig on the chemical blood-picture. It is certain that induced malaria therapy will yet pose many worthwhile problems for research to explain.

From Julius Wagner-Jauregg, "The Treatment of Dementia Paralytica by Malaria Inoculation" Nobel Lecture, 13 December 1927, http://nobelprize.org/nobel_prizes/medicine/laureates/1927/wagner-jauregg-lecture.html. With permission of The Nobel Foundation.

Hermann Simon
(1867–1947)

Active Therapy in the Lunatic Facility
(1929)

Hermann Simon was a German psychiatric reformer, who made his reputation during the first three decades of the twentieth century developing what he called "active therapy." He happened upon the idea in 1905, when, because of a staff shortage, he set patients to work on the asylum grounds at Warstein. To his surprise, he found that patients were subsequently calmer and more orderly. Assuming the directorship of the psychiatric facility at Gütersloh in 1919, Simon implemented his form of occupational therapy throughout the asylum there, and soon, 90 percent of its eight hundred residents were working. Under his charge, Gütersloh became a model institution, visited by more than seven hundred guests between 1925 and 1933 and inspiring replicas throughout Europe. Simon held strong conservative and nationalist beliefs and was admittedly influenced by social Darwinism and eugenics.

From his experience in his own treatment halls, every attending physician is familiar with the tendency of many of the ill to constantly pull their blankets over their heads, day and night lying there rigid and motionless, rejecting any attempt to approach them. The simplest physiological consideration leads us to the realization that the continued inhalation of the stuffy air under the blanket must be having a detrimental effect on the gaseous exchange and metabolism. A sufficient, normal metabolism must be the most elementary basis for any kind of therapy for all illnesses, including psychoses associated with brain disorders.

Another, perhaps most important, failing of this much touted bed rest treatment in our system I see lying in the very fact that the one-sided therapeutic esteem that is still to this day bestowed upon it prevents us from taking timely action against the effects of the illness. This is especially the case for many newly afflicted patients. To be sure, bed rest . . . is extraordinarily easy for doctors and staff, just like some other schemes in therapy. If every newly arriving patient is placed in bed for weeks or months without any attention to the type and course of their illness, if the bed has become the sovereign cure for all sorts of problems that arise in the course of a psychosis (agitation, anti-social tendencies, refusal to eat, etc), then the therapeutic thinking of the physician as well as that of the staff becomes very simplified. At that very moment where the bed rest treatment appears to demonstrate marked success—when, for instance, a formerly agitated and disruptive patient is quieted under its influence—the danger of perpetual bed rest exists for the patient, since supposedly "it's better to be in bed than outside" and (if the effort is ever made at all) it is often hard for a patient who has become accustomed to constant bed rest to get used to a new lifestyle.

The root of all the evils that I have described to you is inactivity. Idleness is not only a vice—with our patients, we refer to it as "unsocial characteristics"—but also the beginning of nonsense. Life is activity! That holds for physical as well as mental life. Powers that are not used diminish, disappear. Liveliness is only conserved through activity; the latter is the basis for all achievement. In the case of some psychoses where there is already a heightened excitability, the lack of activity serves to channel this excitability in a deviant direction, in manners, stereotypes, mischief, collecting, aimless running around, pestering others. An experienced psychiatrist once put it this way, "A human being never does nothing—if he does nothing useful, then he will do something useless." We can add to this, he will at least think something useless, something deviant. Successful activity breeds satisfaction, internal and external calm; inactive loafing around breeds bad moods, moroseness, irritability. These, in turn, lead again and again to frequent conflicts with others, to quarrels in words and actions, to continued and loud grumbling and talking. The awful milieu of our earlier "disruptive units," about which more will be said later, arose out of concentrating numerous of these inactive patients together.

In the foreground of patient activity must be, as it has always been, activity in the open, with garden and field work. I don't need to justify this here. Along with this, the second most important activity and involving the largest number of patients is work toward the maintenance of the patient ward and facility, i.e., in the kitchen, laundry, the estate, poultry breeding, and offices. Whatever task can be done by someone who is sick is not to be done by someone who is healthy. Every psychiatric facility has had workshops and craftwork rooms of various kinds for quite a long time. There is hardly a single skilled trade that cannot be carried out on the premises. . . .

The therapeutic moment must stand at center stage in all the activities for patients, and for the physician, the economic value of the work is not the thing that matters in the first instance. But an attending physician will always make sure that the labor force is, as much as possible, being put to good use. It is also therapeutically important that most patients have a feel for whether the work they are assigned serves a purpose or not. Only in the former case will they be able to arrive at and attain a mental relationship with and interest in the work. Moreover, the entire treatment plan must start with the assumption of reintroducing a healthy logic into the life and mental world of the patient; and a first principle of a healthy logic is, that what one does must have a sense and purpose.

On the other hand, in order to move them forward, the patient must be pushed to the upper limits of their abilities in their activities. For only in this way can we gradually achieve progress. . . . The work assigned a patient, therefore, should be real and serious. It is better and more beneficial to press a patient to do two hours a day of serious, genuine labor than allowing him to stand or run around as a dawdling member of a work detail. On the one hand, the need to not strain the patient's existing energies and capabilities, and, on the other, to maintain a high standard together determine a careful individualization of the entire occupational therapy. Herein lies one of the most important as well as most difficult tasks for the psychiatrist. Every aspect of mental life needs to be taken into consideration: the degree of mental clarity or confusion, liveliness or inhibition, the coherence or distractedness of thought, the attention, the fatigability, and lastly—be careful with this one—the affective attitude. . . . The physician must, above all else, take into consideration all the mental abilities that are still within the patient which can be used and developed in order to school the patient from purely mechanical tasks to once again more independent thinking and action, to attentiveness, concentration and finally again to a certain measure of responsibility—to be precise, through goal-oriented training and practice in all aspects of mental life. And even after going to such lengths to get individual patients to work, this is not the end, but rather the beginning, of psychological therapy for us.

This effort at leading each patient to higher stages of achievement and capability is reminiscent of the way in which schooling is organized, whereby pupils are distributed according to their different levels of progress and ability. . . .

First Stage: simplest tasks not requiring any particular degree of independence and concentration. Lending a hand by helping to carry a basket or other object; also, for physically robust patients, routine help in getting meals, carrying laundry. Gradually letting the patients get an object on their own and to bring it to a particular place alone. The simplest domestic work, such as dusting of furniture, doors, and windows and polishing. . . .

Second Stage: mechanical work making minimal demands on attention and vigor. Simple work details in landscaping, that last for a longer period of time, so that the patients have time to get used to being part of a "training colony." [Also] . . . straightforward basket weaving. Spooling for weaving. . . . Simple, feminine, physical labor, such us darning and hemming of clothes, towels, etc. . . .

Third Stage: work demanding moderate attention, vigor, and intelligence. This involves most of the work in details in agriculture and gardening as well as in institutional maintenance (field cultivation, harvesting, cleaning stalls, transporting coal, walkway construction and upkeep); garden work with the exception of special tasks for which lengthier training is necessary. . . .

Fourth Stage: work demanding good attention and a measure of normal ability to reflect. Skilled agricultural and garden work, planting and raising of vegetable cuttings, glasshouse work, servicing of lawnmowers. Weed work, where attention and care are required, as in the case of young plants. Independent feeding and tending of animals (pig stalls, poultry pens).

Mowing. Skilled work in workshops. Preparing new laundry and clothes in the seamstress shop; more refined physical labor of all kinds. . . .

Fifth Stage: full, normal work capacity of a healthy person from the same background. Here belongs the rehabilitation of acute illnesses, some moderate imbeciles, epileptics in an asymptomatic phase, as well as many paranoids (insofar as their outlandish thinking does not hinder their ability to perform and control themselves). . . . It is best to give such patients independent responsibility and appropriate positions of trust, as far this can be tolerated, e.g., as leader of a small work detail, for errands and tasks outside the facility, telephone and front desk service. Also the "unit elders" in "staff-free units" belong here.

From Hermann Simon, *Aktivere Krankenbehandlung in der Irrenanstalt* (Berlin: Walter de Gruyter, 1929), 6–7, 16–27. With kind permission of Walter de Gruyter Press. Translated by Greg Eghigian.

Anonymous
"Insulin and I"
(1940)

Insulin coma therapy (also known as insulin shock therapy) was developed by the Austrian neurophysiologist and psychiatrist Manfred Sakel (1900–1957) around 1930. The labor-intensive treatment generally involved giving psychotic patients daily injections of ever higher doses of insulin until they fell into a hypoglycemic coma. Patients would then be brought back to consciousness with a sugar solution. A typical regimen might involve prompting five or six comas a week for several weeks or even months, with psychiatrists reporting that many patients' symptoms gradually disappeared. While various theories were put forward to explain the phenomenon, there was no agreement on the mechanism behind the treatment's efficacy. By 1941, 72 percent of all American psychiatric facilities reported using the treatment. The following first-person narrative comes from a former patient's description of her experience with insulin shock therapy; the statement was given before a medical meeting of the then Westchester Division of New York Hospitals (formerly known as Bloomingdale).

When you pick up the New York Times and read that you are one of four insane patients completely cured by insulin treatment in an important mental hospital, you can assume three attitudes. You can be indignant at being called insane; you can stick out your chest and say: "Well, I see I made the Times this morning, even if I did have to go crazy to do it!" Or you can say: "What a lucky girl am I—hooray for insulin!"

I couldn't take the first attitude, for I should not be hurt at all to be called insane; having lived for nearly a year among the mentally ill. I have found most of them interesting, some quite entertaining, and I don't think I missed a great deal away from the mentally balanced. To take the second, would only be the Irish in me. The third, of course, would be easy. I am a lucky girl and do say "Hooray for insulin!"

There has been so much written about insanity that for me to add anything would be like telling the old, old story. Clifford Beers found his mind and let us know it.* Seabrook came out of the alcohol into the here, and the process, I guess, wasn't much fun; it never is. There have been "Outward Rooms" and "Closed Doors" and they were not tales by idiots signifying nothing.† They were vital experiences of sensitive people who had the courage to publish their worst. If you bought the books and read them because you wanted a new thrill I could very peacefully see you hanged. If you read them because you wanted to go on a maudlin sentimental binge at the expense of the ineffective other half, I think I should be nauseated if I ever met you. If, however, reading them made you think a little more of the important things in life and a little less of those not so much so, if you

---

*Editor's note: The American Clifford Beers (1876–1943) published *A Mind that Found Itself* in 1908, an autobiographical book about his institutionalization for and his recovery from manic depression. Following the book's success, Beers became a leading advocate for people with psychiatric disabilities.

†Editor's note: The author is referring here to William Seabrook's *Asylum* (1935), Millen Brand's *The Outward Room* (1937), and Margaret Prescott Montague's *Closed Doors* (1934).

remembered to send a flower to a friend occasionally and could tear your-self away from the stock market long enough to really listen to the troubles of your office boy, then I think these writers made no mistake in baring their souls to you. Insanity is certainly a disease of the mind, but more truly a disease of the soul. I can't say I ever thought it did one much good if he had a soul to go flaunting it about. If it was good, some one would just try to take it away, and if it was rotten, there would always be some one around to make it a little more decadent. I have always thought the best thing to do about souls is to shut up and bear them in peace or pain depending, of course, on the kind you have. If yours is particularly painful you do need a doctor, and a good one. Don't ask advice of your friend who reads Freud or buys mentally helpful periodicals at the newsstand. He will tell tales to make your hair stand on end, and what to do if it does. He will toss off Schizophrenia, Dementia Praecox, and Manic Depressive like so many A, B, C's, then run into the opposite direction when you need real help. For me to dissertate on symptoms, progress, and convalescence of these diseases would be like calling in a craftsman to do an artist's work. I have no techni-cal knowledge of mental illness and too much respect for those who have, to take pot-shots and besides, I don't like to talk about my operations. I have always felt the same way about them as I do about labor pains or digging a trench for the peonies. 'Twas "feelthy" work, but peonies are so beautiful.

The peonies are particularly beautiful today. So is the blue Long Island Sound which laps peacefully at my garden's edge. The red geraniums in the pots on the terrace are flaming in the sun. I have found the world just as beautiful as when I left it ten months ago. I would much rather talk about your garden and mine, but I can't: I must talk about insulin—a magic drug, and about the intelligence of those who had the foresight to use it.

I did lose my mind—people do. I don't think it would be particularly interesting to anyone beside my friend the doctor—how I did, and why. Suffice it to say that I do not remember being taken to the hospital, nor did I recognize I was in one for eight months. I lived an Alice-in-Wonderland sort of existence in a world of my own hallucinations, traveled in many lands, and had so many vivid experiences that when I did get well, I don't see why I wasn't a complete wreck.

One morning when a nurse said I was to go downstairs for treatment my heart went down into my boots. What more horrible things could they have to offer? Continuous baths and cold packs were things to beg to be taken out of. Another treatment could only be worse. I tried to influence a young student nurse to get my clothes out of the closet and dress me, thinking they all might forget me, but ah no, things are not done that way in my hospital and when the appointed time came, down I went with a special nurse, flapping along the corridors in my dilapidated mules. There were two beds in the treatment room, two nurses, and a man sitting at a desk. When they took me over to him, he said, "Put her in a pack," and I did not think he could ever be a friend. So the biggest and smallest nurse came and wrapped me in swaddling clothes. I thought I smelled chloroform and was floating away to be delivered of a child, and was quite sure of this when they injected the insulin in my hip. It was just another dose of pituitrin to me. I shall never forget the little nurse who finally released me from the pack and put me back in a nice dry bed. Large cups of lemonade were given me and finally lunch came in on a tray. The patient in the other bed sat up and ate all her lunch, but I was terrified to eat mine and needed a lot of help from the nurse. By this time I was simply drenched in perspiration and couldn't have felt more like a clam. This, caused by the insulin, is one of the most unpleasant things about it. I was rubbed with alcohol and my special nurse took me upstairs.

During the afternoon I was fed milk chocolate and huge glasses of orange juice filled with glucose to replace the sugar content which the insulin removes. Every day, except Sunday, for six weeks I went down to that room to repeat the same treatment, and every day I dreaded it just as much, if not more. I was never given another pack, but I had so many distorted ideas about insulin that the effect of it was horrible to me. I would get into the bed very quietly thinking that if I could stay like that nothing would happen, but soon little beads of perspiration would begin to come out on my arms and I would know that I was lost. I was dissolving away into nothingness. The soap with which I bathed was oozing out of my pores and making me deathly sick; my distorted mind was taking me through most harrowing experiences. I would often come out of this to find myself tied in bed and would count her my guardian angel who untied the knots and released me.

The man, whom I soon learned to call doctor, would come over to my bed and ask if I didn't want to go out and play ping-pong or badminton. I would have played football to get out of there. And I did go out and play badminton every afternoon with a pocket-full of milk chocolate. At four in the afternoon my nurse and I would go back to the treatment room for nourishment. More orange juice with glucose and more chocolate. Sometimes the nurses would have boxes of bonbons that patients had given them. I remember on Valentine's Day being offered a gay candy heart from one of the boxes and being so thrilled over it.

It was about this time that, with some misgiving, I was transferred to another hall. What would it be like? Who would be there and what would they do to me?

I found it to be a hall with beautiful flowers, kind and helpful nurses, and a patient I once knew. Even though she did not remember me, my recognizing her helped me a little to place myself and be aware of where I was. Insulin treatments still went on, and I was still trying to devise ways in which to get out of them. Some mornings, like a school child, I would carry a few flowers in my hand to bribe the teacher. But doctors and nurses are made of sterner stuff. The insulin was never forgotten and my mornings were hell. Into a rocking, rolling sea of intangibles to come up out of it shivering and shaking and freezing to death. A hot bath and clean clothes, the joy of all joys. I spent my afternoons playing badminton or walking with my nurse. When I was on the hall I sat in a chair and stayed there, being afraid to move until someone called me to meals. I didn't make anything in the occupation therapy department, but sat and looked at the baskets they hoped I might weave. Every time the door-bell rang in the building, I prayed it was a gymnasium instructor calling for me to play games. These girls were bright, gay, and well dressed. The sight of normal people in good clothes does much for the morale of the mental patient. In the gym, my nurse would sit on one of the window seats while I played badminton or ping-pong. I played very badly, but liked being there so much more than on the hall where I never seemed to know what to do, or in occupation where I certainly did not occupate.

February 22, when I went to the insulin room, my doctor said I was to have one more dose of insulin on the twenty-third. This horrible business was to be over next day! I heard that a doctor I knew in New York was coming to see me. It seemed strange that I might go upstairs to see if he were real. I heard them talking about a tea-dance, and I asked to go. I wanted to see if it were real too.

That day after the insulin my nurse bathed and dressed me and the two little nurses from the insulin room came running into my room with rouge, lip-stick, and powder. If I were going dancing, they were going to see that I went with my best face forward. They were laughing and full of fun and as interested as a mother sending her daughter to her first dance. I never quite believed I was going to this party until I stepped into the ball-room where an orchestra was playing good dance music and the room was filled with gaily dressed people. It was the first time in seven months I had seen so many men. We sat along the wall and had tea and sandwiches. My doctor from the insulin room asked me to dance. He danced beautifully, but I felt heavy and stiff. He said "Star Dust" was one of his favorites. All this music was unfamiliar to me. Things that people had been dancing to all winter, I supposed. I don't know that I distinguished one from another, but I liked the orchestra and I have always liked to dance.

I danced with a young nurse who told me about taking his patient to hear the trials at the county court. He said he had always wanted to be a lawyer.

After dancing I would go back to my nurse and sit with her and my sister who had driven over to see me. She kept telling me very definite things about my own family. This was all surprising to me, as I had believed everyone I had ever known was dead. Every time I would launch off into one of my witless hallucinations, she would tell me that she would have to go home if I couldn't talk sense.

The thing I wanted to talk about most was the last insulin treatment the next day. Was it really true? She assured me it was; the doctor had told her I was to have no more. I could certainly endure the next treatment if it was to be the last.

We finally found our hostess, one of the head nurses, and said good-bye. Back on the hall I was given my supper from a tray and had just as many strange complexes about food as I had six months ago, and certainly must have tried the patience of the little student nurse who fed me. I went to bed happy, thinking of tomorrow.

It must be understood that insulin does not affect every patient the same way. It is not a dose of salts. Some of the patients who took it seemed very sick, others were on halls that were not considered "bad." They played games well, did good work in occupation, and seemed alert. I was badly confused until February 23.

That day when I woke up, there was no sleepy fluttering of the eyelids, no yawning or stretching to pull myself awake. I just came alive with all cylinders in perfect working order. I went down for the last insulin injection, and it was just as horrible as it had always been. When it was over, I came upstairs with my nurse, feeling as though I had had three glasses of champagne. After a bath and clothes, we went out to walk. The world never looked so beautiful. I couldn't breathe enough of the air or look enough at the sky. We walked and walked with the cool wind whipping my hair about my face. It was like sailing on a September day when the blue water is full of sun glint. We sat in one of the arbors while I smoked a cigarette, and I talked and talked, making up for lost time. It seemed so strange to see cars on the road beyond the fence. The world going on about its business as usual. I felt well, I liked what I saw, and I was happy. That state of mind never left me. My special nurse soon left and I was on my own. Saturdays and Tuesdays I went out to tea with some member of my family and those were gala days. It was such fun to go to the different shops to tea and be brought up to date on all the news. I found I had missed a hurricane and a war scare, and that Hitler had taken Czechoslovakia. All my conversations started with "tell me." I was soon moved to an open hall, which meant no locked doors, more exercise, and more privileges. Here I was hailed by my first name when I entered the dining room and was taken on for bridge and Chinese checkers in the evening. I had a very attractive room and liked taking care of my own clothes again. It was nice having powder, perfume, and lipstick where I could get at it. On the other halls everything is locked away, and one must ask a nurse for everything. This never bothered me very much, but I appreciated the change. In other words, I didn't know what I had missed until I was given something better. I began to knit socks and went into the art room at occupation. Here in the next two months I made two belts embroidered in wool, a wooden salad bowl, polished to a beautiful patina, a pair of painted book-ends and some pottery. I loved this room. The woman in charge was a charming person, helpful and encouraging, and the patients turned out some excellent work.

In the afternoons we all went to the gymnasium and I began to play a good game of badminton, getting into games with more seasoned players which I certainly enjoyed. I would get back on the hall in time for a tub before dinner. After dinner it was bridge or knitting, watching the others play. Twice a week I went to the choral classes and enjoyed the singing. I also began to play the piano again and found I played better than before I was sick. Life on the hall was very pleasant. People were friendly and hospitable to newcomers. Voices were soft, gentle, and low, and consideration of others seemed to be the main theme.

I left here soon to go to one of the cottages on the grounds. I was sorry to go, but glad to know it meant advancement. This was a charming little house, and I was teased a lot when I got what they called the royal suite, a delightful room with green walls and rose damask curtains, maple furniture, and pewter lamps. Those who planned my welfare couldn't have been more thoughtful.

At the cottage life went on much as before. There were ten patients and one nurse in charge. Some of the patients had been on the other halls with me, some had taken insulin and some had not. We had lots of fun talking about the weird things we had done when we were very sick. In the mornings we went to occupation, took a long walk, and had lunch. In the afternoon it was badminton from three-thirty till five. Evenings were given over to bridge. We were well-fed and well exercised. We were rubbed with salt, put under the sun lamp and baked, then showered with hot and cold hoses. Our social life was taken care of. Every day would bring more buds out on trees, and I would look at the forsythia and make bets as to when it would burst forth.

With all this we should have gotten well, and many of us did. We do have a feeling of affection for those who went through it with us and those who brought us out. Insulin did make me well, but the hospital and the doctors and nurses connected with it are entirely responsible for my well-being. One thinks of a hospital as a machine, of white linen efficiency and disinfectants. The works are all there in my hospital. It is run by men and women of intelligence and profound knowledge. They conduct their affairs with grace and charm. If it is an insane asylum, it is one that I am proud to have been in.

Insulin and I say hooray!

From Anonymous, "Insulin and I," *American Journal of Orthopsychiatry* 10 (1940): 810–814. (© American Orthopsychiatric Association), reprinted with permission of the American Orthopsychiatric Association.

Walter Freeman
(1895–1972)
and James W. Watts
(1904–1994)
"Psychosurgery during 1936–1946"
(1947)

If nineteenth-century neurology had helped convince many that mental disorders were by and large brain diseases, neurologists, often seemed unable to offer many treatment alternatives for dealing with this reality. That began to change when the Portuguese neurologist Egas Moniz (1874–1955) developed a surgical procedure he called a "prefrontal leukotomy." Evidence from pathological anatomy, experiments on mammals, and wartime head injuries convinced Moniz that the destruction of tissue in the prefrontal lobes of the brain might cause the health of psychiatric patients to improve. Designing a special wire knife, which he dubbed a "leukotome," he operated on his first patient on 27 December 1935. Years later, in 1949, he received a Nobel Prize for his innovation.

Moniz's work was closely followed by that of a professor of neurology at George Washington University in the United States, Walter Freeman. Freeman and his colleague James Watts created their own procedure and gave it the name *lobotomy*, in order to distinguish it from Moniz's leukotomy. Until 1945, however, Freeman himself actually had never performed a lobotomy. After first practicing on cadavers, he developed a new technique, one that he believed would not require the assistance of a neurosurgeon. This was the transorbital lobotomy, by which an ice pick was inserted into the skull through the eye socket, tapped with a hammer, and then moved around in order to destroy tissue. By the early-1950s, Freeman was traveling the country, visiting asylums and teaching the technique to eager staff. In the period between 1939 and 1951 alone, around eighteen thousand lobotomies were performed in the United States.

Psychosurgery was introduced into this country ten years ago, amid rumblings of disbelief and thunderings of disapproval. Its seems appropriate now that a survey of results of the first decade be presented.

It was the experimental work of a group of investigators in Yale University that started Egas Moniz on the surgical treatment of mental disorders. Jacobsen, in association with Fulton, noted a profound alteration in response to frustration in the chimpanzee with both front poles excised. Before operation, if the animal made a few mistakes, he would scream with rage, urinate and defecate in the cage, roll in the feces, shake the bars and refuse to continue the experiments. After the operation the same animal would continue in the experimental situation long beyond the patience of the examiner, making mistake after mistake, without the least indication of being upset emotionally.

At about the same time Brickner published an extensive report on the case of a man whose frontal lobes had been removed several years before because of a tumor. This man was of average intelligence, as shown by various tests following the operation, but the striking thing about him was his complete lack of self consciousness and his obliviousness to the seriousness of his own predicament. While Brickner did not mention worry by name, his patient was obviously incapable of exercising this most human of intellectual-emotional exercises.

Egas Moniz had theories of his own, but they tied in well with the findings of Fulton and Jacobsen and of Brickner; therefore he and Almeida Lima commenced operating on psychotic patients and first reported their results in the spring of 1936. Fulton called our attention to these reports, and by the end of 1936 we completed our first series of operations on 20 patients. Seven of these patients had to have a second operation because of relapse, and 2 of them underwent three operations before the psychosis could be overcome. However, a recent check on this first series revealed that 1 patient died after operation and 5 more since, including 1 by suicide. Of the 14 living patients, 4 are employed and 4 are keeping house; 4 are living at home, and only 2 are in institutions (appendix).

At the time of our first reports we emphasized the need of a long period of observation before definitive conclusions could be drawn. Up to the present time we have kept in touch with all our patients, now numbering well over 400, and the results in succeeding years are on the whole similar to those in the first series. By means of refinements in the technic of prefrontal lobotomy, we are able to secure a higher percentage of successful results in relatively favorable cases; and, knowing what could be accomplished in these, we have undertaken operation in a large number of unfavorable cases. Consequently, the percentages in the various categories of social adequacy have remained about the same over several years.

In prefrontal lobotomy the surgeon incises the white matter in both frontal lobes in such a way as to sever the connections between the thalamus and the frontal pole. From the time of our first operations we have asked ourselves what the operation does to the psychosis to make it clear up. We vividly recall the case of a young woman who was responding with intense fear to her hallucinations. They were of the most disagreeable kind, the voice calling her a dog and threatening her with hell fire. She was in a panic, and her attention could hardly be gained. Within a few hours after operation she described the same experiences but in a subdued tone of voice, as though they were hardly worth mentioning. A few days later, when questioned about the voices, she replied: "Voices? No. My ears have gone dead." This case illustrates the bleaching of the emotional tone and the quieting of anxiety that almost always accompany prefrontal lobotomy. In fact, of all the symptoms of mental disorder, emotional tension has undergone the most profound alteration after prefrontal lobotomy. This does not mean that these patients are apathetic, lacking all emotion. As a matter of fact, as they recover from the post-operative inertia, they are fairly responsive, sometimes more than they were before they became sick; but the emotion attaches itself to external happenings rather to inner experiences. Patients who have been operated on are usually cheerful, responsive, affectionate, and unreserved. They are outspoken, often critical of others and lacking in embarrassment. For the first few weeks or months they are rather childlike in their attitudes and behavior. They require more than the ordinary motivation to accomplish and are satisfied with something less than perfection. They tend to procrastinate, to make up their minds too quickly and to enunciate opinions without considering the various implications. Some patients are distractible, others have single track minds; some are indolent, others are human dynamos. The most striking and constant change from the preoperative personality lies in a certain unselfconsciousness, and this applies both to the patient's own body and to his total self as a social unit. The patient emerges from operation with an immature personality that is at first poorly equipped for maintaining him in a competitive society; but with the passage of time there is progressive improvement, so that in about one-half the cases earning a living again becomes possible.

On the basis of these experiences, we have advanced the hypothesis that the frontal lobes are especially concerned with foresight and insight and that the emotional component associated with these functions is supplied by the thalamus. When the thalamic connections are severed, the functions of foresight and insight suffer temporary obliteration, and even in the later course of recovery are never as completely endowed with feeling tone as they were before. A modicum of function is preserved, because the direct connections are not completely severed and because indirect connections probably also exist. Foresight and insight are two very important functions for any person living in a complex society. One may well ask whether the surgeon is justified in depriving a patient of these functions even for the sake of relieving his psychosis. We believe the surgeon would be entirely justified if it could be shown that the patient became psychotic because of perversions of these same functions of foresight and insight, together with the attachment of an abnormal emotional tone.

When one studies a psychotic patient with these functions in mind, it is not so difficult, if the case is not so far advanced, to determine the fact that many of the symptoms of the psychosis may indeed be attributed to pathologic selfconsciousness. Why otherwise would a patient believe that *he* was being kept under surveillance by the F.B.I.; that German spies were entering *his* room, using thought control on *him*, putting dope in *his* food or accusing *him* of sexual perversions? These ideas are intensely personal to him and preoccupy his mind to the exclusion of all rational, coherent thought process. Or take a patient who has a string of complaints as long as his arm concerning *his* stomach and *his* bowels, *his* heart and *his* head. Here is a person, also, whose function of consciousness of the self has gone beyond normal limits into a state of hypochondriasis. His attention becomes concentrated on his various organs to the exclusion of everything else. In both cases there is also a distressing concern for the future; not only what "they" are going to do to him, but also in regard to the prospects of the ulcer, cancer, or heart trouble. Above all, there is the emotional component which invests the symptoms and the ideas with a disabling force and completely prevents the patient's adaptation to the realities of existence. Such persons are sentient rather than rational beings. They live with their emotion concentrated on themselves, with an admixture of self pity or guilt that induces invalidism or, at the last extremity, suicide.

Prefrontal lobotomy cuts off the emotional component concerned with these ideas. It relieves the symptom of mental pain. In temporarily abolishing foresight and insight, the operation breaks the vicious circle of preoccupation, emotional tension and imagination that makes the suspected disease or persecution much more serious than any reality could be. It brings the patient back to earth and the enjoyments thereof.

The past decade has seen a certain vindication of our ideas on the subject of prefrontal lobotomy. Even in our first papers we cautioned against going to extremes. Now, at the beginning of the second decade, we would reiterate these cautions. Prefrontal lobotomy is an operation of last resort. It should be performed only on those patients who no longer have a reasonable hope of spontaneous recovery. It should be done only in cases of threatened disability or suicide, and only after conservative measures have failed. It should be done with the full appreciation of the changes in personality that will inevitably be brought about in the patient if the operation is to succeed, and with a knowledge of possible unfavorable results, such as persistent inertia, convulsive seizures, incontinence, and aggressive misbehavior. At the same time, prefrontal lobotomy should be performed while the patient is still fighting his disease, in other words, while the emotional tension is still present to a considerable degree. When emotion subsides and the patient accepts his dream world in lieu of reality, surrenders to his fantasies, then there is little that surgery can accomplish. It has been suggested that if a patient with dementia praecox fails to improve after a year prefrontal lobotomy should be considered. In view of the poor prognosis of dementia praecox, we should be inclined to accept this idea. In our cases in which operation was performed within the first two years of illness the percentage of good results was 85, whereas of those cases in which operation was done after two to thirty years of illness good results were only obtained in 31 per cent.

The types of patients who respond best to prefrontal lobotomy are those with the obsession-tension states, with or without compulsions, and the chronic anxiety syndromes, with or without hysterical conversion. Twenty years of invalidism can vanish in a few weeks. Involutional depressions also clear up in a goodly percentage. Schizophrenic states are strikingly modified if the patient is excited, resistive, assaultive, and disturbed.

The quiet, deteriorated patients are usually unchanged. Alcoholic, psychopathic, and epileptic patients, criminals and patients with organic diseases of the brain are seldom benefited.

Prefrontal lobotomy is being adopted in many parts of the world. The war interfered with the development of the procedure in continental Europe, so that the United States and Great Britain got a head start especially so far as detailed studies are concerned. Portugal and Italy, which had been in the forefront, dropped behind. Scattered reports have come from various Latin American republics; from Sweden and Czechoslovakia; from India, New Zealand, and Hawaii. More enthusiasm seems to be present in England than anywhere else. McKissock states in April 1946 that he had personally performed 500 operations, and in the June 1946 issue of the *Proceedings of the Royal Society of Medicine* there are statistics on more than 800 cases. In this country, we should estimate that up to the present time approximately 2000 lobotomies have been performed. A recent survey by Brody and Moore called attention to the rather great similarity of reports from various clinics in the percentage of patients who derive benefit from the operation. In round figures, one-third recover, one-third improve, and one-third fail to improve. There are variations from one investigator to another and from one disease to another, but the results are sufficiently good to warrant the use of prefrontal lobotomy on a large scale for the relief of the very serious and chronic forms of mental disease that keep the back wards of the psychiatric hospital filled to capacity and beyond.

We would close this review of prefrontal lobotomy by calling attention to its use in the treatment of pain due to organic disease. In case of an incurable illness, such as cancer, or of persistent pain in a phantom limb, intractable causalgia or the lightning pains of arrested tabes, the physician is likely to give up too easily and to prescribe narcotics, to the ultimate detriment of the patient with long-standing illness. A year ago we reported experiences in the relief of long-standing pain with prefrontal lobotomy. It would seem that in cases of this condition, as in the cases of purely mental disorders, it is the emotional component, the consciousness of the part and the anticipation of the future disability and death that contribute to the distress of the patient. In many cases the attitude of the patient toward his disease is more disabling than the disease itself; the fear of pain, greater than the pain. With prefrontal lobotomy the physician now has it in his power to relieve the fear, the anticipation, and to render the illness more tolerable to the patient. Since this can be done without significant impairment of intellectual capacity, it would seem that prefrontal lobotomy might be a very considerable boon to the large number of patients whose life will not be long but will, nevertheless, be made miserable by suffering. The physician cannot be criticized for recommending prefrontal lobotomy in order to secure a certain euphoria for those patients who have only pain and death to look forward to.

Appendix

The 20 cases in which operation was performed in 1936 were reported in 1938. A brief follow-up report as of September 1946, approximately ten years after the first lobotomy, is now given. All the patients have been kept under rather close observation at intervals of a year or less. The same case numbers are used.

Case 1.—A housewife aged 63 had a history of agitated depression of one year's duration, with two previous nervous breakdowns. After prefrontal lobotomy she quieted down, went out socially, drove her car, kept the household accounts, enjoyed her home but took little responsibility. She had several epileptic seizures, fracturing one of her wrists in one of them. In 1941 she died of pneumonia. Her husband wrote that the last five years were the happiest of her life.

Case 2.—A woman aged 59, a bookkeeper, had agitated depression of six months' duration, probably complicated by intoxication with sedatives. Prompt recovery followed prefrontal lobotomy, with return to work in three months. She continued this work for eight years, until her retirement because of age, and then returned to her office to help out during the war. She finally retired in June 1946 and has been living comfortably at home.

Case 3.—A housewife aged 34 had obsessive preoccupations, depression, and suicidal ideas of three years' duration. The first lobotomy was performed in December 1936, with little improvement; the second, in September 1937, with no change, and the third, in 1941, with extreme flattening of emotional life. She presents extreme indolence, petulance, and puerility and assumes no responsibility for the care of the home. She presents a rather pleasant front but has a sterile intellectual life. She is cared for at home by her mother.

Case 4.—A housewife aged 49 had involutional depression of one years' duration (with a history of three previous attacks) and organic changes caused by a nearly successful suicidal attempt with gas. After lobotomy she continued to show apathy, loss of memory and other signs of organic disease of the brain. She had frequent convulsion and incontinence. She died in status epilepticus in 1944. Autopsy showed minimal operative lesions (all lobotomies in 1936 were done by the Egas Moniz "core" technic), but there were extensive cortical softening at the base of the frontal and temporal lobes and necrosis of the globus pallidus.

Case 5.—A housewife aged 35 had a history of depression and agitation of four years' duration and three suicidal attempts. She benefited only temporarily from the operation, failed to make a satisfactory adjustment at home or on the farm and finally committed suicide in 1940. Autopsy was not performed.

Case 6.—A housewife aged 60, with agitated depression, died on the sixth post-operative day of hemorrhage. Autopsy was not performed.

Case 7.—A business man aged 59, with a history of involutional depression of nine years' duration, improved briefly after lobotomy but relapsed before he could return to his office. A second lobotomy was undertaken by a different surgeon in 1938, and the patient emerged permanently relieved of his depression but with a boisterous, arrogant, and extravagant nature that required institutionalization. His condition remains unchanged, after eight years.

Case 8.—A housewife aged 62 had a history of hypochondria of seventeen years' duration with superimposed agitated depression for two years. A year after operation she found part-time employment as a practical nurse and continued in this work until 1945, when she went to live with her daughter. She is fat, jolly, and outspoken and is said to be "quite a worker for her age." The visceral complaints cleared up.

Case 9.—A housewife aged 48, with involutional depression of two years' duration, had had many admissions to the hospital for abdominal complaints. No improvement followed the first lobotomy, in November 1936. The second operation was performed in March 1937, with relief. However, the patient was indolent and sarcastic and was subject to outbursts of anger, which made it necessary to confine her in an institution for eighteen months. After this she resumed her household duties, cared for her grandchildren during the war and still performs most of the domestic work in her daughter's home. On several occasions she has had fleeting depressions, only one of which was sufficiently severe to require treatment; two electroshocks were sufficient.

Case 10.—A housewife aged 60, with agitated depression of seven years' duration, had transitory improvement after the first lobotomy, in November 1936. At the second operation, in March 1937, severe bleeding was encountered, and the operation was not completed. The patient remained unimproved and died of a heart attack the following July. Autopsy was not performed.

Case 11.—A secretary aged 32, with catatonic schizophrenia of two months' duration and a history of a previous attack in 1934, lasting only a month, recovered rapidly, and apparently completely, after lobotomy and returned to her position. She was unable to continue because of return of emotional tension, followed by another catatonic attack, for which she was hospitalized in July 1937. Insulin and metrazol shock treatments failed to induce recovery; her family refused permission for further operation, and she remains in the hospital, greatly deteriorated, fat, and inaccessible.

Case 12.—A stenographer aged 25 entered a catatonic state in July 1936 and showed no change after unilateral prefrontal lobotomy. When operation was performed on the opposite side, she "woke on the table." She improved slowly; in a year she took a course in interior decorating but did nothing constructive with it, then returned to work as a stenographer and continued in this until 1942, when she again lapsed into a catatonic state. More extensive prefrontal lobotomy again abolished the condition, but she made a slow and imperfect recovery and was rather hostile to her family. After two years she found a clerical position and a separate domicile and continued living in this way for over a year; but when her parents became ill she returned home and has cared for them in small ways for the past year.

Case 13.—A cement finisher aged 33 had obsessive preoccupation with his heart and general exhaustion of eighteen months' duration. After prefrontal lobotomy he was euphoric but soon relapsed. Two years later, however, he was able to resume laboring work part time. His adjustment improved with time, and for the past four years he has been steadily employed as janitor at a school, where he is highly thought of.

Case 14.—A housewife aged 30 had agitation, feelings of unreality and probably hallucinations of six years' duration. After prefrontal lobotomy she made an erratic adjustment and was in and out of hospitals for four years. After that she was divorced, and since remarried and writes enthusiastically of her new life.

Case 15.—A stenographer aged 42 had an acute onset of catatonic stupor in the course of rheumatic heart disease of many years' duration. Both the mental symptoms and the cardiac irregularity cleared up briefly after prefrontal lobotomy, but the improvement was not sustained. She died of congestive heart failure in April 1937 with recrudescence of mental symptoms.

Case 16.—A housewife aged 60 had a history of obsessive-compulsive neurosis dating back thirty-six years, with intervals of good health, but with complete disability of four years' duration. Prefrontal lobotomy was followed by temporary euphoria and later return of symptoms. The second lobotomy, in March 1937, was followed by immediate disappearance of the emotional toning, but with persistence of the compulsive washing and brushing for at least three years. She presented marked increase in weight and was outspoken, tactless, and disagreeable with her family. There has been steady improvement over the years, although she still shakes her skirt at imaginary dirt. She recently celebrated her seventieth birthday and is cheerful, outspoken, and rolypoly.

Case 17.—A telephone operator aged 33, with obsessive syphilophobia of twelve years' duration, obtained partial relief from operation and was able to return to work. After a broken engagement her fears returned, and a second lobotomy was performed in 1938. She immediately lost her fears but became indolent and talkative in a silly, vapid way, was too distractible to continue at her work, helped out on a farm for a year or two and for the past two years has been steadily employed in a mill. She writes in a rather childish way of her plans for getting married.

Case 18.—An attorney aged 37 had a history of severe psychoneurosis complicated with alcoholism of many years' duration. Prefrontal lobotomy relieved his fears but not his alcoholism, and he made an erratic adjustment for several years, enlisting in the Army and serving with the military police until his active service was terminated, after the third court-martial, with a psychiatric discharge. Since then he has been performing legal work for the Government, with increasingly less frequent alcoholic bouts.

Case 19.—A bookbinder aged 40 had been hypochondriacal since girlhood, with a record of twelve to eighteen abdominal operations. She had been bedridden for two years. She walked on the third post-operative day and thereafter recovered slowly, but surely. She has been employed for the past seven years at her old job. She still complains when asked about her symptoms but never mentions them otherwise.

Case 20.—A housewife aged 40, with attacks of manic-depressive psychosis at long intervals, recovered in about a year from an episode in 1929 and was free for seven years. During the attack in 1936 she attempted suicide, sustained severe internal injuries but had only fleeting relief from depression. Prefrontal lobotomy was carried out in December 1936, with fleeting improvement. The following spring she again attempted suicide and sustained extensive burns. The clinical picture was decidedly schizoid at that time, and she was maintained in a psychiatric hospital for over a year. Finally, she received a brief course of metrazol shock therapy and recovered promptly. She has been taking care of her household satisfactorily for the past five years in spite of major domestic difficulties.

Psychiatric Eugenics in Nazi Germany

Fritz Lenz
(1887–1976)

Human Selection and Race Hygiene
(1921)

Adolf Hitler (1889–1945) and the Nazi Party borrowed heavily from earlier racist and eugenic thinkers. Social Darwinism and eugenics advocates had begun to consider what they believed to be the racial implications of natural selection already in the nineteenth century. In Germany, Alfred Ploetz (1860–1940) and Wilhelm Schallmayer (1857–1919) developed the idea of "race hygiene," a program calling for the use of science, medicine, and public policy to promote what they considered to be racial health. And in 1921, Erwin Baur (1875–1933), Eugen Fischer (1874–1967), and Fritz Lenz published *Outline of Human Genetics and Race Hygiene*, a highly acclaimed synthesis of genetics, anthropology, and medicine. The multivolume work quickly became the standard textbook in German race hygiene throughout the 1920s and 1930s, going through five editions between 1921 and 1940. We know that Hitler himself read the second edition while he was serving a prison sentence in the early 1920s.

Fritz Lenz, who authored volume 2 of the book, was a onetime student of Alfred Ploetz. During World War I, he served as a hygienist at a prisoner-of-war camp. He eventually rose to become head of the department of eugenics at the Kaiser-Wilhelm Institute for Anthropology, serving as adviser to the government in the drafting of the 1933 sterilization law (see the following document in this volume). Lenz survived World War II and was hired afterward as a professor of human heredity at the University of Göttingen.

Regarding the truly mentally ill, natural selection is also today still effective, if only not to the same degree as in primitive cultures, where the mentally ill regularly die early. And among native people today, one happens upon the mentally ill far more seldomly than with us, where the insane are cared for and protected. Without this care, most mentally ill would soon fall victim to all sorts of perils, particularly suicide, to which most of them are inclined. A significant number of those predisposed to mental illness are also released from facilities as cured or improved. They then often have the opportunity to reproduce—apparently it has been assumed that this would result in a steady increase in mental illnesses.

Whether the hereditarily mentally ill among us are increasing in number has not been statistically proved or disproved up to this point. The growth in the number of intakes in asylums—for instance, in Bavaria, the figure has risen from 24 per 100,000 residents in 1880 to 50 per 100,000 in 1910—can be explained primarily by the better care in facilities over time. To be sure, paralysis has increased markedly over the past decades; but this is of little interest to us here, since it comes from syphilis, an external cause. At the same time, alcohol-related mental disorders were obviously not as prevalent in earlier times as they were in the decades before the war. It is hardly probable, in fact just the opposite is likely the case, that hereditary mental illnesses are on the rise. There is no valid, statistical evidence for the contention that parents of the mentally ill or the mentally ill themselves have relatively large numbers of children. Among the mentally ill who are accommodated in facilities, two-thirds are single. From the perspective of selection, their institutionalization has an overwhelmingly positive impact; it takes away from the insane the very opportunity to reproduce that they would have outside the facility.

It may be that conditions in simple peasant life may provide more opportunities for the spread of predispositions to mental disorders than is the case for us. My experience during the war with Russian and French prisoners of war appears to provide support for this. Among the Russians, around 9 out of every 10,000 men fell ill with symptoms of schizophrenia every year; but with the French, the figure was only 1.7. Since all told around 14,000 prisoners were observed for three years, it could be only a case of coincidence. The difference may also only be a result of the small numbers that were examined in France, especially since the percentage of those who were not [sic?] let into the army was fairly small. I would like to accept that schizophrenic constitutions can be maintained and propagate more easily under the simpler living conditions of the Russian peasant than in western Europe. Of particular importance in this regard might be the sig-nificant difference in the average age of marriage. Since in central and west-ern Europe, the individual tends to enter into marriage around the end of the third decade, at a time when the majority of cases of schizophrenia have already broken out, only a small portion of those who are predisposed reproduce. In eastern Europe, however, where marriage is entered into already at the end of the second decade, carriers of this predisposition marry in greater number; it is also that case that the state of mind of some peasants leads a woman, even if she is feeble-minded due to illness, to have more children.

Even if in past centuries numerous mentally ill fell victim to a barbaric legal system, and still more simply degenerated into fools, I nevertheless believe that under our present living conditions, natural selection (as it has to do with predispositions to mental illness) is more intensive as it was then. At any rate, present degeneration is frighteningly widespread. According to the national census of 1910, 392 mentally ill and feeble-minded per 100,000 residents were tallied, resulting in more than a quar-ter million for the entire empire; and that naturally counted only those known cases, whereas a tally according to general medical examination of the population would have obviously resulted in a much higher figure. In Switzerland, where surveys have been conducted under medical supervi-sion, 800 to 1,000 mentally disturbed per 100,000 residents were found; and the great majority clearly involve hereditary conditions, since those arising from external causes like paralysis or delirium either quickly lead to death or are generally soon neglected.

Actual idiocy will also certainly be wiped out as it was centuries ago. A large segment among idiotic children die already during the first years of life, and also those idiots who reach an older age naturally never marry and hardly reproduce out of wedlock. The reproduction of clearly feeble-minded persons is also certainly lower than the average; sexual selection in this regard is more effective in males than females. In general, the man must perform a trade in order to be able to marry. Feeble-minded girls, however, are often married without any concern for their mental makeup; in addition, they disproportionately often have illegitimate children, since they are insufficiently able to foresee the consequences of sexual relations. In the entire German Reich, there are 100,000–200,000 feeble-minded and more than 75,000 idiots. Since a large share of the feeble-minded die relatively early in life, the feeble-minded make up a greater portion of newborns than of those later in life. At least 1–2 percent of all births might be feeble-minded and 1/4 percent idiotic.

The lesser degrees of feeble-mindedness pose a greater danger to the fitness of the race than those of a higher degree. Here the reason is the same as with some organic nervous maladies. Due to their predisposition, the moderately feeble-minded are directed toward taking on simple, physical trades, and they have an above-average reproduction. The feeble-minded are naturally the least accessible to deliberate birth control, and the high mortality of their children is being more and more undermined by social welfare measures. Thus, one must reckon with a continuing rise in partial feeble-mindedness.

A share of the epileptics become feeble-minded already early on in their youth, so that reproduction is out of the question. Another share has only isolated attacks, however, and can propagate their predisposition. According to Echeverría, decades ago, the marriage of an epileptic brought only around 3.3 children, of which 1.4 died early; thus, only 1.9 per marriage grew to adulthood. And since many others never even enter into marriage, their propagation is even less likely. Still, however, epilepsy today is extraordinarily widespread. One must expect one epileptic per 300–400 residents, and among newborns, still more.

The selection circumstances of psychopaths are quite involved. Among prisoners of war, I observed pronounced hysteria decidedly more frequently among Russians than among the French. Here a similar train of thought as relates to schizophrenia might be appropriate. "The intensification and accelerated tempo of the modern work process, the noise, the haste, and the heightened responsibility, all this forces countless nerves to collapse, also among the lower classes" (Rüdin). It can be rightly said, then, that natural selection works more toward the decline of nervous tendencies, the more that external living conditions trigger predispositions.

When we hear reports from the Middle Ages of mass mental epidemics, child crusades, flagellations, dance epidemics, and epidemics of possession, we mostly tend to believe that such things are no longer possible in our enlightened age. In Russia, however, "possession" is still fairly common; there it is commonplace for someone to imagine that a snake or some other reptile is inside him. In just the past centuries, Russia has experienced horrible mental epidemics: self-mutilation, numerous self-immolations, strangulation of co-religionists, and child murder based on superstition were an integral part of Russian sects. And when we look around us with open eyes, we can recognize, in some of the mental crazes during and after the war, the effects of similar states of mind.

A significant number of all psychopaths die by their own hand. In the German Reich before the war, around 20 suicides per 100,000 residents annually were counted. Since numerous other cases occurred besides those included in the statistics which were either hidden or counted as accidents, it might have been that around 2–4 percent of all men died by their own hand, whereas suicide was three times less frequent among women. Although that segment of the population in which most suicides take place is noteworthy for its higher intelligence (more advanced students, academics, artists), the selection effect of this phenomenon—one that is considerably co-determined by modern living conditions—is, all told, certainly overwhelmingly positive. Especially predispositions to manic-melancholic mental disturbances, epilepsy, neurasthenia, and other psychopathies are eradicated in this manner. Selection through suicide, therefore, tends in the direction of strengthening the will to live and of a sanguine temperament within the population.

Hardened criminals, who are almost consistently psychopathically predisposed, on average today leave behind fewer offspring. According to Goring, habitual offenders in England married no less frequently than the rest of the population (63 percent versus 62 percent), but they had only 3.5 offspring versus an average of 5.7. Moreover, 31.5 percent of their infants died versus 15.6 percent within the general population. On the other hand, the comparatively milder legal treatment today, in comparison with earlier times, allows for the preservation of unsocial predispositions to a greater extent than earlier.

Those character anomalies that express themselves in sexual perversions have naturally been strongly self-destructive during all historical periods. An entirely peculiar case at present is the case where homosexuals are enlightened by others of their ilk through extensive recruitment. The resulting holding back of this type of person from marriage might work toward a general decrease in psychopathic predispositions.

From Fritz Lenz, *Grundriß der menschlichen Erblichkeitslehre und Rassenhygiene, Bd. 2: Menschliche Auslese und Rassenhygiene* (Munich: J. F. Lehmanns Verlag, 1921), 15–20. Translated by Greg Eghigian.

Germany
"The Law for the Prevention of Hereditarily Ill Offspring"
(14 July 1933)

In January 1933, Adolf Hitler was named chancellor of Germany, and the Nazi Party entered a governing coalition. Within six months, Hitler and the party effectively turned the German government into a one-party system. With a much firmer hold on power, the National Socialists moved to address their domestic policy goals. After first passing a set of laws restricting the rights of German Jews, the new regime established a law in July calling for the compulsory sterilization of those deemed "hereditarily ill." With the law's taking effect in 1934, authorities moved swiftly. In the first year alone, eighty thousand were sterilized. All told, estimates are that around four hundred thousand people were sterilized under the 1933 law, 75 to 80 percent under the diagnosis of "moral feeble-mindedness." In contrast to Sweden, where a similar law was applied almost exclusively to women, the German law was used against both sexes equally.

The Reich government has passed the following law, and hereby announces

§ 1

(1) Anyone who is hereditarily ill can be sterilized, if, according to the experience of medical science, it can be expected in all probability that his [sic] offspring will suffer from severe physical or mental hereditary defects.

(2) Hereditarily ill is, according to this law, anyone suffering from one of the following illnesses:

     congenital feeble-mindedness
     schizophrenia
     manic depression
     hereditary epilepsy
     Huntington's chorea
     hereditary blindness
     hereditary deafness
     severe hereditary physical deformity.

(3) In addition, anyone suffering from severe alcoholism can also be sterilized.

§ 2

(1) Authorized to make a request is anyone who should be sterilized. If this person is legally incompetent or is legally incapacitated because of a mental weakness or has not yet reached age eighteen, then the legal guardian is authorized to make the request. He [sic] requires the permission of the legal guardian court. In all other cases of limited competence, the application requires the consent of the legal guardian. If an adult has a professional caretaker, then his [sic] consent is necessary.

(2) A certificate from a licensed physician in Germany is to be attached, confirming that the individual to be sterilized has been informed about the nature and consequences of the sterilization.

(3) The application can be rejected.

§ 3

For inmates of a hospital, psychiatric or nursing facility, the state physician, or for inmates of a penal facility, the warden, can also apply for sterilization.

§ 4

The application is to sent to the local office of the Hereditary Health Court in written form or dictated as a statement. A medical examination report or something similar must lend credibility to the relevant facts in the application. The local office has to inform the state physician of the application.

§ 5
The District Hereditary Health Court that has general jurisdiction over the individual to be sterilized is responsible for the decision.

§ 6
(1) The Hereditary Health Court is to be affiliated with a regional court. It consists of regional court judge as chair, a state physician, and another physician licensed in Germany who is especially familiar with eugenics. A deputy is to be appointed for each member.

(2) A chair may not be anyone who has decided over an application for permission to guardian rights according to §2, Par. 1. If a state physician has made the application, then he [sic] may not be involved in the decision.

§ 7
(1) The proceedings of the Hereditary Health Court are not public.

(2) The Hereditary Health Court must carry out the necessary investigation. The court can examine witnesses and experts as well as order the personal appearance and medical examination of the individual to be sterilized, and in cases of unexcused absences, to demand his [sic] appearance. Civil court procedure regulations are to be applied as it relates to the examination and the swearing in of witnessing and experts as well as the exclusion and rejection of court personnel. Physicians who are questioned as witnesses or experts are obligated to maintain their professionalism in making a statement. Court and administrative authorities as well as treatment facilities must respond to the Hereditary Court's request for information.

§ 8
The court must come to its own decision on the basis of the entire results of the proceedings and the evidence. The decision is reached following verbal discussion and requires a majority. The decision is to be written up and to be signed by all those members participating in its formulation. It must cite the reasons for which the sterilization has been approved or rejected. The decision is to be sent to the original applicant, the state physician, as well as to that person for whom the sterilization was applied, or, in the case they are not legally capable, to his [sic] legal representative.

§ 9

Persons identified in §8, Sentence 5 can submit a written or dictated appeal of the decision before the local office of the Hereditary Health Court within a period of one month after its delivery. The appeal postpones any decision. The Hereditary Health Court decides on the appeal. If the appeal deadline is missed, then restitutio in integrum in keeping with the guidelines of civil proceedings is permissible.

§ 10

(1) The Superior Hereditary Health Court is affiliated with the Regional Superior Court and has jurisdiction over the same district. It consists of a member of the Regional Superior Court, a state physician, and a physician licensed in Germany, who is especially familiar with eugenics. A deputy is to be appointed for each member. §6, Par. 2 obtains, as appropriate.

(2) Procedures before the Superior Hereditary Court are governed by §§7, 8.

(3) The decision of the Superior Hereditary Court is final.

§ 11

(1) The necessary surgical procedure for the sterilization may only be carried out in a treatment facility by a physician licensed in Germany. This physician may only first undertake the operation, once the order for sterilization is finalized. The highest authority in the federal state determines the treatment facilities and physicians who are authorized to perform the sterilization. The operation may not be undertaken by the physician who made the application or served as a member of the committee in the proceedings.

(2) The physician performing the operation must file a written report to the state physician about the performance of the sterilization, with information about the procedures applied.

§ 12

(1) If the court has made a final decision in favor of sterilization, it is to be carried out even against the will of the person to be sterilized, as long as this individual has not filed an appeal. The state physician is to enlist police authorities to carry out necessary measures. If other measures are not sufficient, then the application of direct force is permitted.

(2) If circumstances exist that demand another examination of the evidence, then the Hereditary Court is to rehear the case, and the sterilization is to be temporarily postponed. If the application was [originally] rejected, then a rehearing is only permissible if new facts have emerged that justify the sterilization.

§ 13
(1) The state carries the costs of the court proceedings.

(2) The costs of the medical operation are covered by the sickness insurance board to which the person belongs, [or] for those in need, the welfare association. In all other cases, the costs are covered by the state and the individual being sterilized, up to the lowest standard rates according to medical fee regulations and the average standard rates for public treatment centers.

§ 14
Sterilization that does not follow the regulations of this law as well as a removal of the gonads are only permissible if a physician carries them out according to governing practices in medicine, in order to avoid a serious threat to the life or health of the individual on whom the operation is being performed and with their consent.

§ 15
(1) Persons taking part in the legal proceedings or in carrying out the surgical operation are obligated to keep these secret.

(2) Anyone violating confidentiality will be sentenced to prison for up to one year or given a fine. Prosecution is initiated only on the basis of an application. The chair can submit the application.

§ 16
(1) The execution of this law is the responsibility of the federal states.

(2) The highest state authorities determine the location and district of the responsible courts, subject to regulation §6, Par. 1, Sentence 1 and §10, Par. 1, Sentence 1. They name the members and their deputies.

§ 17
The Reich Minister of Interior, in agreement with the Reich Minister of Justice, issues the necessary legal and administrative regulation for executing this law.

§ 18

This law comes into force on 1 January 1934.

The Reich Chancellor Adolf Hitler

The Reich Minister of Interior Frick

The Reich Minister of Justice Dr. Gürtner

From Gesetz zur Verhütung erbkranken Nachwuchses vom 14. Juli 1933, www.documentarchiv.de. Translated by Greg Eghigian.

Documents on the "T-4" and "14f13" Programs
(1939–1945)

Using the outbreak of World War II as a pretext, Hitler directed his personal physician, Karl Brandt, in 1939 to initiate a program that would carry out the medical killing of individuals deemed to be living a "life unworthy of life." Asylum directors, pediatricians, psychiatrists, nurses, and hospital staff were recruited for the operation, which became known as the T-4 Program. Officially running from October 1939 until August 1941, the program was responsible for the killings of around one-third of the institutionalized psychiatric population—men, women, and children—by means of starvation, medication overdose, or gassing. Although the program was supposed to be clandestine—lies were concocted to tell relatives about the fate of their loved ones—rumors spread. By fall 1941, the T-4 Program was formally discontinued. The killings went on, however, shrouded in more secrecy than ever. In addition, many T-4 personnel were transferred to eastern Europe, where their experience was used to run a new SS operation aimed at killing concentration camp inmates incapable of hard labor or suffering from incurable diseases—the 14f13 Program. During the years 1939–1945, roughly two hundred thousand people were killed under the two programs.

The following texts give us a glimpse into the thinking and logistics behind the killing operations and what staff and patients knew about them. The first is a letter by Dr. Irmfried Eberl, the director of the gassing facilities in Brandenburg and Bernburg, in which he discusses his views on a draft of a possible euthanasia law (the law was never enacted). The second is an internal T-4 document that shows just how informally directives were transmitted to personnel. The third text represents a report by a former patient at the asylum in Grafeneck, entered into evidence during the 1949 trial of staff who had been involved in the T-4 operations there. The final document is postwar testimony from Dietrich Allers, the former head of the Central Euthanasia Office (a German court later found him to be involved in at least thirty-four thousand deaths).

Position of Dr. Irmfried Eberl on the Draft of a Planned Euthanasia Law (with Reference to Mercy Killing and the Elimination of "Life Unworthy of Life")

6 July 1940

To Reich Committee for the Scientific Registration of Severe
    Hereditary and Constitutional Afflictions

Berlin W 9

Post Box 101

Re: Your Letter of 3 July 1940

On the naming of the law, I can say nothing more on the subject, for it is my opinion that the title "Law on the Killing of Those Incapable of Living" would be the most sensible, but it had to be abandoned. The term "assistance in dying" [Sterbehilfe] is unfamiliar, but it will doubtless gain relevant content through the law itself.

The demarcation of registered cases according to the law is clear in §1. In §2, under these cases would fall:

a) all schizophrenics, as long as they are capable of no or only mechanical occupational activity;

b) all feeble-minded who are no longer capable of any productive activity, including within the facility;

c) all syphilitic patients for whom the course of the disease is so advanced that they are no longer capable of productive work;

d) all epileptics who either have frequent seizures or manifest significant changes in character;

e) all cases of senile dementia who are considerably unclean and also require constant commitment in a therapeutic or nursing home facility and, in their earlier years, made no notable contributions to the benefit of the people or the nation;

f) in addition, all remaining mental disturbances that are not suited to productive activity.

Productive activity refers to the fact that the patient in question does not simply perform mechanical activities, but rather he, for example, in agriculture, works with others and is capable of making appropriate contributions. Patients who, for instance, run around in field details, but there do nothing or very little, are obviously to be included. Furthermore, all criminals who require psychiatric institutionalization naturally fall under this law.

As to the substantive content, I have the following to say:

Re: §2, Par. 2. Here, acquired afflictions that are caused by war injury or factory accident are to be excluded. I would like to restrict this exception in sofar as such a patient can be given assistance in dying, if he expressly wishes it.

Re: §4, Par. 4. Here I would like to broach the question of whether two years of institutional observation suffices in order to determine that a chronic mental illness is incurable.

. . . .

The medical community will welcome this law, particularly §1, since the physician is often in the situation where severely ill, incurable patients long for death, yet he is not in the position today to provide this help; in this case, the killing must fall to his own conscience.

It is also the case that the people will absolutely understand and welcome §1, apart from the absolutely Catholic-oriented part of the population. The impact of the second part of the law will be another matter, i.e., the elimination of life unworthy of life. Even if it's the case that this kind of law is already in the air to some extent—thus, a part of our people will understand it—a not insignificant part will offer considerable resistance, in particular when it come to the family members of the mentally ill. The further consequence of this will be that it will become much harder to get the mentally ill into institutions, as long as they have the slightest possibility of accommodation and care at home. What consequences this can have for public health and criminality is hard to assess. Nevertheless, I believe that this law will gain acceptance just as the marriage health law and the law for the prevention of hereditarily ill offspring themselves have over time and that, with appropriate enlightenment—which would have to be done at the same time or, better yet, before its announcement—the law will meet with appropriate approval. . . .

Heil Hitler!

Eberl

"Removal According to a Strict Standard": Medical Examination Report Standards of Bouhler/Brandt—an Internal T-4 Document

Decisions about euthanasia-authorized personnel with regard to medical examination reporting (taking into account the results of the conversation at Berchtesgaden on 10 March 1941)*

1. The removal of all those who are incapable of performing productive work (including in institutions), in other words, not only the mentally dead.

2. Not to be included are those war veterans who have served on the front, were wounded, or have received decorations. In evaluating the value of merits on the front, particularly decorations, Herr Jennerwein makes the decision.[†] Questionable upcoming cases that appear in our facilities are to be returned there until Herr Jennerwein has made a decision on the basis of the records. Otherwise, war participation does not protect one from being included in the operation.

3. With seniles, the greatest restraint, only in pressing circumstances, e.g., criminality or asociality, inclusion. In both of these last cases, records are to be consulted in each case and copies of excerpts from the documents are to be attached.

---

*Editor's note: Philipp Bouhler was head of the Office of the Chancellery. Karl Brandt was Hitler's personal physician. Both men acted as Hitler's authorized representatives in the killing program, taking orders directly from the Führer himself, often from his retreat in Berchtesgaden.

[†]Editor's note: "Jennerwein" was the pseudonym of Viktor Brack, an engineer working in Hitler's chancellery office who later became involved in the construction of a number of death camps.

4. Only German nationals are to be included in the operation, in other words, no Poles. A concentration of all Poles in purely Polish facilities in the eastern districts is foreseen. Outside of the Protectorate, institutionalized Czechs of German nationality can be included. Czechs of Czech nationality are supposed to be deported to the Protectorate.

If citizenship cannot be determined, this should be determined by our authorized personnel, if possible.

In cases where citizenship still cannot be determined, the case should be rejected until a conclusive conversation with State Secretary Frank.

Enemy foreigners may also not be included in the operation. Of those who have no citizenship whatsoever, only those for whom it can be proved they have had no one looking after them for a longer period of time.

5. For the time being, do not work in Alsace, Lorraine, Luxemburg, Eupen, Malmedy, the Protectorate and [General] Government.

6. Foreign and stateless Jews are to be placed in a Jewish facility built for them, insofar as deportation to their homeland—thinking here in particular of Switzerland—is not possible.

For Jews from overseas, a notification is not to take place.

7. The children who fall within the large operation will be medically examined and reexamined by the national consortium of psychiatric and nursing care facilities. Those cases that are positively evaluated will be given over to the national committee for removal.

The children in Bethel should be treated with special care.

Otherwise, just as before, removal according to a *strict standard*!

"I fear that the Führer's book *Mein Kampf* represents the foundation": Copy of a Report of the Patient Richard H. (Zwiefalten)

The rumor—that in Grafeneck people were being turned into angels and the corpses were being burned, so that graves could not be dug, no cause of death determined—did not come from me. I made the sole mistake of *speaking openly* about what others recount, in the presence of nurses, to repeat it, in order to give them the possibility of denying the rumor. This rumor comes from multiple outside sources, I cannot be made responsible for what is common knowledge in Stuttgart and in other cities.

Proof.

1. A patient who is no longer here told 15 patients, he himself witnessed how two children ages 5 and 6 were given an injection in another ward, after which they died. So that no examination would be possible, both were taken to G. and burned. It is clear that I could not say anything, since all the patients know that I was not on such a ward, but the 15 patients heard this.

2. Another patient recounted, he himself overheard a staff person ask another, "What did you see in Grafeneck?" This one answered, "You don't see anything of the operations, that's a lie, you can only see how the smoke from the cremations rises." I didn't tell anyone about it, I did not see any smoke and didn't hear any staff people.

3. A visitor (I did not have the visit myself) brought the news that a teacher by the name of Sch. arrived from Weissenau to Gr. and there disappeared. Family members inquired and finally it was admitted he died shortly after arrival in G., that is well known in the entire town. I know nothing about that, I didn't tell anyone.

4. Many patients say they themselves have seen that the car, when it arrives empty in order to pick up patients, each time brings 4–5 large bags full of old clothes and shoes that come from those cremated. I myself have seen no bag, no clothes, no shoes, I didn't tell anyone.

5. A patient who shortly returned, but is no longer here, told 15 patients, he met a painter on a transport in the Munich police jail, who 2 years earlier had worked on the paintings from the old monastery in the facility, and this guy told him, he was now in preventive detention, on his way to Dachau, because he spoke *truthfully* about the fact that various patients in the facility here died an unnatural death, and, so that a cause of death could not later be determined, corpses were brought to G. and burned. I didn't tell anyone about this, I was not on the transport, I have not been in Munich for 6 years.

6. Many report that transports arrive at G. every week, from Weissenau, Reichenau, Wiesloch, Schussenried, Winnenden, Zwiefalten, etc. [ ] these transports were kept secret, one can ask the nurses, drivers, etc. where the others went, but nobody says anything.

7. One patient said, he was sent to G. and was given a stamp on the shoulder like the others, later the doctor saw this mark and, in the presence of the patient, scolded the staff person responsible for the stamp, [saying] he had said this man is to be set free, he does not belong with the others,

this one is not supposed to be stamped. After that, the mark was removed with a strong liquid.

8. Paul R. got a letter that was widely read, R. let lots of others read it, his wife wrote, "Are you still in Zwiefalten, are you still alive, we hear so much these days."

9. A patient said in front of many others that a staff person told him R. and U. had also been removed.

10. Another patient recounts, Herr Tr. was removed.

11. A patient recounts and repeated that: Two months ago, his mother visited him, got to know a woman whose was visiting her son here at the time. Shortly after, his mother wrote this [second] woman, asking when she was going to Zwiefalten next, and the answer she received was, unfortunately she can no longer visit her son, he left Zwiefalten, [but] she cannot find out where to, he probably is no longer alive.

12. I fear that the Führer's book *Mein Kampf*, that lies here, represents the foundation for such rumors, for there on page 144 it states, one is supposed to raise many children, but one must also be sure those who are raised eliminate all mental and physical weakness, in order to prevent overpopulation, all wishy-washy humanitarianism here is only cowardice, etc.

Difficulties in Keeping Secrets:
Statement of Dietrich Allers, Manager of T4

On taking on my position [January 1941] with the National Consortium [of Psychiatric and Nursing Care Facilities], the situation was such that only the relatives of patients who were subject to euthanasia were informed about the death. The original facility and the local welfare association looking after the patient were simply told that, with the patient being transferred to a transitional facility, their responsibilities were over. Questions involving the whereabouts of the patient were supposed to be answered with reference to the order of the responsible national defense commissar and all mail for the patients as well as all other questions directed to the national consortium.

For everyone who knew about the collaboration of various state authorities, quasi-governmental agencies as well as economic organizations, it is clear that considerable confusion arose. The first consequence was naturally that all the national defense commissars were flooded with questions from relatives and interested service providers. In principle, the national defense commissars were provided with the transfer orders and were also informed about the course of the euthanasia measures, but were naturally not given specific details. Thus, after an initial response, they sent questions, etc. on to the National Consortium. The welfare agencies had to know what became of the patients, since they had contested patient costs and, to some extent, had taken on pensions and other patient benefits. They demanded reimbursement for earlier benefits, partly the personal effects, partly they wanted to follow up on the reimbursement claims on behalf of responsible relatives. For many patients, there were insurances of various kinds. The insurance companies appeared and demanded information, since, in the meantime, the inheritors were making insurance claims. The finance offices demanded information because the registry offices that were solely created for the purpose of euthanasia, as a result of not knowing the regulations, failed to inform the former about the patient's demise. In part, inheritance courts popped up with questions directed at the National Consortium. This was especially the case for what was called at the time the Ostmark, where surviving family member hearings were required according to Austrian law. Finally, quasi-governmental agencies, under whose authority patients in state hospitals were institutionalized, needed to be informed. Military draft authorities, who were also interested in male residents in the facilities, were to be informed. In different cases, local welfare organizations and municipal welfare authorities were among those asking questions. And finally, there was the notification of the health offices. That was important because of existing marriage laws at the time.

I believe, with this, I have detailed what kind of work I had before me. If you imagine that the euthanasia program ran for more than a year, you can get a sense of the extent of my activities.

From Ernst Klee, ed., *Dokumente zur "Euthanasie"* (Frankfurt: Fischer Taschenbuch Verlag, 1985), documents no. 25 (pp. 87–91), no. 32 (pp. 100–103), no. 41 (pp. 112–114), no. 55 (pp. 140–141). © 1985 Fischer Taschenbuch Verlag GmbH, Frankfurt am Main. Translated by Greg Eghigian.

Mental Illness, Psychiatry, and Communism

Thea H.
(b. 1923)
An Experience of Psychosis
in Post–World War II Germany
(1949)

The experience of hallucination (perceiving someone or something that is really not there) has long been recognized in Western society as a characteristic feature of mental disorder. While ethnopsychiatrists and historians have noted some striking similarities in the form that hallucinations have assumed over history, it is also clear that the content of psychotic experiences differs across societies and time periods. The following is an excerpt from a letter written by a German woman, Thea H. (her name has been changed to protect her identity), to her doctors in the spring of 1949, shortly after she was checked into the psychiatric clinic at the Charité Hospital in East Berlin. It offers us a unique glimpse into the mind of a person still actively hallucinating.

Thea H.'s case is particularly instructive in that it takes place against the backdrop of the end of World War II. Following the war, both Germany and the city of Berlin were divided into zones of military occupation (American, British, French, and Russian). Thea H. was a student living in West Berlin at this time. Hospital records indicate that she was a devout communist, a fact that apparently led to her being arrested by the Nazis and held in a concentration camp during the years 1943–1945. Over the course of the four years following her release from the camp, she found herself in and out of psychiatric institutions, including the facility at Haldensleben, under the direction of Dr. Ziegelrot. There, doctors may well have administered electroshock to her, this being a common form of treatment for schizophrenia at the time.

28 May 1949

So, you want to know everything—from the point of the events, so to speak, up to this present moment when my powers have left me? I will now try again to make visible the order of events and all those powers that affect being and consciousness—external events, perception, thoughts into words—will words be enough to convey an alien consciousness? I don't know, but I will nevertheless demonstrate my good intentions.

It was already there in those days and in those thoughts that circled around in my head. Its central point was that paper about transportation, its statistics, and the question about to what extent it served as a mirror image of economic development. Economic development—how varied are its factors and how pathetic, by contrast, are the indicators of transportation statistics. I had rummaged around, combined, rejected and could not recognize the standard picture of simple production numbers in correlation with the track lengths and shipping. The organic structure of capitalism appeared to me much more significant. It must provide the basis for the connection of the real relationships between the transportation process and the normal production processes.

On this question of a mistaken assessment of the matter of organic structure, I went to Lenin and Stalin for advice. Suddenly the wonderful conceptual formulation of the organic structure fell into place. . . . After having finished the reassessment and formulation of the basic thinking of my essay in my paper "Costs and Prices," which hardly struck me in the end as my own product, I chatted with Stalin about the question of the dialectic in connection with the immortality of the human soul. I explained to him that I could not believe in the immortality of the soul on the basis of the theory of dialectics alone. . . . Dialectical materialism teaches that the highest form of living material is the brain as the organ of consciousness. If this highest form of living material dies as a consequence of the death of the human body and, in its wake, the brain is transformed into its inorganic parts, then a qualitative change must result that we cannot yet pursue in reality, in the sense of the Leninist approach to human knowledge.

Stalin replied to this: "My dear child, naturally you are right, for those invisible unities of consciousness are just the very things that are at the disposal of our active and developing consciousness in order to point out those processes of the past that still have an effect in the present."

. . . In the course of the argument I was having, a terrible doubt about the adequacy of my capacity for judgment now overcame me. I raised a great many objections against the right to influence my thought in this unreal form, such that by the end, it was no longer clear to me what remained of my own mental properties. With that, I was once again with Stalin. "But my little child," he grinned at me, "we are simply giving you [questions], in association with your inner complex of questions that have emerged out of the confrontation with the world around us—these are relevant preconditions for your further development, for as everyone knows, questions emerge wherever in real life a solution is needed. As an intellectual worker—something you want to become—you will solve these questions to a certain extent as part of your training. And how this looks within the scope of the constantly working collective consciousness, we will show you one day. First, you will get to know your own capabilities; second, we will get to know you, something even more important; and third, you will learn how you have to work as a part of the intellectual collective production process, as soon as it becomes a question of peace and the future existence of this world." With these words, he looked at me sadly, smiled, and disappeared.

In his place appeared Prof. Ziegelrot, who once posed the question to me in [the psychiatric facility at] Haldensleben, "And do you really know whether you were schizophrenic?" This time he said very seriously and measured, "You don't believe that we exist, we who are speaking with you. We will prove it to you. And since this question so desperately interests you, you will do what we recommend. You are now a part of a scientific experiment intended to answer the question, 'What is schizophrenia?'" Since I still did not know whether everything was merely an apparition or reality, I submitted to this instruction, but decided in the meantime to not accept it as reality and made notes in my gray notebook about the instructions of the collective. These notes, in which I acted as an experimental subject for an experiment in suggestion, . . . had to have something to say about the question posed at the beginning. Over the course of the night, however, the experiment took a strange turn. I was told there is not only organic, living material on the earth, but also that this material is subject to laws of development that extend beyond the earth. Organic life has the function of setting off a process on this earth that has long since taken place on other stars. We now had to carry this out on our star using atom splitting. I despairingly challenged this line of thinking. "You have to ask all human beings before I perform such an insane act." I wrung my hands.

Like a pale death's head, it grinned at me. "But you are located at such a low level of intellectual development, that you can't conceive it," was the reply.

"But no," I retorted, "every human being comprehends life, some more instinctively, others more unconsciously. The present action is determined by two different spheres. . . . For every human being, [these spheres] can be developed in a harmonious, interconnected fashion."

The skulls widened their grins: "No," said one of them, "we suspect that in your head is located the highest level of processed subconscious. [And since] we know your family, we want to observe your consciousness level while you sleep. Very slowly, we will force you to fall asleep, so that we can eavesdrop. Your consciousness level is the final life process on earth that remains unknown to us. But we want this other world, of which we know nothing, and for this, we must destroy this world of human maggots."

That was too much for my heart, which was full of joie de vivre and kindness. I decided to refuse to go along. . . . Dead eyes watched me and waited for my murderous sleep. I followed the hand of the clock till about 8 a.m. and trembled with my notebook in hand as my sole piece of evidence of this criminal experiment. I then quickly dressed. Where should I now go? I packed up my work from the past few weeks in my bag and left the house. In the thaw of the morning, I marched the streets, not knowing my goal, finally ending up at my friend's.

. . . . .I finally sought out a doctor I trusted, Dr. Erdmann, and told him of my dilemma. There, suddenly, as I tried to explain to him the events of the past few days, it hit me like a hammer, the knowledge of clarity rejoiced in me. Two powers have been wrestling in the world, and now, at this moment, contact was established. Your inner wrestling is only a reflex of outward reality. . . .

Once again on the streets, I didn't know the way I should go. Slowly I turned in the direction of the zone border Berlin-Brandenburg. Suddenly a harsh voice said, "We know that this world must be destroyed. Destroyed will be the world of suffering, of hate, of death, of dearth, and in its place will be built a world of life and joy." And then softer, "Do you believe that?" Sad and exhausted after a sleepless night, I sank to the ground and looked at the radiant evening sky. "I can't believe what I don't know," I answered. "Don't you see that I am a German? For us, death was cloaked as life, and belief murdered loved ones. I can no longer believe." Suddenly, Einstein shook his gray head, looked around, and spoke to an assembly of learned men: "We have to teach her to believe." And then he looked me in the eye just like the evening sky had radiated earlier. "Lay your two hands together," he spoke in a friendly way, "and tell us in whom you believe. You are to receive a treasure from us and to bring it to those in whom you have faith, so that the world can live in peace." "Ach," I lamented, "it's not so much faith, but I have always had the experience in my life that they have been right, and I have constantly felt safe in their hands. I know I could be wrong, but I believe in the Russians." These words provoked a peal of laughter, and it was as if the leaves of the trees shook in the dying evening wind.

"But, little thing," Einstein finally uttered, "then you are a Bolshevik, and you belong in the Russian zone. Now see to it that the CIC [American counterintelligence] does not get you! But as a sign that you may believe in us, we are giving you something that you are to carry over. It is a power. It can destroy or create. You trust in the people and in the SED [the East German Communist Party]. Now go there, and when you arrive at the [Communist] party school with the gift we now give you, then you and your faith have won, then you have convinced us. And so that you know, we are the collective consciences of the world." And with these words, I sensed something heavy in my hands and could not pry them apart. As I now crossed the border, my limbs were heavy and I sensed how the weight of the power in my hands changed. "Slowly," a voice warned me, "in your hands, you hold the contact. If it tears, then the unity of the world is destroyed. You must protect it."

I informed the border police jubilantly that the unity of the world had been prepared. . . . The policemen led me into a house, which I believed was the party school. On the walls hung Karl Marx and a motto "Freedom Is Insight into Necessity." They then called the Karl-Marx-School. As they all grouped around me and then more came, I started trusting. And then one of them spoke in a quiet voice: "You have reached your goal. Pry your hands apart." I believed him and did what I was directed. I then determined, how- ever, that this was only the police, and that made me sad. They then led me back to the zone border. Everything was still as it had been. Beams stared over the street, and I was told to make my way home in the Ami [Ameri- can] sector. I traveled a bit in a car that happened to pass by. I found every- thing so gloomy and dead, as if it was the night before the end of the world. But upon the first rays of the rising sun, I staggered back across the zone border into the Russian zone, to my friend's, until I fell exhausted at her feet.

This then was schizophrenia—atomic physics felt in one's own body? My friend brought me here in this madhouse, and here I live until today and ask myself: "How can a human being live in a world with a divided world-consciousness without herself suffering from a split consciousness???"

From Bundesarchiv Berlin DQ1/5571. Translated by Greg Eghigian.

Records in the Case of Pyotr Grigorenko
(1969–1970)

Pyotr Grigorenko (1907–1987) was a decorated major general in the Soviet Red Army, who, by the 1960s, came to believe that the USSR was no longer living up to its ideals. Grigorenko became involved in founding a dissident organization and distributing fliers calling for more democratic governance. Arrested in 1964, he was sent to the Serbsky Institute for Forensic Psychiatry in Moscow for psychiatric evaluation. Clinicians there determined that his reformist views reflected "a paranoid personality development with delusions," and he was committed to a psychiatric institution. He was soon released, but over the following four years he continued speaking out on human rights issues. Arrested again, he was examined by a psychiatrist, who declared him sane. Unsatisfied, the KGB sent him one more time to the Serbsky Institute for an evaluation, which took place in November 1969. The experts at the institute once again declared him insane, and Grigorenko was committed to a psychiatric facility for the following several years. In 1991, four years after his death, a special Russian panel of psychiatric experts reexamined the files in Grigorenko's case and declared him to have been clinically sane.

Grigorenko's was only the most famous of numerous cases in which sane Soviet political dissidents were committed to psychiatric facilities beginning in the early 1960s. Studies conducted after the fall of the USSR indicate that the practice involved party and state officials, hospitals, and psychiatrists. One conservative estimate is that between 1960 and 1985 around 300–675 dissidents were being held in Soviet psychiatric institutions at any given time.

Grigorenko's Account of His Psychiatric Examination
at the Serbsky Institute, Written Immediately after the Examination
by the Committee of Experts, in the Period 20–25 November 1969

There is a large room, solidly crammed with office desks. One of these is in the middle of the room, with four persons seated at it. In the chairman's place is a fairly young-looking, plump man with brown, slightly curly hair. I learned afterwards that this was the director of the Serbsky Institute and an associate member of the U.S.S.R. Academy of Medical Sciences, Morozov. To his left is Lunts and on his right in a brown suit, the only one not wearing a white coat. Maiay Mikhailovna sits opposite the chairman. They show me a place across from the desk, near the chairman. I sit down, I look around.

"Do you see many acquaintances?" I am asked.

"Yes, but of my old acquaintances there is only Daniel Romanych and the doctor who sits over there by the window. I met him in Leningrad in 1964 when the question of my discharge from the Lenin Special Psychiatric Hospital was decided. The others," I say pointing to the doctors of the fourth section, "are current acquaintances."

I realize that the commission is at the central desk, the others present being students. They are settled at desks placed by the wall. . . . Please note that Lunts is the only one whom I call by his family name: this is a peculiarity of the system. According to the law they are obliged to give me the full names of everyone on the commission, and I even have the right to reject some and solicit for the inclusion of others. That is how it was in Tashkent, but here we have high priests who act with pomp and ceremony, and I, worthless being that I am, do not even have the right to know who they are. But let us return to the commission. The chairman begins the discussion:

"Well, how do you feel?"

"I do not know how to answer you. Probably like a guinea pig would feel if he were able to realize his situation."

"I am not talking about that. I would like to know if you feel differently from how you did at the session here in 1964."

"Yes."

"How?"

"You see, at that time such a method of investigation, transforming a defendant into a madman, was something for which I was completely unprepared. I was literally shocked by this discovery and looked upon the staff at this place as specially selected, hardened criminals. I believed that I had been brought here to 'give official sanction' to my confinement in an insane asylum for the rest of my days. Therefore, I despised all the employees and was extremely overwrought and irritable. I did not want to follow any of the rules and gave much time to the political enlightenment of the psychiatric experts. All this obviously made a terrible impression on those around me and might have given some sort of grounds for pronouncing me insane."

"As Daniel Romanovich told me, you said to him in a conversation that what had happened then seemed as though it was happening in a fog."

"I say the same thing now. My discovery was such a great shock that I still regard what happened then as a terrible nightmare."

"And now."

"Now my position is different. First of all, the examination by a commission of experts was no surprise for me. Secondly, I have known many very decent psychiatrists, and I have tried to remember, even when dealing with a criminal institution, that among the people who work there might be some completely honest individuals. So I have decided in all my personal contacts to concentrate my attention precisely on those decent ones. Now I am completely calm and see around me, not simply doctors, but people. I hope that the experts will try to see me as a human being too." (I smiled at him.)

"Yes, but all you say is related to the events of the examination itself, whereas there were actions which even without the doctors, raised doubts about your sanity."

"I do not know of any such actions."

"But here in the record of the proceedings of the commission which determined the possibility of ceasing your confinement in the Leningrad Special Psychiatric Hospital, it is stated that you admitted that your actions were wrong."

"And I admit it now."

"How can you co-ordinate your two statements?"

"It is very simple. Not every mistake a person makes is the result of a disturbed mind. My mistakes were caused by my incorrect political development—I was too much of a rugged, straightforward Bolshevik-Leninist by education. I had become accustomed to thinking that only what Lenin taught is correct. Therefore, when I came up against the discrepancy between what Lenin wrote and how it was in real life, I saw only one way out: back to Lenin. But this was a mistake. Irreversible changes have taken place in our life and no one can turn life back to 1924, or even to 1953. Further accomplishments can be achieved only by starting from the present day, using Lenin's theoretical heritage creatively, and taking into account all past experience. When I acknowledge the error of my actions, I was thinking above all of this lack of understanding. I did not reveal this then because they did not require this from me. Therefore, the fact that my mistakes had nothing to do with those being corrected by psychiatric interference remained unexplained."

"How do you explain the fact that after psychiatric intervention you acted normally for a year and a half and then went back to your old ways?"

"The psychiatrists had nothing to do with my so-called 'normal' behavior. I presume you are referring to the fact that I wrote nothing for distribution." (The chairman nodded affirmatively.) "I wrote nothing in 1965 and 1966 for two reasons, which were beyond my own or the psychiatrists' control. The first reason was there was no time. I worked as a loader in two stores in order to earn a living for myself and my family. I earned 132 roubles in total, which is almost as much as I paid income tax for my salary at the Military Academy. The work was very hard. The working day was twelve hours and there was no day off. I was exhausted when I got home and had only enough strength to get into bed. I lost so much weight that my clothes hung on me as they would on a hanger. The second reason for my silence is that during this first year and a half I still hoped that they would restore my hard-earned pension, which had been unlawfully taken away from me. If this had happened, I would not be talking to you now. While I was in the Leningrad Hospital I had already planned that I would write a history of the Great Patriotic War [World War II] when I was released. My heart was set on this work. But experience showed that illegal repressions do not cease, but instead piled up with time. The fact that I was barred from any kind of work, which forced me and my family to live in a state of semi-starvation, together with the never-ending insolent and illegal shadowing, demonstrated graphically that the time had not yet come for me to climb into an ivory tower and pursue 'pure science.' As long as our country is not provided with a reliable shield against tyranny it is the duty of every honest man to participate in creating this shield, whatever the threats to him. But you are mistaken when you say that I went back to my old ways. What I have done in the past two years does not even superficially resemble my old ways." . . .

"Do you definitely want to be brought to trial?"

"Unfortunately it is not up to me to decide this question. Of course, I would prefer to have the case discontinued at the preliminary investigation stage. But, I repeat, this does not depend on me."

"But treatment could save you from being brought to trial."

"There is nothing for me to be treated for, and I have no intention of feigning illness in order to be spared responsibility. I am prepared to answer fully for my actions."

"But if they convict you, you will lose your pension."

"There is a good Russian proverb: 'If they cut off your head, you don't cry over your hair.' Whether I am convicted or put in a prison called a special psychiatric hospital, I have still lost my freedom. And a pension cannot take the place of freedom. Why should I grieve over my pension? Why assume I will be convicted without fail? I do not consider myself guilty and I will try to prove this to the court."

"So you plan to defend yourself regardless of everything?"

"I do not quite understand what you mean by 'regardless of everything.' I do not plan to lie or shift. I will speak about my activities frankly and honestly and give my motives for them. All in all, I will face the truth as I see it. But even if I do not succeed in proving my innocence, the maximum sentence I could get, according to the article under which I am charged, is three years. This means that by the time the sentence takes effect I will have about two years left to serve. A so-called cure would take no less time. Moreover, I would not spend these two years in a closed prison, but in a labor camp, where I would work in fresh air among normal people. Furthermore, they could give me less than three years, or even exile—there are precedents for this—in which case I would not lose my pension. Finally, there is always the possibility of an amnesty on the occasion of Lenin's birth centenary. If I am convicted this amnesty could apply to me. If I receive 'treatment,' the possibility is excluded. They don't give a madman amnesty from his illness."

With that my second forensic psychiatric examination for the year and my second encounter with the Serbsky Institute came to an end. I still do not know the results of the Serbsky commission. When I find out it will finally be clear to me whether this Institute is merely a criminal establishment left over from the accursed past or if the people there are also foul criminals, dangerous to society, who hide themselves behind white coats.

Report No. 59/S on the In-Patient Forensic
Psychiatric Examination of P. G. Grigorenko

On 19 November 1969 in the Serbsky Central Scientific Research Institute of Forensic Psychiatry, an examination was made of P. G. Grigorenko, born in 1907, and charged under Article 190–1 of the Russian Criminal Code. Grigorenko entered the Institute in compliance with an order of 13 October 1969 from the Investigator of Especially Important Cases of the Uzbeck Procuracy in connection with doubts about the psychological soundness of the patient.

From statements by the patient, medical records and documents of the case, it is known that he lost his mother at an early age, grew up in difficult material circumstances and began to do heavy physical labor while staying quite young. He was a weak unhealthy child. He began school at the age of eight. In character he was lively, sociable, inquisitive, easily carried away and candid. He always stood up for his own opinions and defended the weak. He was a good student After completing the fourth form, he went to work as a metal worker's apprentice. From this time onwards he took an active part in public life and entered the Komsomol [a Soviet youth organization]. He studied at the Workers' Faculty of the Kharkov Technological Institute. In 1931 he was enlisted in the army and sent to the Military Engineering Academy. . . .

He later graduated from the General Staff Academy and served in Kharbarovsk until 1943. He worked, in his own words, with enthusiasm and tried to investigate every matter thoroughly, always looking for what, in his opinion, had significance for the solution of the given problem.

In the early years of the war he received a Party reprimand for critical remarks about the state of the Soviet armed forces. From 1943, he took part in the Patriotic War. In 1944, he was wounded in the leg and suffered a contusion with brief loss of consciousness. He was not hospitalized.

After the war he was employed at the Frunze Military Academy as a senior instructor, and in 1949 defended his master's thesis. . . . In 1959, he was appointed head of the Faculty of Military Administration. At this time he had no complaints about his health, was active, conducted scientific work, published articles, and followed the social and political events in the country. He pondered a great deal over the occurrences at the twentieth Party Congress and came to the conclusion that the consequences of the "personality cult" had not yet been eliminated completely and that there were still "Bonapartist methods of work" in the Party.

In 1961, he expressed "critical remarks" at a district Party conference and was afterwards dismissed from his post. He took this very hard, was convinced of his innocence and tried to restore his rights. At this time, he suffered headaches, noises in the head, and pains in his heart. He became more quick-tempered and irritable and could not stand contradiction. In 1962, Grigorenko was assigned to the post of chief of the Operations Department of the army in the Maritime Territory.

As is evident from Report No. 25/S of the forensic psychiatric examination in 1964, which contains information about his period of service in the Maritime Territory, Grigorenko, in addition to being energetic and exceptionally industrious, suffered from conceit; overestimated his knowledge and capabilities, was quick-tempered, unrestrained, and did not have authority. He says that he was offended by his transfer from Moscow and thought that they had deliberately "sent him away." He then concluded that the government was "decaying" and had departed from Leninist norms and principles. He thought it was essential to conduct a campaign of instruction and explanation among the people aimed at "destroying" the existing order. While studying Marx and Lenin, he had thought a great deal about the mistakes of the leadership and tried to outline the correct course. He was engrossed in these thoughts and considered that for him this was a "matter of conscience and honor."

In 1964, while on leave in Moscow, he distributed leaflets containing these views. Criminal charges were brought against him under Article 70, paragraph 1, of the Russian Criminal Code. He underwent an inpatient forensic psychiatric examination at the Serbsky Institute from 12 March to 18 April 1964.

His psychological condition was described as manifesting reformist ideas, in particular that of the reorganization of the state apparatus combined with an overestimation of his personality reaching messianic proportions. He was emotionally caught up in his own experiences and was unshakeably convinced of the rightness of his actions. In addition, elements of pathological reactions to his surroundings were noted, as well as unhealthy suspiciousness and a sharply expressed emotional excitability.

The conclusion of the team of experts of 17 April 1964 was that: "Grigorenko suffers from a mental illness in the form of a paranoid (delirious) development of his personality, accompanied by early signs of cerebral arterio-sclerosis. He is not of sound mind and needs compulsory treatment in a special psychiatric hospital."

Grigorenko underwent compulsory treatment at the special psychiatric hospital in Leningrad until 22 April 1965. While in the hospital he at first behaved with self-confidence and was obstinate and persistent in his demands. He was easily irritated and then became malicious and irate, and dwelt on emotionally colored experiences. He exhibited a tendency to interpret facts broadly and to overestimate his own capabilities. He did not look critically at his own condition and at the situation that had developed. Subsequently, he became calmer and his behavior seemed more normal. . . .

On 16 March 1965, the commission reached the conclusion that Grigorenko had been suffering from mental illness in the form of a paranoid development of the personality with an early cerebral arterio-sclerosis. At that time, however, Grigorenko had recovered from this illness and was in a state of steady equilibrium which did not require hospital treatment. He only showed signs of cerebral scleroris.

After his discharge from the hospital, as the patient tells it, he learnt that he had been deprived of his rank and pension. He took this very hard, and thought that he had been treated unjustly and "inhumanely." He wrote letters and statements, but did not achieve anything. He found himself in difficult material circumstances because, having being classified as an invalid of the second category, he could not find work. . . .

In 1965, after sending a series of letters and statements to various departments, he was allotted a pension of 120 roubles. However, he did not consider the decision fair and continued to send letters and applications requesting a review of the decision. But he received no answer. As he notes, this made him take offense and become irritable. . . .

Around 1967, he began to engage himself once more in "general political" questions and to direct all his energy toward the struggle for truth. He quickly became acquainted with people whose views were acceptable to him, readily consorted with them and worked on articles in which he set forth his views on various events taking place within the country. At the same time, he wrote letters to government leaders openly criticizing their activities and expressing his own opinions. He was enthusiastic about this work and considered it useful and necessary; it gave him an escape from the inactivity, which he believed, the KGB was trying force upon him. Though his character continued to be lively and active, he became even more hot-tempered and emotionally vulnerable. He considered it necessary to respond to any events which he thought were unjust, even though they had no relation to him. It was by precisely these strivings that he explains his activity during the trials of certain person charged under Articles 70 and 190–1 of the Russian Criminal Code and the active help he gave the Crimean Tatars who were trying to return to the Crimea . . .

On 18 August 1969, Grigorenko underwent an outpatient forensic psychiatric examination under the chairmanship of Professor F. F. Detengof in Tashkent. The commission did not discover any psychopathological disorders and reached the conclusion that Grigorenko showed no symptoms of mental illness, just as he had shown no such symptoms during the time when he committed the incriminating offense (1965–69). They concluded that he is of sound mind.

In the documents of his criminal case there is testimony from witnesses, including his relatives, in which Grigorenko is described as honest, with high principles, well-balanced and affable, and no strangeness in his behavior is noted. At the same time, other witnesses testified that he had "dictatorial ways," talked much and heatedly, and when he was arguing his point of view, tried to force it upon the person with whom he was conversing. Witnesses who saw Grigorenko outside the courthouse on 9–11 October 1968, during the trial of persons indicted under Article 190–1 of the Russian Criminal Code, observe that he "stood out" by his conduct, that he was active, expressed his view on the trial loudly and used abusive language, insulting the *druzhinniki* (voluntary militia) by calling them fascists and members of the Black Hundred [a far-right monarchist movement]. He drew a crowd of people around him, told them about himself and shouted that he would fight for democracy and truth. During the period of investigation, as the documents in his case show, Grigorenko would shout in answer to reproofs and insult the prison staff when he took exercise or was in his cell. He was agitated during the interrogation and for a time refused to eat.

The examination at the Institute has revealed the following:

Neurological Condition: Right pupil is larger than the left, mesolabila skin creases symmetrical. Tongue deflects slightly to the left when thrust out. Lumbar lordosis flattened, flexibility of the spine in the neck and lumbar regions somewhat limited. Reflex of right knee is less than with his left knee, slight positive Marinesko symptom on both sides. All types of sensation are normal. Steadiness in Romberg position. Wasserman reaction in the blood is negative. An examination of the optic fundi shows traces of a partial disturbance in the circulation in the upper branch of the central vein in the right eye.

The electro-encephalographic examination showed: disruptions of the bio-electrical activity of a diffusive character and a persistent asymmetrical amplitude by means of the presence of synchronic flashes of alpha-oscillations and pathological forms of activity, more clearly on the left, and a lowering lability of the brain structure. Accent of changes in the left cerebral hemisphere.

Psychological Condition: Upon his arrival and during the first days of his stay at the Institute, the patient protested against the forensic psychiatric examination. He was agitated, spoke in loud tones and asserted that his placement in the Institute for an examination was "tyranny," all the more so since the previous outpatient commission had pronounced him psychologically healthy. Subsequently the patient became calmer and readily made contact with the doctor. During the conversations he behaved with self-respect and willingly gave information about himself, but then would dwell on an emotional experience and begin to raise his voice. His face would turn red, his hands would begin to shake and he would get into a state of emotional agitation. . . .

He views his struggle as absolutely legitimate and the path which he has followed as the only correct one. When attempts were made to dissuade him he became angry and malicious, and declared to the doctor that his entire life has been a struggle, that he foresaw the possibility of arrest but this has never stopped him since he cannot repudiate his ideas. At present he considers himself mentally healthy.

He formally declared in a conversation with doctors that he does not rank himself among prominent people and claims that he does not think his activity has historical significance. He said that he acted according to the dictates of his own conscience and hopes that his struggle will have some effect.

His letters, which are among the documents of the case, reveal a blatant overestimation of the importance of his activity and of the significance of his personality, as well as reformist ideas, which he is unshakeably convinced are right. He also manifests a distinct tendency to write numerous long letters. These show that, although his critical faculty is disturbed, he has preserved his previous knowledge and skills, as well as his former ability to present formally a consistent account of the facts. In his section of the Institute the patient tries to remain calm, is polite and sociable with those around him and reads literary works.

CONCLUSIONS

Grigorenko is suffering from a mental illness in the form of a pathological (paranoid) development of the personality with the presence of reformist ideas which have arisen in his personality, together with psychopathic character traits and the first signs of cerebral arterio-sclerosis.

This is corroborated by his psychopathic state in 1964, which arose during an unfavorable situation and expressed itself in highly emotional ideas of reformism and persecution. Later, as is evident from documents in his criminal case and data from the present clinical examination, he did not fully recover from his paranoid condition. Reformist ideas have become persistent and determine the patient's behavior. Moreover, the intensity of these ideas increased periodically as a result of various external circumstances which have no direct relation to him. This is accompanied by an uncritical attitude towards his own statement and actions. This mental illness excludes the possibility of the patient being responsible for his actions or having any control over them; hence, the patient must be pronounced of unsound mind.

The commission cannot agree with the diagnosis of the outpatient forensic psychiatric examination conducted in Tashkent because of the presence of pathological changes in Grigorenko's psyche which have been set forth in this report. These changes could not be revealed in the course of an outpatient examination since the patient's behavior is outwardly normal, his statements are formally consistent, and he has preserved his former knowledge and skills—all of which is characteristic of a pathological development of the personality. Grigorenko requires compulsory treatment for his psychological condition in a special psychiatric hospital, since the paranoid ideas of reformism described above are of a persistent nature and determine the patient's behaviour.

Signed by Corresponding Member of the U.S.S.R. Academy of Medical Sciences, G. V. Morozov; Corresponding Member of the U.S.S.R. Academy of Medical Sciences, Professor V. M. Morozov; Professor D. R. Lunts; Senior Research Officer Z. G. Turova; Lecturer and Junior Research Officer M. M. Maltseva

World Psychiatric Association "Declaration of Hawaii"

(1977)

The political abuse of psychiatry in the Soviet Union first began to be widely publicized in the Western media in the 1970s. At the Fifth World Congress of the World Psychiatric Association (WPA) in 1971, critics demanded an end to the practice of institutionalizing dissidents in psychiatric facilities. It was not until the Sixth World Congress of the WPA in Hawaii in 1977, however, that the organization publicly condemned the USSR. In addition, the Congress unanimously adopted a code of ethics known as the Declaration of Hawaii. The declaration was subsequently updated at the 1983 Congress in Vienna, and in 1996, the WPA General Assembly in Madrid approved a comprehensive statement of psychiatric ethical guidelines.

Ever since the dawn of culture ethics has been an essential part of the healing art. Conflicting loyalties for physicians in contemporary society, the delicate nature of the therapist-patient relationship, and the possibility of abuses of psychiatric concepts, knowledge, and technology in actions contrary to the laws of humanity all make high ethical standards more necessary than ever for those practicing the art and science of psychiatry.

As a practitioner of medicine and a member of society, the psychiatrist has to consider the ethical implications specific to psychiatry as well as the ethical demands on all physicians and the societal duties of every man and woman.

A keen conscience and personal judgment is essential for ethical behaviour. Nevertheless, to clarify the profession's ethical implications and to guide individual psychiatrists and help form their consciences, written rules are needed.

Therefore, the General Assembly of the World Psychiatric Association has laid down the following ethical guidelines for psychiatrists all over the world.

(1) The aim of psychiatry is to promote health and personal autonomy and growth. To the best of his or her ability, consistent with accepted scientific and ethical principles, the psychiatrist shall serve the best interests of the patient and be also concerned for the common good and a just allocation of health resources.

To fulfill these aims requires continuous research and continual education of health care personnel, patients, and the public.

(2) Every patient must be offered the best therapy available and be treated with the solicitude and respect due to the dignity of all human beings and to their autonomy over their own lives and health.

The psychiatrist is responsible for treatment given by the staff members and owes them qualified supervision and education. Whenever there is a need, or whenever a reasonable request is forthcoming from the patient, the psychiatrist should seek the help or the opinion of a more experienced colleague.

(3) A therapeutic relationship between patient and psychiatrist is founded on mutual agreement. It requires trust, confidentiality, openness, co-operation, and mutual responsibility. Such a relationship may not be possible to establish with some severely ill patients. In that case, as in the treatment of children, contact should be established with a person close to the patient and acceptable to him or her.

If and when a relationship is established for purposes other than therapeutic, such as in forensic psychiatry, its nature must be thoroughly explained to the person concerned.

(4) The psychiatrist should inform the patient of the nature of the condition, of the proposed diagnostic and therapeutic procedures, including possible alternatives, and of the prognosis. This information must be offered in a considerate way and the patient be given the opportunity to choose between appropriate and available methods.

(5) No procedure must be performed or treatment given against or independent of a patient's own will, unless the patient lacks capacity to express his or her own wishes or, owing to psychiatric illness, cannot see what is in his or her best interest or, for the same reason, is a severe threat to others.

In these cases compulsory treatment may or should be given, provided that it is done in the patient's best interests and over a reasonable period of time, a retroactive informed consent can be presumed, and, whenever possible, consent has been obtained from someone close to the patient.

(6) As soon as the above conditions for compulsory treatment no longer apply the patient must be released, unless he or she voluntarily consents to further treatment. Whenever there is compulsory treatment or detention there must be an independent and neutral body of appeal for regular inquiry into these cases. Every patient must be informed of its existence and be permitted to appeal to it, personally or through a representative, without interference by the hospital staff or by anyone else.

(7) The psychiatrist must never use the possibilities of the profession for maltreatment of individuals or groups, and should be concerned never to let inappropriate personal desires, feelings, or prejudices interfere with the treatment.

The psychiatrist must not participate in compulsory psychiatric treatment in the absence of psychiatric illness. If the patient or some third party demands actions contrary to scientific or ethical principles the psychiatrist must refuse to co-operate. When, for any reason, either the wishes or the best interests of the patient cannot be promoted he or she must be so informed.

(8) Whatever the psychiatrist has been told by the patient, or has noted during examination or treatment, must be kept confidential unless the patient releases the psychiatrist from professional secrecy, or else vital common values or the patient's best interest makes disclosure imperative. In these cases, however, the patient must be immediately informed of the breach of secrecy.

(9) To increase and propagate psychiatric knowledge and skill requires participation of the patients. Informed consent must, however, be obtained before presenting a patient to a class and, if possible, also when a case history is published, and all reasonable measures be taken to preserve the anonymity and to safeguard the personal reputation of the subject.

In clinical research, as in therapy, every subject must be offered the best available treatment. His or her participation must be voluntary, after full information has been given of the aims, procedures, risks, and inconveniences of the project, and there must always be a reasonable relationship between calculated risks or inconveniences and the benefit of the study.

For children and other patients who cannot themselves give informed consent this should be obtained from someone close to them.

(10) Every patient or research subject is free to withdraw for any reason at any time from any voluntary treatment and from any teaching or research programme in which he or she participates. This withdrawal, as well as any refusal to enter a programme, must never influence the psychiatrist's efforts to help the patient or subject.

The psychiatrist should stop all therapeutic, teaching, or research programmes that may evolve contrary to the principles of this Declaration.

World Psychiatric Association, "Declaration of Hawaii," *British Medical Journal* 2 (1977): 1204–1205. With the kind permission of the WPA Executive Committee.

Antipsychiatry, Social Psychiatry, and Deinstitutionalization

Frantz Fanon
(1925–1961)

"The 'North African Syndrome'"
(1952)

Frantz Fanon, the son of an upper-middle-class Indian Martinican father and an Alsatian mother, was born and raised on the Caribbean island of Martinique. It was in Martinique, a French colony until 1946, that Fanon first became conscious of the ways in which a colonial setting shaped people's identities. In 1947, he went to France, studying psychiatry in Lyon. Working there, he became concerned about the numerous North African migrant workers he encountered who complained of a variety of seemingly inexplicable ailments. In 1953, he arrived in Algeria, then a French colony, to better understand the limits of European medicine for non-Western individuals. His experience in Algeria quickly convinced him that colonialism possessed its own pathological psychology, which it passed on to those under its rule. Believing that Western psychiatry was, therefore, incapable of understanding and remedying the problems facing the colonized, Fanon left psychiatry in 1956 to become a political revolutionary and a spokesperson for armed, anti-colonial insurrection. "The 'North African Syndrome,'" written at times in poetic style, is his attempt to analyze psychiatry's inability to come to terms with the plight of North African migrant workers in France.

It is a common saying that man is constantly a challenge to himself, and that were he to claim that he is no longer he would be denying himself. It must be possible, however, to describe an initial, a basic dimension of all human problems. More precisely, it would seem that all the problems which man faces on the subject of man can be reduced to this one question:

"Have I not, because of what I have done or failed to do, contributed to an impoverishment of human reality?"

The question could also be formulated in this way:

"Have I at all times demanded and brought out that man that is in me?"

I want to show in what is to follow that, in the specific case of the North African who has emigrated to France, a theory of inhumanity is in a fair way to finding its laws and its corollaries.

All those men who are hungry, all those men who are cold, all those men who are afraid . . .

All those man of whom *we* are afraid, who crush the jealous emerald of our dreams, who twist the fragile curves of our smiles, all those men we face, who ask us no questions, but to whom we put strange ones.

Who are they?

I ask you, I ask myself. Who are they, those creatures starving for humanity who stand buttressed against the impalpable frontiers (though I know them from experience to be terribly distinct) of complete recognition?

Who are they, in truth, those creatures, who hide, who are hidden by social truth beneath the attributes of *bicot, bounioule, arabe, raton, sidi, mon z'ami?**

FIRST THESIS.—*That the behavior of the North African often causes a medical staff to have misgiving as to the reality of his illness.*

Except in urgent cases—an intestinal occlusion, wounds, accidents—the North African arrives enveloped in vagueness.

He has an ache in his belly, in his back, he has an ache everywhere. He suffers miserably, his face is eloquent, he is obviously suffering.

"What's wrong, my friend?"

"I'm dying, *monsiuer le docteur.*"

His voice breaks imperceptibly.

---

*Translator's note: Terms of contempt applied in France to Arabs in general and to Algerians in particular.

"Where do you have pain?"

"Everywhere, *monsieur le docteur*."

You must not ask for specific symptoms: you would not be given any. For example, in pains of ulcerous character, it is important to know their periodicity. This conformity to the categories of the time is something to which the North African seems to be hostile. It is not lack of comprehension, for he often comes accompanied by an interpreter. It is as though it is an effort for him to go back to where he no longer is. The past for him is a burning past. What he hopes is that he will never suffer again, never again be face to face with the past. This present pain, which visibly mobilizes the muscles of his face, suffices him. He does not understand that anyone should wish to impose on him, even by way of memory, the pain that is already gone. He does not understand why the doctor asks him so many questions.

"Where does it hurt?"

"In my belly." (He then points to his thorax and abdomen.)

"When does it hurt?"

"All the time."

"Even at night."

"Especially at night."

"It hurts more at night than in the daytime, does it?"

"No, all the time."

"But more at night than in the daytime."

"No, all the time."

"And where does it hurt now."

"Here." (He then points to his thorax and abdomen.)

And there you are. Meanwhile patients are waiting outside and the worst of it is that you have the impression that time would not improve matters. You therefore fall back on a diagnosis of probability and in correlation propose an approximate therapy.

"Take this treatment for a month. If you don't get better, come back and see me."

There are then two possibilities:

1. The patient is not immediately relieved, and he comes back after three or four days. This sets us against him, because we know that it takes time for the prescribed medicine to have an effect on the lesion. He is made to understand this, or more precisely, he is told. But our patient has not

heard what we said. He *is* his pain and he refuses to understand any language, and it is not far from this to the conclusion: It is because I am Arab that they don't treat me like others.

2. The patient is not immediately relieved, but he does not go back to the same doctor, nor to the same dispensary. He goes elsewhere. He proceeds on the assumption that in order to get satisfaction he has to knock at every door, and he knocks. He knocks persistently. Gently. Naively. Furiously.

He knocks. The door is opened. The door is always opened. And he tells about *his pain*. Which becomes increasingly his own. He now talks about it volubly. He takes hold of it in space and puts it before the doctor's nose. He takes it, touches it with his ten fingers, develops it, exposes it. It grows as one watches it. He gathers it over the whole surface of his body and after fifteen minutes of gestured explanations the interpreter (appropriately baffling) translates for us: he says he has a belly-ache.

All these forays into space, all those facial spasms, all those wild stares were only meant to express a vague discomfort. We experience a kind of frustration in the field of explanation. The comedy, or the drama, begins all over again: approximate diagnosis and therapy.

There is no reason for the wheel to stop going around. Some day an X-ray will be taken of him which will show an ulcer or a gastritis. Or which in most cases will show nothing at all. His ailment will be described as "functional."

This concept is of some importance and is worth looking into. A thing is said to be vague when it is lacking in consistency, in objective reality. The North African's pain, for which we can find no lesional basis, is judged to have no consistency, no reality. Now the North African is a man-who-does-n't-like-work. So that whatever he does will be interpreted *a priori* on the basis of this.

A North African is hospitalized because he suffers from lassitude, asthenia, weakness. He is given active treatment on the basis of restoratives. After twenty days it is decided to discharge him. He then discovers that he has another disease.

"My heart seems to flutter inside here."

"My head is bursting."

In the face of this fear of leaving the hospital one begins to wonder if the debility for which he was treated was not due to some giddiness. One begins to wonder if one has not been the plaything of the patient whom one has never too well understood. Suspicion rears its head. Henceforth one will mistrust the alleged symptoms.

The thing is perfectly clear in the winter; so much so that certain wards are literally submerged by North Africans during the severe cold spells. It's so comfortable within hospital walls.

In one ward, a doctor was scolding a European suffering from sciatica who spent the day visiting in the different rooms. The doctor explained to him that with this particular ailment, rest constituted one half of the therapy. With the North Africans, he added, for our benefit, the problem is different: there is no need to prescribe rest; they're always in bed.

In the face of this pain without lesion, this illness distributed in and over the whole body, this continuous suffering, the easiest attitude, to which one comes more or less rapidly, is the negation of any morbidity. When you come down to it, the North African is a simulator, a liar, a malingerer, a sluggard, a thief.*

SECOND THESIS.—*That the attitude of medical personnel is very often an a priori attitude. The North African does not come with a substratum common to his race, but on a foundation built by the European. In other words, the North African, spontaneously, by the very fact of appearing on the scene, enters into a pre-existing framework.*

For several years of medicine has shown a trend which, in a very summary way, we can call neo-Hippocratism. In accordance with this trend doctors, when faced with a patient, are concerned less with making a diagnosis of an organ than with a diagnosis of a function. But this orientation has not yet found favor in the medical schools where pathology is taught. There is a flaw in the practitioner's thinking. An extremely dangerous flaw.

We shall see how it manifests itself in practice.

I am called in to visit a patient on an emergency. It is two o'clock in the morning. The room is dirty, the patient is dirty. His parents are dirty. Everybody weeps. Everybody screams. One has the strange impression that death is hovering nearby. The young doctor does not let himself be perturbed. He "objectively" examines the belly that has every appearance of requiring surgery.

---

*Author's note: *Social security? It's we who pay for it!*

He touches, he feels, he taps, he questions, but he gets only groans by way of response. He feels again, taps a second time, and the belly contracts, resists . . . He "sees nothing." But what if an operation is really called for? What if he is overlooking something? His examination is negative, but he doesn't dare to leave. After considerable hesitation, he will send his patient to a center with the diagnosis of an abdomen requiring surgery. Three days later he sees the patient with the "abdomen requiring surgery" turn up smilingly in his office, completely cured. And what the patient is unaware of is that there is an exacting medical philosophy, and that he has flouted this philosophy.

Medical thinking proceeds from the symptom to the lesion. In the illustrious assemblies, in the international medical congresses, agreement has been reached as to the importance of the neurovegetative systems, the diencephalon, the endocrine glands, the psychosomatic links, the sympathalgias, but doctors continue to be taught that every symptom requires a lesion. The patient who complains of headaches, ringing in his ears, and dizziness, will also have high blood-pressure. But should it happen that along with these symptoms there is no sign of high blood-pressure, nor of brain tumor, in any case nothing positive, the doctor would have to conclude that medical thinking was at fault; and as any thinking is necessarily thinking about something, he will find the *patient* at fault—an indocile, undisciplined patient, who doesn't know the rules of the game. Especially the rule, known to be inflexible, which says: any symptom presupposes a lesion.

What am I to do with this patient? From the specialist to whom I had sent him for a probable operation, he comes back to me with the diagnosis of "North African syndrome." And it is true that the newly arrived medico will run into situations reminiscent of Molière through the North Africans he is called upon to treat. A man who fancies himself to be ill! If Molière (what I am about to say is utterly stupid, but all these lines only explicate, only make more flagrant, something vastly more stupid), if Molière had had the privilege of living in the twentieth century, he would certainly not have written *Le Malade Imaginaire*, for there can be no doubt that Argan is ill, is actively ill:

"*Comment, conquine! Si je suis malade! Si je suis malade, impudente!*"*

---

*Translator's note: "What, you hussy! You doubt if I'm sick! You doubt if I'm sick, you impudent wench!"

The North African syndrome. The North African today who goes to see a doctor bears the dead weight of all his compatriots. Of all those who had only symptoms, of all those about whom the doctors said, "Nothing you can put your teeth into." (Meaning: no lesion.) But the patient who is here, in front of me, this body which I am forced to assume to be swept by a consciousness, this body which is no longer altogether a body or rather which is doubly a body since it is beside itself with terror—this body which asks me to listen to it without, however, paying too much heed to it—fills me with exasperation.

"Where do you hurt?"

"In my stomach." (He points to his liver.)

I lose my patience. I tell him that the stomach is to the left, that what he is pointing to is the location of the liver. He is not put out, he passes the palm of his hand over that mysterious belly.

"It all hurts."

I happen to know that this "it all" contains three organs: more exactly five or six. That each organ has *its* pathology. The pathology invented by the Arab does not interest us. It is a pseudo-pathology. The Arab is a pseudo-invalid.

Every Arab is a man who suffers from an imaginary ailment. The young doctor or the young student who has never seen a sick Arab *knows* (the medical tradition testifies to it) that "those fellows are humbugs." There is one thing that might give food for thought. Speaking to an Arab, the student or the doctor is inclined to use the second person singular. It's a nice thing to do, we are told . . . to put them at ease . . . they're used to it . . . I am sorry, but I find myself incapable of analyzing this phenomenon without departing from the objective attitude to which I have constrained myself.

"I can't help it," an intern once told me, "I can't talk to them in the same way that I talk to other patients."

Yes, to be sure: "I can't help it." If you only knew the things in my life that I can't help. If you only knew the things in my life that plague me during the hours when others are benumbing their brains. If you only knew . . . but you will never know.

The medical staff discovers the existence of a North African syndrome. Not experimentally, but on the basis of an oral tradition. The North African takes his place in this asymptomatic syndrome and is automatically put down as undisciplined (cf. medical discipline), inconsequential (with reference to the law according to which every symptoms implies a lesion), and insincere (he says he is suffering when we know there are no *reasons* for suffering). There is a floating idea which is present, just beyond the limits of my lack of good faith, which emerges when the Arab unveils himself through his language:

"Doctor, I am going to die."

This idea, after having passed through a number of contortions, will impose itself, will impose itself on me.

No, you certainly can't take these fellows seriously.

THIRD THESIS.—*That the greatest willingness, the purest of intentions require enlightenment. Concerning the necessity of making a situational diagnosis.*

Dr. Stern, in an article on psychosomatic medicine, based on the work of Heinrich Meng, writes: "One must not only find out which organ is attacked, what is the nature of the organic lesions, if they exist, and what microbe has invaded the organism; it is not enough to know the 'somatic constitution' of the patient. One must try to find out what Meng calls his 'situation,' *that is to say, his relations with his associates, his occupations and his preoccupations, his sexuality, his sense of security or of insecurity, the dangers that threaten him; and we may add also his evolution, the story of his life. One must make a 'situational diagnosis.' "*

Dr. Stern offers us a magnificent plan, and we shall follow it.

1. *Relations with his associates.* Must we really speak of this? Is there not something a little comical about speaking of the North African's relation with his associates, in France? Does he *have* relations? Does he *have* associates? Is he not alone? Are they not alone? Don't they seem absurd to us, that is to say without substance, in the trams and the trolleybuses? Where do they come from? Where are they going? From time to time one sees them working at some building, but one does not *see* them, one perceives them, one gets a glimpse of them. Associates? Relations? There are no contracts. There are only bumps. Do people realize how much that is gentle and polite is contained in this word, "contact?" Are there contacts? Are there relations?

---

*Author's note: Dr. E. Stern, "Médicine psychosomatique," *Psyché*, Jan.–Feb. 1949, p. 128. Editor's note: Emphasis added by author.

2. *Occupations and preoccupations.* He works, he is busy, he busies himself, he is kept busy. His preoccupations? I think the word does not exist in his language. What would he concern himself with? In France we say: *Il se préoccupe de trouver du travail* (he concerns himself with looking for work); in North Africa: he busies himself looking for work.

"Excuse me, Madame, but in your opinion, what are the preoccupations of a North African?"

3. *Sexuality.* Yes, I know what you mean; it consists of rape. In order to show to what extent a scotomizing study can be prejudicial to the authentic unveiling of a phenomenon, I should like to reproduce a few lines from a doctoral thesis in medicine presented in Lyon in 1951 by Dr. Léon Mugniery:

"In the region of Saint Etienne, eight out of ten have married prostitutes. Most of the others have accidental and short-time mistresses, sometimes on a marital basis. Often they put up one or several prostitutes for a few days and bring their friends in to them.

"*For prostitution seems to play an important role in the North African colony.** . . . It is due to the powerful sexual appetite that is characteristic of those hot-blooded southerners."

Further on:

"It can be shown by many examples that attempts made to house North Africans decently have repeatedly failed.

"These are mostly young men (25 to 35) with great sexual needs, whom the bonds of a mixed marriage can only temporarily stabilize, and for whom homosexuality is a disastrous inclination. . . .

"There are few solutions to this problem: either, in spite of the *risks*[†] involved in a certain invasion by the Arab family, the regrouping of this family in France should be encouraged and Arab girls and women should be brought here; or else houses of prostitutions for them should be tolerated . . .

"If these factors are not taken into account, we may well be exposed to increasing attempts at rape, of the kind that the newspapers are constantly reporting. Public morals surely have more to fear from the existence of these facts than from the existence of brothels."

---

*Translator's note: Emphasis added by author.

[†]Translator's note: Emphasis added by author.

And to conclude, Dr. Mugniery deplores the mistake made by the French government in the following sentence which appears in capitals in his thesis: "THE GRANTING OF FRENCH CITIZENSHIP, CONFERRING EQUALITY OF RIGHTS, SEEMS TO HAVE BEEN TOO HASTY AND BASED ON SENTIMENTAL AND POLITICAL REASONS, RATHER THAN ON THE FACT OF THE SOCIAL AND INTELLECTUAL EVOLUTION OF A RACE HAVING A CIVILIZATION THAT IS AT TIMES REFINED BUT STILL PRIMITIVE IN ITS SOCIAL, FAMILY AND SANITARY BEHAVIOR."

Need anything be added? Should we take up these absurd sentences one after the other? Should we remind Dr. Mugniery that if the North Africans in France content themselves with prostitutes, it is because they find prostitutes here in the first place, and also because they do not find any Arab women (who might invade the nation)?

4. *His inner tension.* Utterly unrealistic! You might as well speak of the inner tension of a stone. Inner tension indeed! What a joke!

5. *His sense of security and of insecurity.* The first term has to be struck out. The North African is in a perpetual state of insecurity. A multisegmented insecurity.

I sometimes wonder if it would not be well to reveal to the average Frenchman that it is a misfortune to be a North African. The North African is never sure. He has rights, you will tell me, but he doesn't know what they are. Ah! Ah! It's up to him to know them. Yes, sure, we're back on our feet! Rights, Duties, Citizenship, Equality, what fine things! The North African on the threshold of the French Nation—which is, we are told, his as well—experiences in the political realm, on the plane of citizenship, an imbroglio which no one is willing to face. What connection does this have with the North African in a hospital setting? It so happens that there *is* a connection.

6. *The dangers that threaten him.* Threatened in his affectivity, threatened in his social activity, threatened in his membership in the community—the North African combines all the conditions that make a sick man.

Without a family, without love, without human relations, without communion with the group, the first encounter with himself will occur in a neurotic mode, in a pathological mode; he will feel himself emptied, without life, in a bodily struggle with death, a death on this side of death, a death in life—and what is more pathetic than this man with robust muscles who tells us in his truly broken voice, "Doctor, I'm going to die"?

7. *His evolution and the story of his life.* It would be better to say the history of his death. A daily death.

A death in the tram,

a death in the doctor's office,

a death with the prostitutes,

a death on the job site,

a death at the movies,

a multiple death in the newspapers,

a death in the fear of all decent folks of going out after midnight.

A death,

yes, a DEATH.

All this is very fine, we shall be told, but what solutions do you propose?

As you know, they are vague, amorphous . . .

"You constantly have to be on their backs."

"You've got to push them out of the hospital."

"If you were to listen to them you would prolong their convalescence indefinitely."

"They can't express themselves."

And they are liars,

and also they are thieves

and also and also and also

the Arab is a thief

all Arabs are thieves

It's a do-nothing race

dirty

disgusting

Nothing you can do about them

nothing you can get out of them

sure, it's hard for them being the way they are

being that way

but anyway, you can't say it's our fault.

—But that's just it, it *is* our fault.

It so happens that the fault is YOUR fault.

Men come and go along a corridor you have built for them, where you have provided no bench on which they can rest, where you have crystal-lized a lot of scarecrows that viciously smack them in the face, and hurt their cheeks, their chests, their hearts.

Where they find no room
where you leave them no room
where there is absolutely no room for them
and you dare tell me it doesn't concern you!
that it's no fault of yours!

This man whom you thingify by calling him systematically Moham-med, whom you reconstruct, or rather whom you dissolve, on the basis of an idea, an idea you know to be repulsive (you know perfectly well you rob him of something, that something for which not so long ago you were ready to give up everything, even your life) well, don't you have the impression that you are emptying him of his substance?

Why don't they stay where they belong?

Sure! That's easy enough to say: why don't they stay where they belong? The trouble is, they have been told they were French. They learned it in school. In the street. In the barracks. (Where they were given shoes to wear on their feet.) On the battlefields. They have had France squeezed into them wherever, in their bodies and in their souls, there was room for something apparently great.

Now they are told in no uncertain terms that they are in "our" coun-try. That if they don't like it, all they have to do is go back to their Casbah. For here too there is a problem.

Whatever vicissitudes he may come up against in France, so some peo-ple claim, the North African will be happier at home . . .

It has been found in England that children who were magnificently fed, each having two nurses entirely at his services, but living away from the family circle, showed a morbidity twice as pronounced as children who were less well fed but who lived with their parents. Without going so far, think of all those who lead a life without a future in their own country and who refuse fine positions abroad. What is the good of a fine position if it does not culminate in a family, in something that can be called home?

Psychoanalytical science considers expatriation to be a morbid phe-nomenon. In which it is perfectly right.

These considerations allow us to conclude:

1. The North African will never be happier in Europe than at home, for he is asked to live without the very substance of his affectivity. Cut off from his origins and cut off from his ends, he is a thing tossed into the great sound and fury, bowed beneath the law of inertia.

2. There is something manifestly and abjectly disingenuous in the above statement. If the standard of living made available to the North African in France is higher than the one he was accustomed to at home, this means that there is still a good deal to be done in his country, in that "other part of France."

That there are houses to be built, schools to be opened, roads to be laid out, slums to be torn down, cities to be made to spring from the earth, men and women, children and children to be adorned with smiles.

This means that there is work to be done over there, human work, that is, work which is the meaning of a home. Not that of a room or a barrack building. It means that over the whole territory of the French nation (the metropolis and the French Union), there are tears to be wiped away, inhuman attitudes to be fought, condescending ways of speech to be ruled out, men to be humanized.

Your solution, sir?

Don't push me too far. Don't force me to tell you what you ought to know, sir. If YOU do not reclaim the man who is before you, how can I assume that you reclaim the man that is in you?

If YOU do not want the man who is before you, how can I believe the man that is perhaps in you?

If YOU do not demand the man, if YOU do not sacrifice the man that is in you so that the man who is on this earth shall be more than a body, more than a Mohammed, by what conjurer's trick will I have to acquire the certainty that you, too, are worthy of my love?

Thomas Szasz

(b. 1920)

"The Myth of Mental Illness"

(1960)

Against the backdrop of the end of World War II, the beginning of postwar prosperity in the United States and Western Europe, and the rise of new social protest movements, a number of public intellectuals, mental health professionals, and psychiatric patients and their relatives began questioning some of the most basic assumptions of psychiatry and psychotherapy. By the mid-1970s, their particular criticisms and activism became known as the antipsychiatry movement. The leading voices of antipsychiatry were often psychiatrists, psychotherapists, and social scientists who themselves had become disillusioned with the conventional values and methods of mental health care. They and their allies took it upon themselves to publicly criticize such things as the treatment of deviant behavior and mental states as diseases, the professional dominance of physicians, the practice of institutionalization, and the use of psychopharmaceuticals in treating personal problems. To this day, antipsychiatry's reception has been marked by both enthusiastic support and resolute dismissal.

In the United States at least, no name is more closely associated with the antipsychiatry movement than that of Thomas Szasz. Born in Budapest, Szasz came to the United States in 1938, where he earned an MD and trained in psychoanalysis. He is a prolific author, and his works—beginning with his book *The Myth of Mental Illness*, first published in 1961—and his libertarian views about psychiatry have made him an influential, yet polarizing, public figure for almost fifty years.

My aim in this essay is to raise the question "Is there such a thing as mental illness?" and to argue that there is not. Since the notion of mental illness is extremely widely used nowadays, inquiry into the ways in which this term is employed would seem to be especially indicated. Mental illness, of course, is not literally a "thing"—or physical object—and hence it can "exist" only in the same sort of way in which other theoretical concepts exist. Yet, familiar theories are in the habit of posing, sooner or later—at least to those who come to believe in them—as "objective truths" (or "facts"). During certain historical periods, explanatory conceptions such as deities, witches, and microorganisms appeared not only as theories but as self-evident causes of a vast number of events. I submit that today mental illness is widely regarded in a somewhat similar fashion, that is, as the cause of innumerable diverse happenings. As an antidote to the complacent use of the notion of mental illness—whether as a self-evident phenomenon, theory, or cause—let us ask this question: What is meant when it is asserted that someone is mentally ill?

In what follows I shall describe briefly the main uses to which the concept of mental illness has been put. I shall argue that this notion has outlived whatever usefulness it might have had and that it now functions merely as a convenient myth.

Mental Illness as a Sign of Brain Disease

The notion of mental illness derives it [sic] main support from such phenomena as syphilis of the brain or delirious conditions—intoxications, for instance—in which persons are known to manifest various peculiarities or disorders of thinking and behavior. Correctly speaking, however, these are diseases of the brain, not of the mind. According to one school of thought, all so-called mental illness is of this type. The assumption is made that some neurological defect, perhaps a very subtle one, will ultimately be found for all the disorders of thinking and behavior. Many contemporary psychiatrists, physicians, and other scientists hold this view. This position implies that people *cannot* have troubles—expressed in what are *now called* "mental illnesses"—because of differences in personal needs, opinions, social aspirations, values, and so on. *All problems in living* are attributed to physicochemical processes which in due time will be discovered by medical research.

"Mental illnesses" are thus regarded as basically no different than all other diseases (that is, of the body). The only difference, in this view, between mental and bodily diseases is that the former, affecting the brain, manifest themselves by means of mental symptoms; whereas the latter, affecting other organ systems (for example, the skin, liver, etc.), manifest themselves by means of symptoms referable to those parts of the body. This view rests on and expresses what are, in my opinion, two fundamental errors.

In the first place, what central nervous system symptoms would correspond to a skin eruption or a fracture? It would *not* be some emotion or complex bit of behavior. Rather, it would be blindness or a paralysis of some part of the body. The crux of the matter is that a disease of the brain, analogous to a disease of the skin or bone, is a neurological defect, and not a problem in living. For example, a *defect* in a person's visual field may be satisfactorily explained by correlating it with certain definite lesions in the nervous system. On the other hand, a person's *belief*—whether this be a belief in Christianity, in Communism, or in the idea that his internal organs are "rotting" and that his body is, in fact, already "dead"—cannot be explained by a defect or disease of the nervous system. Explanations of this sort of occurrence—assuming that one is interested in the belief itself and does not regard it simply as a "symptom" or expression of something else that is *more interesting*—must be sought along different lines.

The second error in regarding complex psychosocial behavior, consisting of communications about ourselves and the world about us, as mere symptoms of neurological functioning is *epistemological*. In other words, it is an error pertaining not to any mistakes in observation or reasoning, as such, but rather to the way in which we organize and express our knowledge. In the present case, the error lies in making a symmetrical dualism between mental and physical (or bodily) symptoms, a dualism which is merely a habit of speech and to which no known observations can be found to correspond. Let us see if this is so. In medical practice, when we speak of physical disturbances, we mean either signs (for example, a fever) or symptoms (for example, pain). We speak of mental symptoms, on the other hand, when we refer to a patient's *communications about himself, others, and the world about him.* He might state that he is Napoleon or that he is being persecuted by the Communists. These would be considered mental symptoms only if the observer believed that the patient was *not* Napoleon or that he was not being persecuted by the Communists. This makes it apparent that the statement that "X is a mental symptom" involves rendering a judgment. The judgment entails, moreover, a covert comparison or matching of the patient's ideas, concepts, or beliefs with those of the observer and the society in which they live. The notion of mental symptom is therefore inextricably tied to the *social* (including *ethical*) *context* in which it is made in much the same way as the notion of bodily symptom is tied to an *anatomical* and *genetic context*.

To sum up what has been said thus far: I have tried to show that for those who regard mental symptoms as signs of brain disease, the concept of mental illness is unnecessary and misleading. For what they mean is that people so labeled suffer from diseases of the brain; and, if that is what they mean, it would seem better for the sake of clarity to say that and not something else.

Mental Illness as a Name for Problems in Living

The term "mental illness" is widely used to describe something which is very different than a disease of the brain. Many people today take it for granted that living is an arduous process. Its hardship for modern man, moreover, derives not so much from a struggle for biological survival as from the stresses and strains inherent in the social intercourse of complex human personalities. In this context, the notion of mental illness is used to identify or describe some feature of an individual's so-called personality. Mental illness—as a deformity of the personality, so to speak—is then regarded as the *cause* of the human disharmony. It is implicit in this view that social intercourse between people is regarded as something *inherently harmonious*, its disturbance being due solely to the presence of "mental illness" in many people. This is obviously fallacious reasoning, for it makes the abstraction "mental illness" into a *cause*, even though this abstraction was created in the first place to serve only as a shorthand expression for certain types of human behavior. It now becomes necessary to ask: "What kinds of behavior are regarded as indicative of mental illness, and by whom?"

The concept of illness, whether bodily or mental, implies *deviation from some clearly defined norm*. In the case of physical illness, the norm is the structural and functional integrity of the human body. Thus, although the desirability of physical health, as such, is an ethical value, what health is can be stated in anatomical and physiological terms. What is the norm deviation from which is regarded as mental illness? This question cannot be easily answered. But whatever this norm might be, we can be certain of only one thing: namely, that it is a norm that must be stated in terms of *psychosocial*, *ethical*, and *legal* concepts. For example, notions such as "excessive repression" or "acting out an unconscious impulse" illustrate the use of psychological concepts for judging (so-called) mental health and illness. The idea that chronic hostility, vengefulness, or divorce are indicative of mental illness would be illustrations of the use of ethical norms (that is, the desirability of love, kindness, and a stable marriage relationship). Finally, the widespread psychiatric opinion that only a mentally ill person would commit homicide illustrates the use of a legal concept as a norm of mental health. The norm from which deviation is measured whenever one speaks of a mental illness is a *psychosocial and ethical one*. Yet, the remedy is sought in terms of *medical* measures which—it is hoped and assumed—are free from wide differences of ethical value. The definition of the disorder and the terms in which its remedy are sought are therefore at serious odds with one another. The practical significance of this covert conflict between the alleged nature of the defect and the remedy can hardly be exaggerated.

Having identified the norms used to measure deviations in cases of mental illness, we will now turn to the question: "Who defines the norms and hence the deviation?" Two basic answers may be offered: (a) It may be the person himself (that is, the patient) who decides that he deviates from a norm. For example, an artist may believe that he suffers from a work inhibition; and he may implement this conclusion by seeking help *for* himself from a psychotherapist, (b) It may be someone other than the patient who decides that the latter is deviant (for example, relatives, physicians, legal authorities, society generally, etc.). In such a case a psychiatrist may be hired by others to do something to the patient in order to correct the deviation.

These considerations underscore the importance of asking the question "Whose agent is the psychiatrist?" and of giving a candid answer to it. The psychiatrist (psychologist or nonmedical psychotherapist), it now develops, may be the agent of the patient, of the relatives, of the school, of the military services, of a business organization, of a court of law, and so forth. In speaking of the psychiatrist as the agent of these persons or organizations, it is not implied that his values concerning norms, or his ideas and aims concerning the proper nature of remedial action, need to coincide exactly with those of his employer. For example, a patient in individual psychotherapy may believe that his salvation lies in a new marriage; his psychotherapist need not share this hypothesis. As the patient's agent, however, he must abstain from bringing social or legal force to bear on the patient which would prevent him from putting his beliefs into action. If his *contract* is with the patient, the psychiatrist (psychotherapist) may disagree with him or stop his treatment; but he cannot engage others to obstruct the patient's aspirations. Similarly, if a psychiatrist is engaged by a court to determine the sanity of a criminal, he need not fully share the legal authorities' values and intentions in regard to the criminal and the means available for dealing with him. But the psychiatrist is expressly barred from stating, for example, that it is not the criminal who is "insane" but the men who wrote the law on the basis of which the very actions that are being judged are regarded as "criminal." Such an opinion could be voiced, of course, but not in a courtroom, and not by a psychiatrist who makes it his practice to assist the court in performing its daily work.

To recapitulate: In actual contemporary social usage, the finding of a mental illness is made by establishing a deviance in behavior from certain psychosocial, ethical, or legal norms. The judgment may be made, as in medicine, by the patient, the physician (psychiatrist), or others. Remedial action, finally, tends to be sought in a therapeutic—or covertly medical—framework, thus creating a situation in which *psychosocial, ethical,* and/or *legal deviations* are claimed to be correctible by (so-called) medical action. Since *medical action* is designed to correct only medical deviations, it seems logically absurd to expect that it will help solve problems whose very existence had been defined and established on nonmedical grounds. I think that these considerations may be fruitfully applied to the present use of tranquilizers and, more generally, to what might be expected of drugs of whatever type in regard to the amelioration or solution of problems in human living.

From Thomas Szasz, "The Myth of Mental Illness," *American Psychologist* 15 (1960): 113–118.

Franco Basaglia
(1924–1980)
"The Problem of the Incident"
(1968)

Like many European countries, Italy of the 1950s continued to have institutions and legal codes governing psychiatric care that dated back to before World War I. As critical voices emerged, the first efforts to reform the existing system began at the local level, outside academia. One of the first and most influential experiments began in 1961 in the northeastern Italian town of Gorizia, where the psychiatrist Franco Basaglia brought his unconventional ideas and a team of like-minded professionals to reform the mental hospital there. Inspired by the philosophies of existentialism, phenomenology, and the therapeutic community, Basaglia moved to realize his ideal of the "open hospital." Under his directorship, Gorizia abolished restraints, patients were allowed to wear street clothes, electroshock was suspended, medications were reduced, and regular staff-patient assemblies were introduced.

Over time, Basaglia came to the conclusion that patients could never be fully reintegrated into society through treatment in an asylum. In 1971, he began a comprehensive reform of psychiatric treatment in Trieste, shifting services from inpatient to outpatient care in the community. By the early-1970s, similar experiments were going on all over Italy under the rubric "democratic psychiatry." These local and regional initiatives eventually culminated in 1978 in the Italian parliament's passage of Law Number 180, which placed strong restrictions on the use of involuntary methods of commitment and treatment and mandated that outpatient services play the primary role in care. The law had its effect: while in 1970, there were 82.5 public psychiatric hospital residents per 100,000 of the adult population in Italy, the figure fell to 30.7 by 1984.

Any violent incident that occurs in a psychiatric institution is immediately attributed to the patient's illness,* the presumed single cause of unpredictable behaviors there. Insofar as psychiatry has defined the mental patient as incomprehensible, the psychiatrist, who is legally bound to supervise and protect the patient, is permitted to abdicate all responsibility for violent or seemingly chaotic behaviors. The psychiatrist is responsible to society, which has delegated to him the control of abnormal and deviant behavior along with the means for transferring to the illness all responsibility for those behaviors, without taking into account therapeutic risks and failures as in all other branches of biomedicine. The psychiatrist's task consists of reducing the patient's subjective experience to a minimum by totally objectifying her within an institutional system oriented to providing against the unanticipated, the unforeseeable. The psychiatrist secures his control of the situation by firmly establishing institutional roles through legal maneuvers (the jurisdiction of the Attorney General), administrative regulations (that concern relations with the Provincial Administration), and scientific nosologies that define the patient's chronic malaise.

In this institutional space where abnormality is normative, the unruly, unbalanced, or disturbed patient is tolerated and excused according to the gross stereotypes of mental illness, just as, in the same way, murder, suicide or sexual assaults in more open institutions are justified and explained as expressions of the unknown, unpredictable mechanisms of psychiatric syndromes. Hence, neither psychiatrist nor the environment can be held accountable for what are defined as *incomprehensible* acts. The abnormal and uncontrollable impulses of the disease are considered sufficiently explanatory.

However, once we become closer to the patient, no longer viewing him as an isolated entity enclosed within an incomprehensible world, but rather as an individual forcibly removed from the social reality to which he once belonged, and uprooted by an institution that assigns him only a passive role, then the institution itself becomes implicated in his behavior. Every event becomes reconnected to the environment in which he lives.

---

*Translator's note: The word *incidente* may be translated as "incident" or "accident." The term used here varies according to context.

The problem of the incident can therefore be considered from two contrasting perspectives, each corresponding to the different ways the institution views the patient.

The primary goal of the classic, closed, custodial institution is *efficiency* and the patient is, therefore, treated primarily as an object. If the patient wants to survive the abuse and destructive power the institution inflicts on her, she must identify with its norms and rules. Whether she conforms to it with servile and submissive behavior or whether she resists it with deviant and insolent behavior, the patient is nonetheless *determined* by the institution. The rigidity of its rules and the one-dimensionality of its reality continue to lock her into a passive and dependent role that allows no alternatives beyond objectification and adaptation.

Thus it is that by establishing a reality with no alternatives other than regimentation and fragmentation that the institution dictates to the patient how she must presumably act. These signals are implicit in the absence of any goals or a future for the patient, which in turn reflects the absence of any alternatives, goals, or future for the psychiatrist, who is appointed by society to control abnormal behavior with a minimum of risk.

Everything in this coercive environment is provided for and controlled in order to avoid *that which must not happen*. In a reality that exists solely to prevent it, freedom can only be experienced as a *forbidden act*, impossible to achieve. The shaft of light from an open door, the unguarded room, the half-open window, the knife left lying about, all present an open invitation to destruction. The patient's identification with the institution means that he can only interpret freedom as an act of violence against himself or others. This is the message and the logic of the institution. Where there are no alternatives and no possibility of autonomous behavior, the only future is death. Death presents itself as a rejection of an unbearable life; as a protest against objectification; as an illusion of freedom; as, in short, the only possible plan. It is far too easy to see this death wish as part of the nature of the illness, as traditional psychiatry would have us believe.

In this context, every action that in some way breaks the iron grip of the institutional regime gives an illusion of freedom, but is nonetheless equivalent to death. The escape from an institution is an attempt to avoid that other future which is death and to experience the sensation of controlling one's destiny. But inevitably the escape ends in capture and continued enslavement or in a death.

Paradoxically, the only responsibility that the institution attributes to the patient is responsibility for the incident which it hastens to blame on the patient and his illness, rejecting any connection to, or participation in, the tragedy. The patient, who has been stripped of all responsibility throughout the long hospital stay suddenly finds himself *totally* responsible for his one "free" act, which almost always coincides with his death. The closed asylum, a dead world that objectifies patients with dehumanizing rules, offers only one clear alternative: death, as the illusion of freedom. In this sense, any accident is merely the expression of a patient's experiencing institutional regulation to the bitter end, taking its message to its most logical final conclusion.

We could shift this discussion from hospitalized mental patients to *any* people without alternatives, without a future, who cannot find a place for themselves in the world. Their exclusion indicates to them the only possible step to take—an act of rejection and destruction.

In the case of the open institution the goal is to try to maintain the patient's subjectivity, even if this is to the detriment of general organizational efficiency. This goal is reflected in every institutional act. When there is a need for patients to identify with the institution, they identify because they see their personal goals and their future reflected in it. It is an open world which offers alternatives and a real sense of possibility to the patients.

In this environment, freedom becomes the norm and the patient becomes accustomed to exercising it, which means taking responsibility, self-control, managing one's life, and understanding one's illness, without the biases of medical science. For this to occur, the institution must be totally involved in the material and psychological support of the patient. This entails breaking the rigidity of roles; ending the objectifying relationships where one person's values are taken for granted, while the other's are not even recognized as values; the creation of alternatives that allow the patient to fight against the closed world of institutional rules, and that give him a sense of existing in a space that fosters continued existence. This means that the only way the institution will now protect itself is through the participation of all its members in developing a community, in which institutional limits are set by the presence of the community and the possibility of reciprocal struggle.

This is, of course, a utopian description of an open institution. There are contradictions within such a reality just as there are outside it. What is essential is that the institution does not try to mask or hide the contradictions, but rather tries to face them with the patients and point them out when they are not immediately obvious.

In this context, the incident is no longer the tragic result of a lack of *supervision*, but rather an indication of the institution's lack of *support*. The actions of the patients, nurses, and doctors can sometimes fail or there can be discontinuities where accidents can still occur. Omissions, commissions, failures, and betrayals of trust have logical consequences, but in all these instances the illness plays a relatively minor role.

The open door becomes a clue to understanding what the door—and the isolation and exclusion of patients—mean in our society. The open door acquires a symbolic value as the patient comes to realize that perhaps he is not after all dangerous to himself and to others. This discovery then leads him to ask why he has been forced into such disgraced and excluded conditions in the first place.

In this way the open institution fosters the patient's recognition that he really *is* excluded. Its sole symbolic function is to demonstrate what has been *done* to the patient and the social significance of the institution that has locked him up.

On the other hand, the open door represents a contradiction in a society that bases its safety and equilibrium on rigid and tight social categories that maintain a division of classes and roles. Psychiatrists and nurses inevitably become aware of this contradiction as they find themselves in situations where they are part accomplice, part victim, forced to uphold a social order they now want to destroy. The open door makes the psychiatrist aware of his own enslavement to a system for which he serves as the silent, unknowing double agent.

What possible meaning do escapes and accidents have in *this* context? They are directly related to the institution's degree of openness to the outside world and to the social nature of that world. The alternatives that the open institution offer can still come up against society's refusal to carry them out. The open door leads, inevitably, to the outside world where society and its violent rules, its discriminations, and abuses continue to reject, deny, exploit, and exclude the mentally ill, who represent one of many disturbing elements for whom public institutions exist.

In such a situation, who is responsible for unfortunate incidents? A mental patient can be released and then find that he is rejected by his family, friends, and co-workers—by a reality that violently dismisses him as superfluous. What can he do except either kill himself or whomever symbolizes that violence against him? When this happens can we *really* speak only in terms of mental illness or of "accidents?"

From Franco Basaglia, "The Problem of the Incident," translated by Teresa Shtob, in *Psychiatry Inside Out: Selected Writings of Franco Basaglia*, edited by Nancy Scheper-Hughes and Anne M. Lovell (New York: Columbia University Press, 1987), 87–91. Translated by Teresa Shtob. Copyright © 1987 Columbia University Press. Reprinted with permission of the publisher.

Department of Health and Social Security, Great Britain
Better Services for the Mentally Ill
(1975)

Deinstitutionalization refers to a process by which large numbers of psychiatric patients are moved out of public asylums and into a variety of other community and institutional settings. Historically, the beginning of deinstitutionalization is often associated with the general introduction of the antipsychotic medication chlorpromazine (also known as Thorazine) in the mid-1950s, which enabled more chronically disturbed patients to be released more easily. But a number of social, institutional, and political changes dating back to World War II led to an emptying of overcrowded asylums across Europe, Australia and New Zealand, and North America. The results were striking. In the United States, for instance, there were around 558,000 patients in public psychiatric facilities in 1955; by 1994, that figure was less than 72,000.

Deinstitutionalization was both a cause and an effect of a change in thinking about how to understand and treat mental disorders. By the 1970s, states began setting up commissions and task forces to both assess progress as well as map future plans in mental health care. In 1975, the British secretary of state for social services issued a white paper, intended to provide the British government with a strategic plan for carrying on the work of previous decades. Three new principles were to serve as orientation points: the integration of mental health services, an emphasis on community care, and the adoption of a team approach.

The Needs of the Mentally Ill

. . . [C]linical labels reveal relatively little about what it means to be mentally ill or to live with someone who is afflicted, or by implication what the needs of the mentally are in terms of services. In one sense it is misleading to attempt any generalised statement about the needs of the mentally ill. The needs of any one mentally ill person are always different from another even though they may have the same diagnostic label. It is not merely that need depends on factors such as age, whether there is home support or a sympathetic employer, but rather that the manifestation of the illness itself will to some extent be coloured by the personality and home environment of the individual. Viewed from the individual level, need is personal and it is important that those working with the patient should see his problems in this way. At the same time these individual perspectives should not mask the significance either of the clinical factors whose identification is fundamental to scientific classification, or of those needs for certain kinds of help which the mentally ill have in common, which are discussed below, and which form the basis of any attempt at national or local planning of services for them. We must aim, therefore, at a range of facilities which can be used by professional staff to provide for each individual the particular combination of care, treatment and support he needs at any point in time.

Not only does need vary qualitatively between different individuals, it varies quantitatively, especially in the length of time for which support and treatment may be required. Much emphasis has been laid, and rightly, on the revolution which has taken place in the treatment of the mentally ill in recent years. This has meant that for many mentally ill people, psychiatric treatment need mean no more than a spell of out-patient or day patient visits or a very few weeks as an in-patient. Nevertheless, there will remain some people who, although their more acute symptoms can be relieved, will need more or less permanent medical, social and nursing support in a sheltered environment. While this group may be relatively few in number their needs must be recognised, especially as the implications in terms of resources are quite disproportionate to their numbers. Another important group are those with mental illness symptoms related to old age. Increasing longevity is bringing its own problems in this respect.

Prevention

In the absence of more precise knowledge primary prevention can only be considered in the rather broad terms of reducing the exposure of individuals to those circumstances and conditions which are likely to place their mental health at risk. Healthy physical, mental and emotional development in childhood is obviously particularly important. Reference has been made already to the wide range of social and environmental conditions which may increase vulnerability to mental illness. The precise weight to be attached to them can rarely be established: poverty, unemployment, lack of job satisfaction and poor working conditions, bad housing, are themselves often a cause of marital stress and breakdown in family life. For some of these central and local authority has a responsibility: but it would be wrong to pretend that we are anywhere near being able to draw up a positive plan for a society conducive to mental health.

Nevertheless we can take some steps to put right some of the clearly unsatisfactory aspects of our social environment. In the field of employment for example, the Employment Medical Advisory Service of the Health and Safety Executive has created a senior appointment in mental health to examine the problems of stress in modern industrial life and offer advice to industry and the unions. It is anticipated that a small team of specialists will be available to undertake surveys and studies, and arrange for appropriate research work with outside bodies such as the Medical Research Council. In this area, the Employment Medical Advisory Service will co-operate closely with the Work Research Unit of the Department of Employment, set up in 1974 to assist organisations in taking practical steps towards increasing the quality of working life by improving the design of jobs and organisation of work. Similarly in its approach to housing problems the Government has taken steps, notably through the Housing Act 1974, to ensure that resources are concentrated on the areas of greatest stress.

Employers, managers, environmental planners all need to bear in mind the potential impact of their decisions on people's mental well-being. The lessons of high rise flats are an illustration: and it to be hoped that local housing authorities in particular will increasingly take into account the question of mental health when considering the effect of new development on existing communities. Rarely will there be easy answers, but it is a dimension of planning which should be acknowledged.

The growth of a wide variety of community development and self help schemes, clubs and societies is particularly encouraging. Such organisations can help provide a whole range of help which though perhaps not specifically directed at mental health have an important part to play in providing those at risk with additional psychological or social resources. Marriage guidance, vocational guidance, clubs and recreational facilities, church and voluntary organisations, education for leisure and retirement, are all relevant. Organisations and services which are specifically aimed to help in particular crises such as marital breakdown, pregnancy, bereavement, retirement or redundancy are of special importance. Collectively and individually we each have a responsibility to be sensitive to the emotional and psychological needs of those who are vulnerable.

Early Recognition

The individual himself may be unaware of his condition. Those around him and even professional staff may not recognise it initially. Mental illness may often be hidden beneath a wide variety of presenting problems: an ostensibly physical complaint, marital and family problems, quarrels with neighbours, accident proneness at work and delinquency may all have their roots in mental illness. Moreover sometimes the person for whom help is apparently sought may not be the only one in need of professional support: the parents, for example, of a disturbed child may themselves require psychiatric help. Service must be organised and professional staff trained to recognise the early stages of psychiatric disturbance and to arrange referral to the appropriate services. Early intervention may often serve to prevent the condition deteriorating to the point at which a severe crisis occurs and hospital admission becomes the only possible solution.

Assessment

Assessment of needs must take account of the effects of mental illness on almost every aspect of a person's life. It should be a continuing process involving all the professions concerned, aimed at reducing as swiftly as possible the damaging effects of illness. The importance of multiprofessional assessment lies not least in the interchange of views between assessors. Not only is this essential in the development of an accurate, broad based assessment, but the assessment by each individual discipline is often influenced by those of others. . . .

Social Rehabilitation

Mental illness often fundamentally affects social adjustment, even after the primary symptoms of the illness have been treated. The sufferer may lack his former energy and drive; and have difficulty in making or resuming personal friendships or family relationships. He may have lost the power of sustained concentration; and the ability to organise even relatively simple daily routines may have to be relearnt. If he is to resume his place in a busy competitive society he will need help in regaining social skills which in the ordinary fit person are taken for granted. The loss of such skills even for a short period of time may have far reaching repercussions. A person recovering from mental illness may well not be able to bear the full responsibility of organising his life.

Social rehabilitation has also to be considered from the standpoint of the community in the wider sense. The pace of development of community service for the mentally ill is dependent partly on changes in attitude by the community. It is also dependent on the community's capacity to adjust to the implications of community care for other groups—for example, the mentally handicapped, the physically handicapped, the elderly mentally infirm. We must ensure that the community is not itself overwhelmed.

Help for the Family

Living with people who have had or who are recovering from mental illness can place heavy strains on a family. The mentally ill do not always fit easily into the family circle or adapt to the family routine: meal times, social activities, entertaining may be disrupted and the family can rapidly become socially isolated. If the mother is ill, the father may find himself having to take time off work and the family income may fall. Special arrangements may need to be made for the care of the children. Research studies have already shown that the children of mentally ill parents are themselves more likely to suffer from mental illness. The family may become afraid to leave a withdrawn and uncommunicative member alone; and they too may become virtually housebound, often giving up sources of income and interest. Under such stresses the family member may become torn between their determination not to reject the individual member, and a desperate need for relief and support. Feelings of guilt may be accentuated where there are brothers and sisters living at home, competing for their parents' attention and resentful of the way in which their own lives and friendships are disrupted.

Some families may be able—and indeed wish—to undertake the demanding task of care. But in these cases it is essential that they receive support and advice from professional staff and that services should be organised to give them effective relief: to enable them to go on holiday and to cope with more urgent domestic crises which may make continued care impractical from time to time, or simply to allow them some respite from the sheer physical and emotional strain.

Development in Services for the Mentally Ill

THE VICTORIAN INHERITANCE

The facilities we have at present to serve the mentally ill are largely an inheritance bequeathed to us by the Victorians. Of the 100 or so hospitals providing treatment solely for the mentally ill now in existence, most were built in the nineteenth century and some have an even longer history. Most are very large—a number were built to accommodate 2000 or more patients; and were deliberately built in areas which were then, and in many cases still are, isolated and remote from centres of population. The aim was twofold; partly to protect society by providing custodial care behind locked doors and high walls and partly to protect the patient by providing him with a secure shelter. A remote site in the country was therefore desirable on both counts, and had the added advantage that it enabled many patients to have the benefit of wholesome work in the open air. In an era which lacked modern medicine, had but the most rudimentary welfare services and no system of social security payments, the large mental hospital was designed to be as far as possible a self-sufficient community meeting the patient's need at once for care and custody.

THE DRUGS REVOLUTION OF THE 1950s

From the time these hospitals were built and right up to the year 1954, the number of resident patients in mental illness hospitals went on steadily increasing save for a small temporary reduction during each of the two World Wars. No new mental illness hospitals were however built after the 1930s and by the early 1950s many were becoming severely overcrowded. Serious thought was then being given to the need to build new mental hospitals; but fortunately the first half of the 1950s saw major developments in drug treatment, in particular with the drug group known as the phenothiazines. The particular significance of these drugs lay in the fact that they enabled doctors to control the disturbed behavior of the psychotic patient. As a result not only was the need for locked doors greatly reduced, but it was also possible for doctors and nurses to develop contact with patients who had hitherto been almost entirely cut off from the real world around them by their psychotic illness. These drugs did not cure illness: but they did enable symptoms to be controlled and relieved and hence made it possible to prevent or at least reduce to a considerable extent the social and personal deterioration accompanying prolonged psychotic illness. The discovery of phenothiazines, and more recently the long acting derivatives, was important but one should not underestimate the significance of other developments: changes in staff attitudes; the introduction of non-physical approaches to treatment; the development of social security and other forms of support outside hospital. Together these developments led to what has been called the "open-door" policy. The function of the hospital was seen increasingly as being for treatment and rehabilitation rather than care and control. With the growing realisation that so many patients could be treated as day patients or out-patients, admission for long term in-patient treatment became less necessary. This changing approach also led to the development of small psychiatric units in general hospitals for treating some mentally ill people locally, instead of at large distant specialist hospitals.

THE ROYAL COMMISSION OF 1957
AND THE MENTAL HEALTH ACT 1959

The Royal Commission on the Law Relating to Mental Illness and Mental Deficiency, and its legislative sequel, the Mental Health Act of 1959, gave formal recognition to the fundamental change in approach which was taking place. The Act made far-reaching changes in the procedures for admission to a mental hospital: for the great majority of patients, admission for psychiatric treatment now entailed no more formality than admission for any other form of hospital treatment. This emphasised the hospital's role as a place for treatment and not merely custody. Directions under the National Health Service Act placed new duties on what were then the health departments of local authorities to provide for the care and after-care of mentally ill people outside hospital.

PROJECTIONS OF DECLINING NUMBERS OF IN-PATIENTS

By the end of the 1950s the repercussions of the new forms of treatment were being dramatically reflected in hospital bed numbers. From 3.4 per 1000 population in 1954, the number of occupied beds had already fallen to 3.1 per 1000 by 1960. Projections made in 1961 by Statisticians at the General Register Office suggested that in the future some 0.9 beds per 1000 population would be needed for patients staying less than 2 years; and that a further 0.9 would be required for newly arising longer stay patients. The projections further suggested that none of the patients then in hospital would still be there in 15 years or so. The 1962 Hospital Plan recognised the place of the short-stay psychiatric unit as a part of the general hospital and envisaged that many of the existing mental hospitals would have no place in the new pattern of service.

THE UNDERLYING MOVEMENT TO COMMUNITY CARE

The underlying movement was becoming clearly discernible, namely of bringing into closer relationship services for the mentally ill whether in hospital or outside it, with services for other forms of illness and handicap. Psychiatry was coming in out of the cold. The report of the Royal Commission commented: "The mental health services would lose much more than they could gain by a return to isolation and separation, and it would be most unfortunate if schemes for co-ordination between hospitals and local authorities were not to be accompanied by correspondingly close contact with other parts of their own services."

HOW FAR HAVE EXPECTATIONS BEEN FULFILLED?

It is now some 15 years since this watershed. How far have hopes been fulfilled: how far frustrated and disappointed? The process of integrating psychiatric with general hospital and community services has gathered strength. There are now a considerable number of general hospital psychiatric units—although varying considerably in size and adequacy of accommodation. There is greater emphasis in undergraduate medical education on psychiatric illness. Only one of the provincial medical schools lacks an Academic Department of Psychiatry. There are however still no such Departments at four of the London medical schools. Social work support and services for the mentally ill are now an integral part of the responsibility of local authority social services departments. The process has not always been smooth. The case, for example, for the integrated social services departments was hotly debated. Both in the medical and social work fields those concerned with the mental illness services still face the very real dilemma of wanting the benefits of integration, yet wishing to retain the different approach to therapy that mental as distinct from physical illness so often requires; of wanting to be an integral part of the general pattern of health and social services facilities, but yet wishing to ensure that the special additional needs of the mentally ill are recognised and provided for.

PHYSICAL AND NON-PHYSICAL METHODS OF TREATMENT

Drug treatments continue to be widely used, and have played a major part in facilitating the decline in length of in-patient stay for many patients and the rapid growth of day and out-patient treatment. It has to be recognised, however, that research has still not shown the precise mechanism by which these drugs have their effect. Some argue that drugs are used too much—particularly in the treatment of neurotic illness; that they treat symptoms only and ignore the underlying social, psychological, and environmental causes of mental illness, for which psychological methods are more appropriate. In particular some stress the importance of family and personal relationships as a factor in causing mental illness and argue that treatment must take account of this. There are those who argue that often it is society or the family which is disturbed rather than the individual patient. Others are equally convinced of the importance of biochemical factors in causation and argue that from this viewpoint drug treatment is the logical remedy. The issues are widely discussed and debated; but what seems beyond doubt is that mental illness is a highly complex phenomenon, taking many forms and caused by a variety of different factors. In recognition of this, the great majority of psychiatrists deliberately adopt an eclectic approach to treatment. While the choice of treatment is a matter of professional judgment, the patient and his family have to find the choice acceptable. Although what doctors say to individual patients about their illness must be a matter for clinical discretion, there would seem to be much to be said, as a matter of principle, for accepting the need to explain to the patient and his family the nature of the illness and the doctor's particular approach to its treatment.

THE "OPEN-DOOR" POLICY

In one sense there has been very considerable progress towards community based services, in that the great majority of psychiatric hospitals and units increasingly see themselves as serving a population that extends far beyond the hospital walls. Out-patient attendances number 1 1/2 million a year, day patient attendances 2 million. Psychiatric nurses are working more and more with patients and their families in their own homes. But by and large the non-hospital community resources are still minimal, though where facilities have been developed they have in general proved successful. The failure, for which central government as much as local government is responsible, to develop anything approaching adequate social services is perhaps the greatest disappointment of the last 15 years. As a result the balance of existing facilities—health and social services—bears increasingly less relation to acknowledged needs. Hospital staff have, rightly in one sense, come to see their role as an active therapeutic one and the hospital as a place for providing medical treatment and nursing care. So they have become unwilling to act as social care custodians for those who would not need to remain in hospital were supporting facilities available in the community. But we have to face the fact that adequate supporting facilities in the community are not generally available. For many years this will pose a continuing problem to which there is no easy answer and it places on the staff of the mental hospitals very real frustrations. Much of their effort in

the past has been directed to developing intensive treatment and rehabilitation leading to discharge back to the community. Largely as a result the
gross overcrowding of earlier years has in general been considerably
reduced. Naturally they wish to see further progress in this direction.
Clearly people should not be admitted to hospital who have no need for
treatment; but admission and discharge policies must be realistic and take
account of the local availability of supporting social services. If they do not,
they put at risk the whole principle of community care in the eyes of the
public. The Government for its part intends to see that over the years the
balance of health and social services is put right.

The frustrations and dilemmas of this situation have been felt no less
by the great majority of local authorities who have been anxious to develop
their services for the mentally ill, but who have been constrained by the
limits on resources and the increasing and competing demands for new
developments throughout the whole social services field.

The term "open-door hospital" has, like "community care" become
with time something of a catchphrase. Such phrases tend to acquire an
oversimplified meaning and it may be worth examining what this concept
means in terms of present day psychiatry. It should clearly be regarded as
signifying an approach to treatment rather than a factual description of the
physical arrangement at the hospital. Wards may be unlocked but professional judgment needs to be exercised as to whether a particular patient at
a particular time should not be sufficiently supervised at least to prevent his
leaving the hospital and abandoning his treatment. The extent to which
physical security is needed is a separate issue discussed [below], but adequate supervision of the relatively few patients who require it, is important
for public trust and confidence in the overall pattern of care.

From Department of Health and Social Security, *Better Services for the Mentally Ill:
Presented to Parliament by the Secretary of State for Social Services by Command of Her
Majesty, October 1975* (London: Her Majesty's Stationery Office, 1975), 6–9,
11–14.

PART IV

The Psychoboom

In the decades following World War II, the fields of psychiatry, clinical psychology, and psychotherapy experienced unprecedented growth. In the United States, membership in the American Psychological Association grew from 2,739 in 1940, to 30,839 in 1970, to around 75,000 by 1993, while membership in the American Psychiatric Association rose from 2,423 to 18,407 between 1940 and 1970. A similar trend took place in Central Europe, where membership in the German Psychological Society went from around 2,500 in 1961 to 20,000 in 1984 and more than 40,000 by 1996. These numbers reflect the fact that, throughout the Western world over the years 1945–2000, psychiatric, psychometric, and psychotherapeutic ideas, services, and professionals became commonplace in mainstream society. It became acceptable among the middle class to see a therapist in order to deal with interpersonal problems; insurance systems began to routinely cover the costs of psychotherapy; clinical testing became a prominent part of educational systems; psychiatric and psychological expertise was frequently called on by government to help advise public policy; and newspapers, magazines, and radio and television outlets recruited counseling professionals for advice columns and shows.

The boom in psychiatric, psychological, and psychotherapeutic work represented a shift in orientation, away from custodial and palliative treatment to outpatient and preventive care. In short, an emphasis began to be placed on mental health care, as opposed to simply treating mental illness. Over the course of the 1950s, 1960s, and 1970s, this trend was particularly evident in

Italy, the Netherlands, Great Britain, West Germany, and the United States.

The simultaneous expansion of the welfare state and the rise of mass consumerism had much to do with this. As both the private and public service sectors grew, there was a concomitant growth in the demand for the knowledge and skills of social workers, nurses, counselors, psychometricians, researchers, and physicians in mental health care. At the same time, self-help, encounter, and patient advocacy groups flourished, their leaders and members taking their cues from consumer and civil rights movements. This was the period when "patients" became "clients."

Attention to the clinical treatment of mental disorders hardly disappeared, though. Soon after World War II, states and private firms began investing resources into scientific research, particularly in the area of pharmacology. In the early 1950s, after a series of experiments, French researchers stumbled upon the antipsychotic properties of a synthetic drug known as chlorpromazine (marketed as Thorazine). Introduced in American asylums in 1954–1955, the drug produced effects that were staggering: there were reports that patients who formerly had been agitated or distracted suddenly became calm and clearheaded. Within months, chlorpromazine became a standard part of the treatment regimen in psychiatric hospitals throughout the United States and Europe. In addition, its implementation encouraged large pharmaceutical companies to see a lucrative market in the development of psychiatric drugs. Over the following fifty years, a host of psychotropic medications made their way into inpatient and outpatient care—amphetamines, barbiturates, benzodiazepines, lithium, MAO inhibitors, tricyclic antidepressants.

The increasing reliance of psychiatry—particularly in the United States—on drug treatment raised questions about standards and efficacy. How could companies, physicians, government officials, and the public be confident that a drug did what developers claimed? Already in the 1950s, clinical researchers had begun employing a method used in other disciplines, testing drug effectiveness by randomly assigning subjects to either an experimental group receiving treatment or a control group not receiving the specified treatment. By the 1980s, randomized clinical trials were accepted by many as the final arbiter in determining the effectiveness of treatments.

Often lost in the popular enthusiasm over drug treatment in psychiatry is the fact that even the most effective medications have treated symptoms, not cured diseases. In fact, one of the questions that rose to prominence during the second half of the twentieth century was exactly how to single out a set of symptoms as constituting a discrete disorder or illness. Contemporary psychiatric professionals and their organizations have spent a great deal of time grappling with this thorny problem. It is, however, only relatively recently that this was even perceived to be a problem.

Until the twentieth century, there were no universally accepted standards of diagnosis for mental disorders. Indeed, historically many physicians believed that a diagnosis was, at best, largely irrelevant to treating a patient or, at worst, restricting and deceptive. Over the course of the late nineteenth and early twentieth centuries, however, governments began demanding statistical data on insanity. In the United States, the lack of uniformity in collecting this data led the American Medico-Psychological Association and the National Committee for Mental Hygiene in 1918 to issue the first standardized nosology: the *Statistical Manual for the Use of Institutions for the Insane*. During World War II, the U.S. Army and Navy developed their own classifications, a system that the American Psychiatric Association (APA) adopted and revised after the war, publishing it as the *Diagnostic and Statistical Manual (DSM)* in 1952. Heavily inflected by psychoanalytic and psychodynamic thinking, the manual was revised and published as the *DSM-II* beginning in 1968.

The content of the *DSM* has always been closely coordinated with that found in the World Health Organization's manual, the *International Classification of Diseases (ICD)*. And since 1968, the United States has had a treaty with the World Health Organization agreeing to accept the *ICD* as the official diagnostic manual in the country. Thus, when it was announced that a ninth revision of the *ICD* was planned for publication in 1978, it was decided to once again revise the American *DSM*. The result was the *DSM-III*, a document that represents a major turning point in the understanding and treatment of mental disorders. Its emphasis on description and behavior and its marginalization of psychodynamic concepts announced a change in the governing consensus within psychiatry. From this point on, biomedical models would come to dominate scholarly and public discussions.

Alcoholics Anonymous
(founded 1935)
"The Twelve Steps" and "The Twelve Traditions"

Concerns over the dominance of professions in psychiatric care helped to fuel the rise and success of patient advocacy and self-help groups during the second half of the twentieth century. One of the most successful and influential self-help organizations has been Alcoholics Anonymous (A.A.). A.A. arose out of a chance encounter in 1935 between two self-professed alcoholics: stockbroker Bill Wilson (known simply as Bill) and surgeon Bob Smith (known as Dr. Bob). Smith, who had become involved in the Oxford Group, an organization begun by Christian missionary Frank Buchman, convinced Wilson that overcoming alcoholism was possible only through turning over one's life to God. Working out of Smith's home in Akron, Ohio, the two men began helping those struggling with alcohol addiction. They soon drafted the "Twelve Steps," and, in 1950, the membership endorsed a statement of group attitudes and principles crafted by the founders and early members (the "Twelve Traditions"). By 1951, the organization claimed a U.S. national membership of one hundred thousand.

A.A.'s twelve-step approach, its regular open meetings, and its dedication to the principle of anonymity have provided a model for countless other mental health support groups, such as Gamblers Anonymous, Narcotics Anonymous, and Overeaters Anonymous. In 2008, it was estimated that there were more than 113,000 groups and more than 2 million members in 180 countries.

The Twelve Steps

1. We admitted we were powerless over alcohol—that our lives had become unmanageable.
2. Came to believe that a Power greater than ourselves could restore us to sanity.
3. Made a decision to turn our will and our lives over to the care of God as we understood Him.
4. Made a searching and fearless moral inventory of ourselves.
5. Admitted to God, to ourselves and to another human being the exact nature of our wrongs.
6. Were entirely ready to have God remove all these defects of character.
7. Humbly asked Him to remove our shortcomings.
8. Made a list of all persons we had harmed, and became willing to make amends to them all.
9. Made direct amends to such people wherever possible, except when to do so would injure them or others.
10. Continued to take personal inventory and when we were wrong promptly admitted it.
11. Sought through prayer and meditation to improve our conscious contact with God, *as we understood Him*, praying only for knowledge of His will for us and the power to carry that out.
12. Having had a spiritual awakening as the result of these steps, we tried to carry this message to alcoholics, and to practice these principles in all our affairs.

The Twelve Traditions

1. Our common welfare should come first; personal recovery depends upon A.A. unity.
2. For our group purpose there is but one ultimate authority—a loving God as He may express Himself in our group conscience. Our leaders are but trusted servants; they do not govern.
3. The only requirement for A.A. membership is a desire to stop drinking.

4. Each group should be autonomous except in matters affecting other groups or A.A. as a whole.

5. Each group has but one primary purpose—to carry its message to the alcoholic who still suffers.

6. An A.A. group ought never endorse, finance or lend the A.A. name to any related facility or outside enterprise, lest problems of money, property and prestige divert us from our primary purpose.

7. Every A.A. group ought to be fully self-supporting, declining outside contributions.

8. Alcoholics Anonymous should remain forever nonprofessional, but our service centers may employ special workers.

9. A.A., as such, ought never be organized; but we may create service boards or committees directly responsible to those they serve.

10. Alcoholics Anonymous has no opinion on outside issues; hence the A.A. name ought never be drawn into public controversy.

11. Our public relations policy is based on attraction rather than promotion; we need always maintain personal anonymity at the level of press, radio and films.

12. Anonymity is the spiritual foundation of all our traditions, ever reminding us to place principles before personalities.

While the Twelve Traditions are not specifically binding on any group or groups, an overwhelming majority of members have adopted them as the basis for A.A.'s expanding "internal" and public relationships.

Carl Rogers
(1902–1987)

"The Attitude and Orientation of the Counselor in Client-Centered Therapy"
(1949)

In two separate surveys of members of the American Psychological Association conducted in 1982 and 2006, individuals were asked to identify which psychotherapists most influenced the field and their own practice. Both times, respondents overwhelmingly agreed on one name: Carl Rogers. Rogers's brand of humanistic psychology is now influencing its third generation of counselors. It is safe to say that most therapists in the United States today are, in one form or another, Rogerian.

After first attending seminary, Carl Rogers received his PhD, in 1931, going on to teach at a number of universities in the United States. Already in the 1940s, Rogers had begun to outline what he initially called "nondirective" therapy, but later dubbed "client-centered" or "person-centered" therapy. He eventually moved to California, where he helped found the Center for Studies of the Person in 1968 and began working closely with encounter groups. The excerpt here provides a good summary of his therapeutic approach shortly before publication of his famous book *Client-Centered Therapy*, published in 1951. It is sometimes easy to forget that, behind the unassuming tone of his prose, Rogers was directly challenging psychiatrists and psychoanalysts about the methods they employed.

The Philosophical Orientation of the Counselor

The primary point of importance here is the attitude held by the counselor toward the worth and the significance of the individual. How do we look upon others? Do we see each person as having worth and dignity in his own right? If we do hold this point of view at the verbal level, to what extent is it operationally evident at the behavioral level? Do we tend to treat individuals as persons of worth, or do we subtly devaluate them by our attitudes and behavior? Is our philosophy one in which respect for the individual is uppermost? Do we respect his capacity and his right to self-direction or do we basically believe that his life would be best guided by us? To what extent do we have a need and a desire to dominate others? Are we willing for the individual to select and choose his own values, or are our actions guided by the conviction (usually unspoken), that he would be happiest if he permitted us to select for him his values and standards and goals?

. . . Perhaps it would summarize the point being made to say that a person can implement, by client-centered techniques, his respect for others only insofar as that respect is an integral part of his personality makeup; consequently the person whose operational philosophy has already moved in this direction of feeling a deep respect for the significance and worth of each person is more readily able to assimilate the client-centered techniques which adequately express this feeling.

A Formulation of the Counselor's Role

At the present stage of thinking in client-centered therapy, there is another attempt to describe what occurs in the most satisfactory therapeutic relationships, another attempt to describe the way in which the basic hypothesis is implemented. This formulation would state that it is the counselor's function to assume, in so far as he is able, the internal frame of reference of the client, to perceive the world as the client sees it, to perceive the client himself as he is seen by himself, and to lay aside all exceptions from the external frame of reference while doing so. . . .

The Difficulty of Perceiving through the Client's Eyes

To try to give you, the reader, a somewhat more real and vivid experience of what is involved in the attitudinal set which we are discussing, it is suggested that you put yourself in the place of the counselor, and consider the following material, which is taken from complete counselor notes of the beginning of an interview with a man in his thirties. When the material has been completed, sit back and consider the sorts of attitudes and thoughts which were in your mind as you read.

> Client: I don't feel very normal, but I want to feel that way. . . . I thought I'd have something to talk about—then it all goes around in circles. I was trying to think what I was going to say. Then coming here it doesn't work out. . . . I tell you, it seemed that it would be much easier before I came. I tell you, I just can't make a decision; I don't know what I want. I've tried to reason this thing out logically—tried to figure out which things are important to me. I thought that there are maybe two things a man might do; he might get married and raise a family. But if he was just a bachelor, just making a living—that isn't very good. I find myself and my thought getting back to the days when I was a kid and I cry very easily. The dam would break through. I've been in the Army four and a half years. I had no problems then, no hopes, no wishes. My only thought was to get out when peace would come. My problems, now that I'm out, are as ever. I tell you, they go back to a long time before I was in the Army. . . . I love children. When I was in the Philippines—I tell you, when I was young I swore I'd never forget my unhappy childhood—so when I saw these children in the Philippines, I treated them very nicely. I used to give them ice cream cones and movies. It was just a period—I'd reverted back—and that awakened some emotions in me I thought I had long buried. (A pause. He seems very near tears.)

As this material was read, thoughts of the following sorts would represent an external frame of reference in you, the "counselor."

> I wonder if I should help him get started talking.
>
> Is this inability to get under way a type of dependence?
>
> Why this indecisiveness? What could be its cause?
>
> What is meant by this focus on marriage and family?
>
> He seems to be a bachelor. I hadn't known that.
>
> The crying, the "dam," sound as though there must be a great deal of repression.
>
> He's a veteran. Could he have been a psychiatric case?
>
> I feel sorry for anybody who spent four and one-half years in the service.
>
> Some time we will probably need to dig into those early unhappy experiences.
>
> What is this interest in children? Identification?
> Vague homosexuality?

Thoughts which might go through your mind if you were quite successful in assuming the client's internal frame of reference would tend to be of this order.

> You're wanting to struggle toward normality, aren't you?
>
> It's really hard for you to get started.
>
> Decision-making just seems impossible to you.
>
> You want marriage, but it doesn't seem to you to be much of a possibility.
>
> You feel yourself brimming over with childish feelings.
>
> To you the Army represented stagnation.
>
> Being very nice to children has somehow had meaning for you.
>
> But it has been—and is—a disturbing experience for you.

If these thoughts are couched in a final and declarative form, then they shift over into becoming an evaluation from the counselor's perceptual vantage point. But to the extent that they are empathic attempts to understand, tentative in formulation, then they represent the attitude we are trying to describe as "adopting the client's frame of reference."

The Rationale of the Counselor's Role

The question may arise in the minds of many, why adopt this peculiar type of relationship? In what way does it implement the hypothesis from which we started? What is the rationale of this approach?

In order to have a clear basis for considering these questions, let us attempt to put first in formal and then in literary terms, a statement of the counselor's purpose when he functions in this way. In psychological terms, it is the counselor's aim to perceive as sensitively and accurately as possible all of the perceptual field as it is being experienced by the client, with the same figure and ground relationships, to the full degree that the client is willing to communicate that perceptual field; and having thus perceived this internal frame of reference of the other as completely as possible, to indicate to the client the extent to which he is seeing through the client's eyes.

Suppose that we attempt a description somewhat more in terms of the counselor's attitudes. The counselor says in effect, "To be of assistance to you I will put aside myself—the self of ordinary interaction—and enter into your world of perception as completely as I am able. I will become, in a sense, another self for you—a mirror held up to your own attitudes and feelings—an opportunity for you to discern yourself more clearly, to understand yourself more truly and deeply, to choose more satisfyingly."

Some Deep Issues

The assumption of the therapeutic role which has been described raises some very basic questions indeed. An example from a therapeutic interview may pose some of these issues for our consideration. Miss Gil, a young woman who has shown deep confusion and conflict, and who has been quite hopeless about herself, has spent the major part of one of her therapeutic hours discussing her feelings of inadequacy and lack of personal worth. Part of the time she has been aimlessly using the finger paints. She has just finished expressing her feelings of wanting to get away from everyone—to have nothing to do with people. After a long pause comes the following.

MISS G.: I've never said this before to anyone—but I've thought for such a long time—This is a terrible thing to say, but if I could just—well, (short, bitter laugh—pause) If I could just find some glorious cause that I could give my life for I would be happy. I cannot be the kind of a person I want to be. I guess maybe I haven't the guts—or the strength —to kill myself—and if someone else would relieve me of the responsibility—or I would be in an accident—I—I—just don't want to live.

C: At the present time things look so black to you that you can't see much point in living—

MISS G.: Yes—I wish I'd never started this therapy. I was happy when I was living in my dream world. There I could be the kind of person I wanted to be—But now—There is such a wide, wide gap—between my ideal—and what I am. I wish people hated me. I try to make them hate me. Because then I could turn away from them and could blame them—but no—It is all in my hands—Here is my life—and I either accept the fact that I am absolutely worthless—or I fight whatever it is that holds me in this terrible conflict. And I suppose if I accepted the fact that I am worthless, then I could go away someplace—and get a little room someplace—get a mechanical job someplace—and retreat clear back to the security of my dream world where I could do things, have clever friends, be a pretty wonderful sort of person—

C: It's really a tough struggle—digging into this like you are—and at times the shelter of your dream world looks more attractive and comfortable.

MISS G.: My dream world or suicide.

C: Your dream world or something more permanent than dreams—

MISS G.: Yes, (a long pause. Complete change of voice) So I don't see why I should waste your time—coming in twice a week—I'm not worth it—What do you think?

C: It's up to you, Gil—It isn't wasting my time—I'd be glad to see you— whenever you come—but it's how you feel about it—if you don't want to come twice a week—or if you do want to come twice a week?—once a week?—It's up to you. (Long pause.)

MISS G.: You're not going to suggest that I come in oftener? You're not alarmed and think I ought to come in—every day—until I get out of this?

C: I believe you are able to make your own decision. I'll see you whenever you want to come.

MISS G.: (Note of awe in her voice) I don't believe you are alarmed about—I see —I may be afraid of myself—but you aren't afraid for me—(She stands up—a strange look on her face).

C: You say you may be afraid of yourself—and are wondering why I don't seem to be afraid for you?

MISS G.: (Another short laugh) You have more confidence in me than I have. (She cleans up the finger-paint mess and starts out of the room) I'll see you next week—(that short laugh) maybe.

Her attitude seemed tense, depressed, bitter, completely beaten. She walked slowly away.

———

This excerpt raises sharply the question as to how far the therapist is going to maintain his central hypothesis. Where life, quite literally, is at stake, what is the best hypothesis upon which to act? Shall his hypothesis still remain a deep respect for the capacity of the person, or shall he change his hypothesis? If so what are the alternatives? One would be the hypothesis that "I can be successfully responsible for the life of another." Still another is the hypothesis, "I can be temporarily responsible for the life of another without damaging the capacity for self-determination." Still another hypothesis is: "The individual cannot be responsible for himself, nor can I be responsible for him but it is possible to find someone who can be responsible for him."

Does the counselor have the right, professionally or morally, to permit a client seriously to consider psychosis or suicide as a way out, without making a positive effort to prevent these choices? Is it a part of our general social responsibility that we may not tolerate such thinking or such action on the part of another?

These are deep issues, which strike to the very core of therapy. They are not issues which one person can decide for another. Different therapeutic orientations have acted upon different hypotheses. All that one person can do is to describe his own experience and the evidence which grows out of that experience.

From Carl Rogers, "The Attitude and Orientation of the Counselor in Client-Centered Therapy," *Journal of Consulting Psychology* 13 (1949): 82–94.

Aaron T. Beck
(b. 1921)
"Cognitive Therapy: Nature and Relation to Behavior Therapy"
(1970)

The 1960s and 1970s witnessed a renaissance in psychotherapy that some have argued compares to the revolution of moral therapy in the eighteenth century. One of the most successful innovations during this time was cognitive-behavioral therapy (CBT). Developed by Aaron Beck and Albert Ellis (1913–2007) independently of one another, cognitive-behavioral therapy is likely the most widely applied form of psychotherapy in the United States today.

Aaron Beck came to the idea of what he originally termed "cognitive therapy" through an early enthusiasm for psychoanalysis. Training first as an analyst, he carried out experiments that he believed would demonstrate the accuracy of psychoanalytic theories of depression. What he found, instead, was that depressed patients tended to be overwhelmed by spontaneous negative thoughts ("automatic thoughts") and that challenging the veracity of these thoughts more often than not led to recovery. In short, contrary to psychoanalytic wisdom, it was not necessary to explore deeply into one's past. The simplicity and replicability of Beck's method has made it amenable to clinical trials and to application for a range of disorders, including personality disorders, eating disorders, and drug abuse.

Two systems of psychotherapy that have increasingly gained prominence have been the subject of rapidly increasing number of clinical and experimental studies. Cognitive therapy, the more recent entry into the field of psychotherapy, and behavior therapy already show signs of becoming institutionalized.

Although behavior therapy has been publicized in a large number of articles and monographs, cognitive therapy has received much less recognition. Despite the fact that behavior therapy is based primarily on learning theory whereas cognitive therapy is rooted more in cognitive theory, the two systems of psychotherapy have much in common.

First, in both systems of psychotherapy the therapeutic interview is more overtly structured and the therapist more active than in other psychotherapies. After the preliminary diagnostic interviews in which a systematic and highly detailed description of the patient's problems is obtained, both the cognitive and the behavior therapists formulate the patient's presenting symptoms (in cognitive or behavioral terms, respectively) and design specific sets of operations for the particular problem areas.

After mapping out the areas for therapeutic work, the therapist explicitly coaches the patient regarding the kinds of responses and behaviors that are useful with this particular form of therapy. Detailed instructions are presented to the patient, for example, to stimulate pictorial fantasies (systematic desensitization) or to facilitate his awareness and recognition of his cognitions (cognitive therapy). The goals of these therapies are circumscribed, in contrast to the evocative therapies whose goals are open-ended.

Second, both the cognitive and behavior therapists aim their therapeutic technique at the overt symptom or behavioral problem, such as a particular phobia, obsession, or hysterical symptom. However, the target differs somewhat. The cognitive therapist focuses more on the ideational content involved in the symptom, viz., the irrational inferences and premises. The behavior therapist focuses more on the overt behavior, e.g., the maladaptive avoidance responses. Both psychotherapeutic systems conceptualize symptom formation in terms of constructs that are accessible either to behavioral observation or to introspection, in contrast to psychoanalysis, which views most symptoms as the disguised derivatives of unconscious conflicts.

Third, in further contrast to psychoanalytic therapy, neither cognitive therapy nor behavior therapy draws substantially on recollections or reconstructions of the patient's childhood experiences and early family relationships. The emphasis on correlating present problems with developmental events, furthermore, is much less prominent than in psychoanalytic psychotherapy.

A fourth point in common between these two systems is that their theoretical paradigms exclude many traditional psychoanalytic assumptions such as infantile sexuality, fixations, the unconscious, and mechanisms of defense. The behavior and cognitive therapists may devise their therapeutic strategies on the basis of introspective data provided by the patient; however, they generally take the patients' self-report at face value and do not make the kind of high-level abstractions characteristic of psychoanalytic formulations.

Finally, a major assumption of both cognitive therapy and behavior therapy is that the patient has acquired maladaptive reaction patterns that can be "unlearned" without the absolute requirement that he obtain insight into the origin of the symptom. . . .

The most striking theoretical difference between cognitive and behavior therapy lies in the concept used to explain the dissolution of maladaptive responses through therapy. Wolpe, for example, utilizes behavioral or neurophysiological explanations such as counter-conditioning or reciprocal inhibition; the cognitivists postulate the modification of conceptual systems, i.e., changes in attitudes or modes of thinking. As will be discussed later, many behavior therapists implicitly or explicitly recognize the importance of cognitive factors in therapy, although they do not expand on these in detail.

Techniques of Cognitive Therapy

Cognitive therapy may be defined in two ways: In a broad sense, any technique whose major mode of action is the modification of faulty patterns of thinking can be regarded as cognitive therapy. This definition embraces all therapeutic operations that *indirectly* affect the cognitive patterns, as well as those that directly affect them. An individual's distorted views of himself and his world, for example may be corrected through insight into the historical antecedents of his misinterpretations (as in dynamic psychotherapy), through greater congruence between the concept of the self and the ideal (as in Rogerian therapy), and through increasingly sharp recognition of the unreality of fears (as in systematic desensitization).

However, cognitive therapy may be defined more narrowly as a set of operations focused on a patient's cognitions (verbal or pictorial) and on the premises, assumptions, and attitudes underlying these cognitions. This section will describe the specific technique of cognitive therapy.

RECOGNIZING IDIOSYNCRATIC COGNITIONS

One of the main cognitive techniques consists of training the patient to recognize his idiosyncratic cognitions or "automatic thoughts" (Beck, 1963).[*] Ellis (1962) refers to these cognitions as "internalized statements" or "self-statements," and explains them to the patient as "things that you tell yourself."[†] These cognitions are termed idiosyncratic because they reflect a faulty appraisal, ranging from a mild distortion to a complete misinterpretation, and because they fall into a pattern that is peculiar to a given individual or to a particular psychopathological state.

---

[*]Author's note: A. T. Beck, "Thinking and Depression: 1. Idiosyncratic Content and Cognitive Distortions," *Archives of General Psychiatry* 9 (1963): 324–333.

[†]Author's note: A. Ellis, *Reason and Emotion in Psychotherapy* (New York: Lyle Stuart, 1962).

In the acutely disturbed patient, the distorted ideation is frequently in the center of the patient's phenomenal field. In such cases, the patient is very much aware of these idiosyncratic thoughts and can easily describe them. The acutely paranoid patient, for instance, is bombarded with thoughts relevant to his being persecuted, abused, or discriminated against by other people. In the mild or moderate neurotic, the distorted ideas are generally at the periphery of awareness. It is therefore necessary to motivate and to train the patient to attend to these thoughts.

Many patients reporting unpleasant affects describe a sequence consisting of a specific event (external stimulus) leading to an unpleasant affect. For instance, the patient may outline the sequence of (a) seeing an old friend and then (b) experiencing feelings of sadness. Oftentimes, the sadness is inexplicable to the patient. Another person (a) hears about someone having been killed in an automobile accident and (b) feels anxiety. However, he cannot make a direct connection between these two phenomena; e.g., there is a missing link in the sequence.

In these instances of a particular event leading to an unpleasant affect, it is possible to discern an intervening variable, namely, a cognition, which forms the bridge between the external stimulus and the subjective feeling. Seeing an old friend stimulates cognitions such as "It won't be like old times," or "He won't accept me as he used to." The cognition then generates sadness. The report of the automobile accident stimulates a pictorial image in which the patient himself is the victim of an automobile accident. The image then leads to anxiety.

This paradigm can be further illustrated by a number of examples. A patient treated by the writer complained that he experienced anxiety whenever he saw a dog. He was puzzled by the fact that he experienced anxiety even when the dog was chained or caged or else was obviously harmless. The patient was instructed: "Notice what thoughts go through your mind the next time you see a dog—any dog." At the next interview, the patient reported that during numerous encounters with dogs between appointments, he had recognized a phenomenon that he had not noticed previously; namely, that each time he saw the dog he had a thought such as "It's going to bite me."

By being able to detect the intervening cognitions, the patient was able to understand why he felt anxious, namely, he indiscriminately regarded every dog as dangerous. He stated, "I even got that thought when I saw a small poodle. Then I realized how ridiculous it was to think that a poodle could hurt me." He also recognized that when he saw a big dog on a leash, he thought of the most deleterious consequences: "The dog will jump up and bite out my eyes," or "It will jump and bite my jugular vein and kill me." Within 2 or 3 weeks, the patient was able to overcome completely his long-standing dog phobia simply by recognizing his cognitions when exposed to a dog.

Another example was provided by a college student who experienced inexplicable anxiety in a social situation. After being trained to examine and write down his cognitions, he reported that in social situations he would have thoughts such as, "They think I look pathetic," or "Nobody will want to talk to me," or "I'm just a misfit." These thoughts were followed by anxiety. . . .

Sometimes, the cognition may take a pictorial form instead of, or in addition to, the verbal form. A woman who experienced spurts of anxiety when riding across a bridge was able to recognize that the anxiety was preceded by a pictorial image of her car breaking through the guard rail and falling off the bridge. Another woman, with a fear of walking alone, found that her spells of anxiety followed images of her having a heart attack and being left helpless and dying on the street. A college student discovered that his anxiety at leaving his dormitory at night was triggered by visual fantasies of being attacked.

The idiosyncratic cognitions (whether pictorial or verbal) are very rapid and often may contain an elaborate idea compressed into a very short period of time, even into a split second. These cognitions are experienced as though they are automatic; i.e., they seem to arise as if by reflex rather than through reasoning or deliberation. They also seem to have an *involuntary* quality. A severely anxious or depressed or paranoid person, for example, may continually experience the idiosyncratic cognitions, even though he may try to ward them off. Furthermore, these cognitions tend to appear completely *plausible* to the patient.

DISTANCING

Even after a patient has learned to identify his idiosyncratic ideas, he may have difficulty in examining these ideas objectively. The thought often has the same kind of salience as the perception of an external stimulus. "Distancing" refers to the process of gaining objectivity towards these cognitions. Since the individual with a neurosis tends to accept the validity of his idiosyncratic thoughts without subjecting them to any kind of critical evaluation, it is essential to train him to make a distinction between thought and external reality, between hypothesis and fact. Patients are often surprised to discover that they have been equating an inference with reality and that they have attached a high degree of truth-value to their distorted concepts.

The therapeutic dictum communicated to the patient is as follows: Simply because he *thinks* something does not necessarily mean that it is true. While such a dictum may seem to be a platitude, the writer has found with surprising regularity that patients have benefited from the repeated reminder that thoughts are not equivalent to external reality.

Once the patient is able to "objectify" his thoughts, he is ready for the later stages of reality testing: applying rules of evidence and logic and considering alternative explanations.

CORRECTING COGNITIVE DISTORTIONS AND DEFICIENCIES

The writer has already indicated that patients show faulty or disordered thinking in certain circumscribed areas of experience. In these particular sectors, they have a reduced ability to make fine discriminations and tend to make global, undifferentiated judgments. Part of the task of cognitive therapy is to help to recognize faulty thinking and to make appropriate corrections. It is often very useful for the patient to specify the kind of fallacious thinking involved in his cognitive responses.

Arbitrary inference refers to the process of drawing a conclusion when evidence is lacking or is actually contrary to the conclusion. This type of deviant thinking usually takes the form of personalization (or self-reference). A depressed patient, who saw a frown on the face of a passerby, thought, "He is disgusted with me." A phobic girl of 21, reading about a woman who had a heart attack, got the thought, "I probably have heart disease." A depressed woman, who was kept waiting for a few minutes by the therapist, though, "He has deliberately left in order to avoid seeing me."

Overgeneralization refers to the process of making an unjustified generalization on the basis of a single incident. This may take the form that was described in the case of the man with the dog phobia, who generalized from a particular dog that might attack him to all dogs. Another example is the patient who thinks, "I never succeeded at anything," when he has a single isolated failure.

Magnification refers to the propensity to exaggerate the meaning or significance of a particular event. A person with a fear of dying, for instance, interpreted every unpleasant sensation or pain in his body as a sign of some fatal disease such as cancer, heart attack, or cerebral hemorrhage. Ellis (1962) applied the label "catastrophizing" to this kind of reaction. . . .

Cognitive deficiency refers to the disregard for an important aspect of a life situation. Patients with this defect ignore, fail to integrate, or do not utilize information derived from experience. Such a patient, consequently, behaves as though he has a defect in this system of expectations: He consistently engages in behavior which he realizes, in retrospect, is self-defeating. This class of patients includes those who "act out," e.g., psychopaths, as well as those whose overt behavior sabotages important personal goals. These individuals sacrifice long-range satisfaction or expose themselves to later pain or danger in favor of immediate satisfactions. This category includes problems such as alcoholism, obesity, drug addiction, sexual deviation, and compulsion gambling. . . .

Therapy of such cases consists of training the patient to think of the consequences as soon as his self-defeating wish arises. Consideration of the long-range loss must be forced into the interval between impulse and action. A patient, for instance, who continually operated his car beyond the speed limit or drove thorough stoplights was surprised each time he was stopped by a traffic officer. On interview, it was discovered that the patient was generally absorbed in a fantasy while driving—he imagined himself as a famous racing-car driver engaged in a race. Therapy at first consisted of trying to get him to watch the odometer—but without success. The next approach consisted of inducing fantasies of speeding, getting caught, and receiving punishment. At first, the patient had great difficulty in visualizing getting caught even though, in general, he could fantasize almost everything. However, after several sessions of induced fantasies, he was able to incorporate a negative outcome into his fantasy. Subsequently, he stopped daydreaming while driving and was able to observe traffic regulations.

In the following case report,* several cognitive techniques directed at modifying anxiety proneness are illustrated.

---

*Author's note: This patient was treated in collaboration with Dr. William Dyson.

Case Report

Mrs. G. was an attractive 27-year-old mother of three children. When first seen by the writer, she complained of periods of anxiety lasting up to 6 or 7 hr a day and recurring repeatedly over a 4-year period. She had consulted her family physician, who had prescribed a variety of sedatives, including Thorazine, without any apparent improvement.

In an analysis of the cause-and-effect sequence of her anxiety, the following facts were elicited. The first anxiety episode occurred about 2 weeks after she had a miscarriage. At that time she was bending over to bathe her 1-year-old son, and she suddenly began to feel faint. Following this episode, she had her first anxiety attack which lasted several hours. The patient could not find any explanation for her anxiety. However, when the writer asked whether she had had any thought at the time she felt dizzy, she recalled having had the thought, "Suppose I should pass out and injure the baby." It seemed plausible that her dizziness, which was probably the result of postpartum anemia, led to the fear she might faint and drop the baby. This fear then produced anxiety, which she interpreted as a sign that she was "going to pieces."

Until the time of her miscarriage, the patient had been reasonably care-free and had not experienced episodes of anxiety. However, after her miscarriage, she periodically had the thought, "Bad things can happen to me." Subsequently, when she heard of somebody's becoming sick, she often would have the thought, "This can happen to me," and she would being to feel anxious.

The patient was instructed to try to pinpoint any thoughts that preceded further episodes of anxiety. At the next interview, she reported the following events:

1. One evening, she heard that the husband of one of her friends was sick with a severe pulmonary infection. She then had an anxiety attack lasting several hours. In accordance with the instructions, she tried to recall the preceding cognition, which was, "Tom could get sick like that and maybe die."

2. She had considerable anxiety just before starting a trip to her sister's house. She focused on her thoughts and realized she had the repetitive thought that she might get sick on the trip. She had had a serious episode of gastroenteritis during a previous trip to her sister's

house. She evidently believed that such a sickness could happen to her again.

3. On another occasion, she was feeling uneasy and objects seemed somewhat unreal to her. She then had the thought that she might be losing her mind and immediately experienced an anxiety attack.

4. One of her friends was committed to a state hospital because of a psychiatric illness. The patient had the thought, "This could happen to me. I could lose my mind." When questioned about why she was afraid of losing her mind, she stated that she was afraid that if she went crazy, she would do something that would harm either her children or herself.

It was evident that the patient's crucial fear was the anticipation of loss of control, whether by fainting or by becoming psychotic. The patient was reassured that there were no signs that she was going psychotic. She was also provided with an explanation of the arousal of her anxiety and of her secondary elaboration of the meaning of these attacks.

The major therapeutic thrust in this case was coaching the patient to recall and reflect on the thoughts that preceded her anxiety attacks. The realization that these attacks were initiated by a cognition rather than by some vague mysterious force convinced her she was neither totally vulnerable nor unable to control her reactions. Furthermore, by learning to pinpoint the anxiety-reducing thoughts, she was able to gain some detachment and to subject them to reality testing. Consequently, she was able to nullify the effects of those thoughts. During the next few weeks, her anxiety became less frequent and less intense and, by the end of 4 weeks, they disappeared completely.

Aaron T. Beck, "Cognitive Therapy: Nature and Relation to Behavior Therapy," *Behavior Therapy* 1 (1970): 184–200. Copyright Elsevier 1970.

Edna I. Rawlings and
Dianne K. Carter

"The Intractable Female Patient"
(1977)

Among the postwar social movements that had a direct impact on psychiatry and psychotherapy, the women's movement was among the most important. Dating back to ancient times, girls and women were singled out as being uniquely predisposed to madness and mental illness. At the same time, men dominated the ranks of medicine, the church, government, and academia and, thus, had a disproportionately greater say in how mental maladies were perceived and treated. The emergence of a new range of social and political possibilities for women, combined with the expanded role of social workers and nurses within social psychiatry, provided women with the opportunity to assume a more directive position in mental health care.

Edna Rawlings and Dianne Carter became involved in a consciousness-raising group at the University of Iowa in the 1970s. This experience led them to begin exploring how feminism could contribute to critically rethinking psychotherapy. In 1977, they published the influential book *Psychotherapy for Women*, in which they argued, among other things, that the chief sources of women's pathology were not personal and internal, but social and external, and that women should not be encouraged to adjust themselves to the unequal social conditions in which they lived. In the following excerpt, the authors critically examine a case history they considered emblematic of the kinds of chauvinistic thinking present in mental health care at the time.

The published case history appeared in the *American Journal of Psychiatry*, 129:1, July 1972, under the title, "The Intractable Female Patient." It was written by H. Houck, M.D., Medical Director of the Institute of Living in Hartford, Connecticut.*

In using the phrase, "intractable female patient," Dr. Houck referred to a category of female patients with similar syndromes, histories, and courses of "illness." "Intractable," according to Houck, means that the patient is not easily governed, managed or controlled. The "illness" exhibited by these women is, therefore, difficult to relieve or cure. This intractability which leads to hospitalization actually appears long before the hospitalization is necessary. Although these patients may have a variety of diagnoses, Houck classifies them all under the category of borderline syndrome described by Grinker.[†]

The patient's presenting problems include anxiety and depression; chronic depression, characterized by anhedonia, is the most prominent feature. However, the patient may not describe herself as depressed, even though she looks and acts unhappy.

> Although they are often attractive, most of these women are socially awkward, sexually naïve, and inhibited (p. 27) . . . She is immature, anxious, and angry, usually aloof, and contemptuous of other women, and demanding and suspicious of men (p. 28).

The early history of the patient reveals poor family relationships. Her mother was probably cold, aloof and dominating; her father, passive and withdrawn. Her husband "tends to be like the father; passive, variably indulent [sic], and easily dominated" (p. 27). Sexual adjustment of the

---

*Authors' note: We asked Dr. Houck's permission to publish his case history verbatim in this book; however, after we sent him material outlining the chapter in which his article would appear, he rescinded permission. He [sic] stated reasons were that our treatment would distort what he intended to say and that he did not wish to be placed, by implication, in either a profeminist or an antifeminist position. The reader will, therefore, have to rely on our summary of Dr. Houck's analysis. We recommend that the reader obtain Dr. Houck's original paper, both to form his/her own opinion of the case and to experience the full impact of Dr. Houck's approach.

[†]Authors' note: The borderline is a syndrome characteristic of arrested development of ego-functions. Some of the symptoms noted are: anger as the main affect, a deficiency in affectional relationships, depressive loneliness, and the apparent absence of self-identity. Although the borderline syndrome appears to be a confusing combination of psychotic, neurotic, and character disturbances with many normal elements, the process itself has a considerable degree of internal consistency and stability and is not merely a response to situational stress (Grinker, Werble, & Drye, 1968).

patient and her husband has always been poor. Child-rearing appears to be the stress that precipitated her hospitalization.

Soon after hospitalization the patient shows remarkable improvement. Houck attributes the improvement to secondary gains obtained by the patient in the form of relief from the demands of home and family. Labeling herself as "sick" legitimizes the patient's escape from her life's responsibilities.

The hospital therapist, particularly a young resident, will immediately judge the patient as an excellent candidate for psychotherapy because, as Houck describes her, she is

> young, intelligent, articulate, psychiatrically sophisticated, well motivated . . . She is, in short, exactly the kind of patient with whom the young resident in particular hopes to work (p. 27).

The resident and the patient quickly generate a lot of relevant case history material. The initial treatment plan includes intensive psychotherapy and, secondarily, some tranquilizing medicine. The patient rapidly develops a dependence on the therapist. Auspiciously, the therapist interprets this as transference.

Soon after therapy begins, a treatment crisis arises. The patient's depression and anxiety return without any apparent precipitating cause. Reassurances from the therapist and increases in medication merely exacerbate the problem. On the other hand, firm limits and control by the therapist lead to improvement. The patient's hostility diminishes, she becomes penitent, and improves. The young therapist may misinterpret the crisis and recovery as a turning point in therapy; however, similar crises continue to occur. The patient uses considerable guile and cunning to undercut the therapist's authority. She appears to derive pleasure from her ability to control therapy by producing a stalemate. In the face of repeated discouragement, the therapist who is committed to psychotherapy, refuses to recognize that the patient is not making progress.

In spite of lack of progress, the husband seldom questions the hospital regarding treatment. He is actually more comfortable with his wife out of the home and he is, as noted above, a very passive person. In cases in which the husband does intervene by removing his wife from the hospital or by threatening divorce, the wife, faced with external conditions over which she has no control, may actually improve. Houck attributes improvement in this instance to the efficacy of environmental manipulation over intensive psychotherapy for this type of patient.

In contrast to the young therapist's treatment, Houck recommends short hospital stays without intensive psychotherapy and without encouragement of childlike dependence or regressive behavior.

> The patient's hospital stay must be comparatively brief, her therapy supportive and aggressively reality oriented, and her attention firmly fixed on home, family, and adult obligations. . . . The pressure throughout the whole of the hospital milieu moves ever toward control, maturity, and independence (p. 30).

In addition, Houck suggest that the therapist concentrate his effort on the husband to assist him in modifying

> lifelong attitudes of passivity and diffidence and to assume a posture of strength and resolution—especially toward his wife (p. 30).

The patient will, of course, be ambivalent about the personality changes occurring in her husband and she will use the ploys to test and undermine his dominance and control similar to those she used with her therapist.

She will not be happy to leave the hospital and return to the home; family stress may result in a return to the hospital. Again, the duration of hospitalization must be limited at the onset. Eventually it may be necessary to block hospitalization as an avenue of escaping her duties as wife and mother. Houck claims that the patient will not make progress until she exerts great pressures on the husband, testing him to take control:

> She will test him to the limit, but if he passes the test she is reassured and comforted. She will keep trying, but she is often aware, at last, that she really hopes she will not win (p. 31).

In the following comparative case analysis, Houck's conception of the problem, his values as a therapist and his approach to treatment will be contrasted with those of feminist therapists. Naturally, we cannot speak for all feminist therapists; thus the ideas expressed in the right-hand column represent our own views as feminist therapists. The concepts listed in the left-hand column represent our understanding or interpretation of what Dr. Houck has said in his article; we also assume full responsibility for that interpretation.

Dr. Houck's Therapy	Feminist Therapy
Conception of the Problem	Conception of the Problem
Terms such as "illness" and "disease" are used in describing the patient.	All the problems described in the paper are of a behavioral nature. The patient has "problems" in living (Szasz 1971).
"Intractable" means that the patient is obstinate toward change and is not easily dominated. She has a strong will and she is not willing to be governed. In a woman these traits are evidence of pathology.	If the patient were male, such traits would be considered evidence of a well-integrated ego. Feminist therapists consider such traits to be healthy for *people*.
Her principal symptoms include depression and anhedonia.	If the patient is suffering from chronic depression, it seems that she is not sufficiently intractable for her own survival. Her intractibility could be interpreted as a positive sign that she is fighting against being submerged as an individual.
The patient does not describe herself as depressed; however, she looks and acts depressed.	If the patient is depressed without awareness, she is out of touch with herself and her feelings; she may be attempting to suppress aspects of herself that are even more unacceptable to others than her present behavior.
The patient is hospitalized because she refuses to meet her adult responsibilities to her home and family.	The patient is hospitalized because of the failure of the traditional feminine sex role. As Bernard (1971) noted: "In truth, being a housewife makes women sick." Since the patient and others in her environment (including her therapists) think that performing the feminine role is the only acceptable behavior for a woman, one of the patient's few alternatives is to "go crazy."
Soon after hospitalization the patient improved remarkably. This suggests that her hospitalization is providing her with	The patient has indeed escaped from the intolerable life situation—one that produced considerable stress for her. We view her behavior

secondary gains in the form of escaping from her home and family. Thus, her behavior is viewed from a moral perspective (shirking her responsibilities).

diagnostically, rather than morally, giving us clues to the nature of her conflict.

The patient's mother is described as cold, aloof, and domineering. Her father is described as passive and withdrawn. Her husband is also described as "passive, variably indulgent and easily dominated." In presenting these descriptions of significant others in the patient's environment, Houck implies that the root of her difficulties is a lack of adequate sex-role models.

We agree that the patient may be having difficulty in adapting to the traditional feminine sex-role. We also believe that the patient's important people, as described, would not provide effective role models for anyone, male or female.

The patient is described as attractive but "socially awkward, sexually naïve and inhibited."

Houck's description fits the traditional female in our society. Appearance, sociability, and sexuality are the dimensions on which women are judged. Other dimensions are assumed to be essentially irrelevant.

The patient is described as "young, intelligent, articulate, psychiatrically sophisticated and well-motivated." She is mistakenly viewed as an ideal candidate for intensive psychotherapy.

The patient fits Goldstein's (1972) description of the ideal patient: YAVIS (young, attractive, verbal, intelligent, sophisticated). This description suggests that she not only is an ideal patient but also has considerable personal strengths to draw upon in spite of the pathonomic diagnostic labels she receives from psychiatrists.

The patient is described as immature. Note: "Immature" is a vague term which is not defined in the text. We assume from the context that Houck means the patient does not have an adequate (traditional) sex-role identification, i.e. she does not do her housework or take care of her children. She also has the audacity to challenge the therapist's authority.

According to our diagnostic formulation the patient does not have an adequate sense of her own personhood, even though she dares to struggle to define herself in the face of strong social and therapist disapproval.

Houck also describes the patient as contemptuous of women and suspicious of men.

In our culture women are trained in these behaviors and in turn are labeled pathological by therapists for exhibiting them.

The patient allegedly yearns for affection and dominance.

Wanting affection seems to us a normal human desire. Wanting to be dominated is the interpretation of a male psychiatrist based upon beliefs concerning appropriate behavior of a woman. We agree that the patient exhibits conflict over the issue of dominance, vacillating between dependency and attempts to assert herself. A basic theme that emerges in this case is one of control: whether the patient will be allowed to decide the course of her life or whether others (therapist or husband) will direct her life.

Houck insists that the core of the patient's syndrome is anger.

We agree, but view her anger as appropriate and healthy. Using sex-role analysis, a feminist therapist could assist the patient in articulating the basis of her anger and channeling it in constructive ways.

The sexual adjustment of this patient is difficult and unsatisfying.

Why attribute the sexual difficulties to the patient? Masters and Johnson (1970) attribute 50 percent of any sexual problem to the wife and 50 percent to the husband. Since we know that the interpersonal relationship between this couple is unsatisfactory, we would be surprised if they reported a satisfactory sexual relationship. Bardwick (1973) observed that the "normal" woman usually engages in coitus not to gratify her own genital sexuality but to satisfy her male partner's needs and to secure his love. Reduced to using sex as barter for affection, this woman, along with many other women, does not derive physical pleasure from sex.

Treatment Goals

Therapy is to be reality oriented; i.e. the patient should be encouraged to assume her adult obligations of housework and motherhood. In sum, the patient should achieve an adequate feminine identity. The focus of treatment should be toward independence and maturity. Note: These words are operationally defined by Houck. He implies that an independent, mature woman carries out her adult obligations as stated above.

The husband should be helped to become dominant in the relationship and to control his wife who should be submissive and dependent in the relationship.

Treatment Goals

Therapy will include sex-role analysis. The therapist will show the woman how the traditional role expectations for women are related to her present conflicts. She will be encouraged to neutralize the effect of others' expectations upon her to decide what she wants for herself, and to take charge of her life to attain her goals. Feminists would not disagree with the goals of independence and maturity, but would define them in a different way. "Independence" implies that a woman has achieved a separate personhood, i.e. she has a sense of identity beyond that of wife, mother, and daughter. She also should have the means to be economically independent if she so chooses. "Maturity" means that she takes responsibility for the direction of her life and is capable of working in a persistent fashion toward achieving her goals.

Feminists oppose the traditional heterosexual relationship model of male dominance and female submission. Healthy relationships are based on equality between the persons involved. A basic inconsistency in the feminine role is that women are expected to be competent and strong, *except* when they are relating to men. The wife cannot achieve independence and maturity if significant males (therapists and husbands) are constantly blocking and punishing her self-assertive responses. Both the husband and wife described in this case history would probably benefit from assertion training to learn how to assert their needs in an appropriate manner.

Style of Treatment

Authoritarian. The therapist is expected to be in control of the patient who is ideally cooperative and docile. The therapist sets the goals of treatment and uses his influence over the patient and her environment to see that his goals are achieved. The therapist is cautioned by Houck to set limits and to exert firm control.

Style of Treatment

Egalitarian. The therapist and woman client will enter into a therapy contract agreeing on the goals of treatment. Feminist therapists assume that a woman can accurately report her own reality. If the therapist observes discrepancies in a woman's behavior or between her behaviors and therapy goals s/he will point out these discrepancies as the therapist's perception, not as reality.

Recommended Treatment Approach

Environmental manipulation. Limited stays in the hospital, training the husband to be more dominant in the relationship, and blocking future hospitalizations in order to prevent the patient from escaping her responsibilities as a wife and mother are the treatment recommendations.

The patient's attempts to control and manipulate the therapist are to be avoided. Note: This suggests suspicion and mistrust of her motives.

Houck opposes intensive individual psychotherapy. Presumably individual therapy will prolong treatment and collude with the patient's attempts to evade her responsibilities to her husband and children.

Recommended Treatment Approach

Environmental analysis including sex-role analysis. This recommended approach would neutralize the patient's feeling "crazy." Any environmental changes that she decides to make after careful examination of the consequences, including divorce or reconciliation with husband, are respected by the therapist.

The therapist and woman enter into a treatment contract which includes mutually agreed on goals and ways of achieving them. This reduces the possibility of manipulation by either party.

Feminist therapists prefer to work in group therapy. A group of women who have faced similar problems provide support and confirmation of the patient's reality. A group will not allow her to evade her responsibilities to herself. The therapeutic contract and feedback from the group will prevent the therapist or the woman from prolonging treatment.

Implied Values	Explicit Values
Acceptance of marriage as the only acceptable life-style for women.	Traditional marriage based on the dominance-submission model is oppressive to women; healthy relationships are based on equality. Many life-styles are acceptable for women.
A woman can be fulfilled only as a wife and mother.	Unless a woman is fulfilled as a person she cannot be fulfilled as a wife and mother.
A woman's mental health depends on her being submissive and having a dominant husband.	A woman's mental health depends on her having personal power—being effective in controlling her own life.

From Edna I. Rawlings and Dianne K. Carter, "The Intractable Female Patient," in *Psychotherapy for Women: Treatment toward Equality*, 1st ed. (Springfield, IL, 1977), 77–86. Courtesy of Charles C. Thomas Publisher, Ltd., Springfield, Illinois.

Diagnostic and Statistical Manual of Mental Disorders-III "Post-traumatic Stress Disorder"
(1980)

In 1974, the American Psychiatric Association formed a task force to coordinate changes in standardized diagnoses in order to keep up with impending revisions of the World Health Organization's *International Classification of Diseases* (ICD). The *DSM-III*, published in 1980, marked a watershed in American and world psychiatry. Influenced by the apparent success of new medications on certain psychiatric disorders and a desire to scientifically demonstrate the effectiveness of categories and treatments in economically trying times, the framers of the *DSM-III* moved away from etiological explanations and psychodynamic vocabulary to stress behavior. The *DSM-III* quickly became indispensable, in that, for the first time, it created a widely accepted, uniform standard for research, publication, funding, and insurance purposes.

The diagnosis of post-traumatic stress disorder (PTSD) was one of the *DSM-III*'s innovations. Inspiration for it was drawn from earlier diagnoses such as "traumatic neurosis" and "shell shock" and was influenced by demands for recognition from Vietnam War veterans and their supporters. In the end, the *DSM-III* framers crafted a diagnosis that proved to be controversial, particularly in the 1980s and 1990s, raising a number of difficult questions. Can memories be traumatic? Can they be repressed? Can repressed memories be reliably recovered? What is the difference between causes of and reasons for a mental illness? And how does one distinguish between a set of symptoms and a disease?

Post-traumatic Stress Disorder, Chronic or Delayed

The essential feature is the development of characteristic symptoms following a psychologically traumatic event that is generally outside the range of usual human experience.

The characteristic symptoms involve reexperiencing the traumatic event; numbing of responsiveness to, or reduced involvement with, the external world; and a variety of autonomic, dysphoric, or cognitive symptoms.

The stressor producing this syndrome would evoke significant symptoms of distress in most people, and is generally outside the range of such common experiences as simple bereavement, chronic illness, business losses, or marital conflict. The trauma may be experienced alone (rape or assault) or in the company of groups of people (military combat). Stressors producing this disorder include natural disasters (floods, earthquakes), accidental man-made disasters (car accidents with serious physical injury, airplane crashes, large fires), or deliberate man-made disasters (bombing, torture, death camps). Some stressors produce the disorder (e.g., torture) and others produce it only occasionally (e.g., car accidents). Frequently there is a concomitant physical component to the trauma which may even involve direct damage to the central nervous system (e.g., malnutrition, head trauma). The disorder is apparently more severe and longer lasting when the stressor is of human design. The severity of the stressor should be recorded and the specific stressor may be noted on Axis IV.

The traumatic event can be reexperienced in a variety of ways. Commonly the individual has recurrent painful, intrusive recollections of the event or recurrent dreams or nightmares during which the event is reexperienced. In rare instances, there are dissociative-like states, lasting from a few minutes to several hours or even days, during which components of the event are relived and the individual behaves as though experiencing the event at that moment. Such states have been reported in combat veterans. Diminished responsiveness to the external world, referred to as "psychical numbing" or "emotional anesthesia," usually begins soon after the traumatic event. A person may complain of feeling detached or estranged from other people, that he or she has lost the ability to become interested in previously enjoyed significant activities, or that the ability to feel emotions of any type, especially those associated with intimacy, tenderness, and sexuality, is markedly decreased.

After experiencing the stressor, many develop symptoms of excessive autonomic arousal, such as hyperalertness, exaggerated startle response, and difficulty falling asleep. Recurrent nightmares during which the traumatic event is relived and which are sometimes accompanied by middle or terminal sleep disturbance may be present. Some complain of impaired memory or difficulty in concentrating or completing tasks. In the case of life-threatening trauma shared with others, survivors often describe painful guilt feelings about surviving when many did not, or about the things they had to do in order to survive. Activities or situations that may arouse recollections of the traumatic event are often avoided. Symptoms characteristic of Post-traumatic Stress Disorder are often intensified when the individual is exposed to situations or activities that resemble or symbolize the original trauma (e.g., cold snowy weather or uniformed guards for death-camp survivors, hot, humid weather for veterans of the South Pacific). . . .

Diagnostic Criteria for Post-traumatic Stress Disorder

A. Existence of a recognizable stressor that would evoke significant symptoms of distress in almost everyone.

B. Reexperiencing of the trauma as evidenced by at least one of the following:

1. recurrent and intrusive recollections of the event
2. recurrent dreams of the event
3. sudden acting or feeling as if the traumatic event were recurring, because of an association with an environmental or ideational stimulus

C. Numbing of responsiveness to or reduced involvement with the external world, beginning some time after the trauma, as shown by at least one of the following:

1. markedly diminished interest in one or more significant activities
2. feeling of detachment or estrangement from others
3. constricted affect

D. At least two of the following symptoms that were not present before the trauma:

1. hyperalertness or exaggerated startle response
2. sleep disturbance
3. guilt about surviving when others have not, or about behavior required for survival
4. memory impairment or trouble concentrating
5. avoidance of activities that arouse recollection of the traumatic event
6. intensification of symptoms by exposure to events that symbolize or resemble the traumatic event

From: "Post-traumatic Stress Disorder," American Psychiatric Association, *Diagnostic and Statistical Manual of Mental Disorders, Third Edition* (Washington, DC: American Psychiatric Association, 1980). Reprinted with permission from the *Diagnostic and Statistical Manual of Mental Disorders, Third Edition.* Copyright 1980. American Psychiatric Association.

Psychiatrists Debate
Osheroff v. Chestnut Lodge
(1990)

Rafael Osheroff was a forty-two-year-old physician with a history of depression and anxiety when he was admitted to the psychiatric treatment center Chestnut Lodge in January 1979. Hospitalized for seven months, Osheroff later filed a lawsuit against the center, in 1982, claiming that by refusing to give him appropriate psychiatric medication, Chestnut Lodge was responsible for his losing his livelihood, his reputation, and the custody of his children. Before a trial took place, both parties reached an out-of-court settlement, in October 1987.

In 1990, two prominent psychiatrists debated the meaning of the case in a now famous exchange in the *American Journal of Psychiatry*. The psychiatrist Gerald Klerman (1928–1992) had been the former head of the federal mental health agency and a witness in the trial on behalf of Osheroff. In the 1970s and 1980s, he had been a leading figure among what he dubbed the "neo-Kraepelinians"—a group of psychiatrists who generally believed that discrete, identifiable mental illnesses existed, that psychiatric research should be oriented toward finding valid diagnostic criteria, and that therapy should be aimed at treating disorders as illnesses. Alan Stone entered the debate a trained psychoanalyst, a professor of law and psychiatry at Harvard University, and a former president of the American Psychiatric Association. As quickly becomes evident in the excerpts below, the Osheroff case raised two important questions: Are drugs more effective than psychotherapy in treating mental disorders? And how should we evaluate the effectiveness of treatments?

Gerald L. Klerman, M.D., "The Psychiatric Patient's Right to Effective Treatment: Implications of Osheroff v. Chestnut Lodge"

The patient, Dr. Rafael Osheroff, a 42-year-old white male physician, was admitted to Chestnut Lodge in Maryland (in the Washington, D.C., metropolitan area) on Jan. 2, 1979. His history included brief periods of depressive and anxious symptoms as an adult; these had been treated on an outpatient basis. He had completed medical school and residency training, was certified as an internist, and became a subspecialist in nephrology. He was married and had three children—one with his current wife and two with his ex-wife.

Before his 1979 hospitalization, Dr. Osheroff had been suffering from anxious and depressive symptoms for approximately 2 years and had been treated as an outpatient with individual psychotherapy and tricyclic antidepressant medications. Dr. Nathan Kline, a prominent psychopharmacologist in New York, had initiated outpatient treatment with tricyclic medication, which according to Dr. Kline's notes, produced moderate improvement. The patient, however, did not maintain the recommended dose, his clinical condition worsened, and hospitalization was recommended.

The patient was hospitalized at Chestnut Lodge for approximately 7 months. During this time he was treated with individual psychotherapy four times a week. He lost 40 pounds, experienced severe insomnia, and had marked psychomotor agitation. His agitation, manifested by incessant pacing, was so extreme that his feet became swollen and blistered, requiring medical attention.

The patient's family became distressed by the length of the hospitalization and by his lack of improvement. They consulted a psychiatrist in the Washington, D.C., area, who spoke to the hospital leadership on the patient's behalf. In response, the staff at Chestnut Lodge held a clinical conference to review the patient's treatment. They decided not to make any major changes—specifically, not to institute any medication regimen but to continue the intensive individual psychotherapy. Dr. Osheroff's clinical condition continued to worsen. At the end of 7 months, his family had him discharged from Chestnut Lodge and admitted to Silver Hill Foundation in Connecticut.

On admission to Silver Hill Foundation, Dr. Osheroff was diagnosed as having a psychotic depressive reaction. His treating physician began treatment with a combination of phenothiazines and tricyclic antidepressants. Dr. Osheroff showed improvement within 3 weeks and was discharged from Silver Hill Foundation within 3 months. His final diagnosis was manic-depressive illness, depressed type.

Although the patient's final diagnosis on discharge from Silver Hill was manic-depressive illness, depressed type, testimony of the treating physician at Silver Hill revealed that, of the two *DSM-II* diagnoses that would subsume a depressive illness as severe as Dr. Osheroff's (manic-depressive illness, depressed type, and psychotic depressive reaction), the diagnosis of manic-depressive, depressed type, was selected because of the potential future complications regarding child custody that could arise from a diagnostic label including the term "psychotic." The Silver Hill physician further testified that she did not find evidence of a narcissistic personality disorder in Dr. Osheroff and that the correct diagnosis according to the *DSM-III* terminology would be major depressive episode with psychotic features.

Following his discharge from Silver Hill Foundation in the summer of 1979, the patient resumed his medical practice. He has been in outpatient treatment, receiving psychotherapy and medication. He has not been hospitalized and has not experienced any episodes of depressive symptoms severe enough to interfere with his professional or social functioning. He has resumed contact with his children and has also become socially active. . . .

According to Chestnut Lodge records, there were differences in medical opinion as to the relative importance to be given the patient's personality conflicts and his depressive diagnosis as they influenced treatment decisions, not over the depressive diagnosis itself. As was the practice at the institution, the patient had two physicians, a psychiatrist-administrator and a psychotherapist. The hospital records suggest there may have been disagreement between these two physicians: the psychotherapist emphasized the need to treat the patient's personality problems as the major condition, and the administrator expressed concern over the continued severity of the patient's depressive symptoms and distressed behavior.

This aspect of the clinical process illustrates the tendency for many psychoanalytically oriented psychotherapists, both in institutional and in community practice, to focus treatment on a patient's personality conflict and character pathology rather than on symptoms. In *DSM-III* terms, there tends to be an emphasis on the axis II diagnosis and relatively little attention given to the axis I diagnosis. The axis I diagnosis, a severe depression in the case of Dr. Osheroff, is often missed, or, even if it is formulated, the personality disorder is chosen as the major target for treatment planning.

SCIENTIFIC EVIDENCE FOR EVALUATING PSYCHIATRIC TREATMENT

With regard to all kinds of therapeutics—pharmacotherapy, surgery, radiation, psychotherapy—the most scientifically valid evidence as to the safety and efficacy of a treatment comes from randomized controlled trials when these are available. Although there are other methods of generating evidence, such as naturalistic and follow-up studies, the most convincing evidence comes from randomized controlled trials.

There have been many controlled clinical trials of psychiatric treatments; most have been conducted to evaluate psychopharmacological agents. These trials were initiated in the 1950s and 1960s in response to the controversy that followed the introduction of chlorpromazine, reserpine, and other "tranquilizers." The application of controlled trials in psychopharmacology expanded after the passage in 1962 of the Kenfauver-Harris Amendments to the Food, Drug, and Cosmetic Act, which mandated evidence of efficacy before a pharmaceutical compound could be approved by the Food and Drug Administration and marketed.

Research on the efficacy of psychotherapy has lagged behind that of psychopharmacology but has, nevertheless, been extensive. Smith et al.* analyzed more than 400 reports of psychotherapy research. Specific reviews of the evidence have appeared with regard to psychotherapy of neurosis, schizophrenia, depression, and obsessive-compulsive disorders.

In view of these developments, a review of the state of evidence regarding the treatments of the two psychiatric conditions for Dr. Osheroff at the time of his hospitalization is in order.

With regard to the treatment of the patient's diagnosis of narcissistic personality disorder, there were no reports of controlled trials of any pharmacological or psychotherapeutic treatment for this condition at the time of his hospitalization. The doctors at Chestnut Lodge decided to treat Dr.

---

*Author's note: M. L. Smith, G. V. Glass, and T. I. Miller, *The Benefits of Psychotherapy* (Baltimore: Johns Hopkins University Press, 1980).

Osheroff's personality disorder with intensive psychotherapy based on psychodynamic theory.

With regard to the treatment of the patient's *DSM-II* diagnosis of psychotic depressive reaction, there was very good evidence at the time of his hospitalization for the efficacy of two biological treatments—ECT and the combination of phenothiazines and tricyclic anti-depressants. The combination pharmacotherapy was the treatment later prescribed at Silver Hill Foundation.

There are no reports of controlled trials supporting the claims for efficacy of psychoanalytically oriented intensive individual psychotherapy of the type advocated and practiced at Chestnut Lodge and administered to Dr. Osheroff. The closest approximation to a controlled clinical trial of this form of intensive individual psychotherapy has been reported with hospitalized schizophrenic patients at two institutions in the Boston area. Contrary to the expectations of the investigators, one of whom was Dr. Alfred Stanton (who had held a senior position at Chestnut Lodge and was one of the authors of *The Mental Hospital*, which describes the Chestnut Lodge institution), the results indicated that intensive individual psychotherapy offered no advantage over standard treatment (hospitalization, medication, and supportive psychotherapy) for these patients.

McGlashan and Dingman* have reported results from follow-up studies of groups of patients treated at Chestnut Lodge. The findings from this naturalistic study do not support the efficacy of long-term psychotherapy and hospitalization for severely depressed patients such as Dr. Osheroff.

It should not be concluded that there is no evidence for the value of any psychotherapy in the treatment of depressive states. Depressive states are heterogeneous, and there are many forms of psychotherapy. There is very good evidence from controlled clinical trials for the value of a number of brief psychotherapies for non-psychotic and nonbipolar forms of depression in ambulatory patients. The psychotherapies for which there is evidence include cognitive-behavioral therapy, interpersonal

---

*Author's note: T. H. McGlashan, "The Chestnut Lodge Follow-Up Study, III: Long-Term Outcome of Borderline Personalities," *Archives of General Psychiatry*, 43 (1986): 20–30; C. W. Dingman and T. H. McGlashan, "Discriminating Characteristics of Suicide: Chestnut Lodge Follow-Up Sample Including Patients with Affective Disorders, Schizophrenia, and Schizoaffective Disorders," *Acta Psychiatrica Scandinavica*, 74 (1986): 91–97.

psychotherapy, and behavioral therapy. However, no clinical trials have been reported that support the claims for efficacy of psychoanalysis or intensive individual psychotherapy based on psychoanalytical theory for any form of depression.

BIOLOGICAL VERSUS PSYCHODYNAMIC PSYCHIATRY

Dr. Stone* raised the possibility that patients who have not improved after prolonged psychotherapeutic treatment may have found a way around their frustrations—a way provided by "biological psychiatrists." Dr. Stone noted that biological psychiatry appears to be on the scientific ascendancy over psychodynamic psychiatry due to the prestige of the neurosciences and the evidence for efficacy of biological treatments.

My conclusion, however, is that the issue is not psychotherapy versus biological therapy but, rather, opinion versus evidence. The efficacy of drugs and other biological treatments is supported by a large body of controlled clinical trials. This body of evidence is all the more relevant to public policy in view of the paucity of studies indicating efficacy for individual psychotherapy.

It is regrettable that psychoanalysts and psychodynamic psychotherapists have not developed evidence in support of their claims for therapeutic efficacy. Twenty years ago, psychodynamic psychotherapy was the dominant paradigm of psychiatry in the United States, particularly in academic centers. A number of European psychiatrists, mostly psychoanalysts, contributed intellectual leadership and imaginative ideas to psychiatry here. Currently, however, psychoanalysis is on the scientific and professional defensive. This situation is, in part, a consequence of the failure of psychoanalysis to provide evidence for the efficacy of psychoanalysis and psychodynamic treatments for psychiatric disorders.

In the period between World War I and World War II, biological psychiatry was in poor repute. Numerous treatments, often of a heroic nature, were advocated: colonic resection, adrenalectomy, excision of teeth, lobotomy. These interventions were based on biological laboratory research of dubious quality and without any systematic studies of safety and efficacy. The situation has changed after World War II, with evidence for the value

---

*Author's note: A. A. Stone, "The New Paradox of Psychiatric Malpractice," *New England Journal of Medicine*, 311 (1984): 1384–1387.

of ECT for depression and insulin coma therapy for schizophrenia and, later, with the introduction of chlorpromazine and other drugs.

THE RESPECTABLE MINORITY DOCTRINE

The Case of *Osheroff v. Chestnut Lodge* prompts the reevaluation of the doctrine of the respectable minority. Until recently, this doctrine held that if a minority of respected and qualified practitioners maintained a standard of care, this was an adequate defense against malpractice. I propose that this doctrine no longer holds if there is a body of evidence supporting the efficacy of a particular treatment and if there is agreement within the profession that this is the proper treatment of a given condition. Moreover, the respectable minority have a duty to inform the patient of the alternative treatments. In an unpublished 1985 paper discussing *Osheroff v. Chestnut Lodge*, K. Livingston wrote,

> Under this review, the respectable minority view would still constitute a defense to a malpractice action where even 10% of practitioners would adhere to the treatment in question. However, the shield of the respectable minority rule would not be available unless the patient had been given informed consent after a disclosure of risk/benefits and alternatives to the therapy.

HOW DO WE PROCEED IN THE ABSENCE OF CONSENSUS?

When there is consensus in the profession as to the appropriate treatment for a given condition (in the case of *Osheroff*, the essential nature of biological treatment for severe depression), then a standard of care can be agreed on and can provide the basis for malpractice action.

However, how are we to evaluate claims for the efficacy of treatments for clinical conditions about which there is no consensus? What are the standards to be applied in diagnostic and clinical situations where there is no consensus within the field with regard to the treatment of the particular disorder? This is a serious policy question that, in the future, may become a legal question. In my opinion, there are three aspects to this issue: 1) What constitutes evidence for efficacy? 2) Who is responsible for generating the evidence? and 3) Who is to make the appropriate evaluation of treatments?

What constitutes evidence of treatment? In my view, the best available evidence as to efficacy comes from controlled trials. I am not taking the position that the only source of evidence for efficacy comes from such trials. Clinical experience, naturalistic studies, and follow-up studies are also sources of relevant evidence. However, when results from controlled clinical trials are available, they should be given priority in any discussion of scientific evidence.

Who should be responsible for generating the evidence? What should be society's policy in regard to treatments for which there is no positive or negative evidence? This issue has not reached resolution, and I feel it merits further discussion within the profession.

My opinion is that the responsibility for generating evidence for efficacy rests with the individual, group, or organization that makes the claim for the safety and efficacy of a particular treatment. In the case of drugs, this responsibility is established by statute. If a pharmaceutical firm makes a claim for efficacy of one of its products, it must generate enough evidence to satisfy the Food and Drug Administration before it can market the drug for prescription use.

No such mandate of responsibility exists for psychotherapy. Anyone can make a claim for the value of a form of psychotherapy—psychoanalysis, Gestalt, est, primal scream, etc.—with no evidence as to its efficacy.

What should be our position toward the claims of the efficacy in certain conditions of multiple treatments for which the evidence varies in quality and quantity? In my view, those treatments which make claims but have not generated evidence are in a weak position.

The efficacy of psychoanalysis and psychoanalytic treatments is in question for conditions for which there is evidence of efficacy with other treatments. For example, how many psychiatrists would justify long-term psychoanalytic treatment of panic disorder and/or agoraphobia when there is no evidence that this treatment works for these disorders but reasonably good evidence for the efficacy of certain drugs and/or forms of behavioral psychotherapy?

Who is to evaluate the evidence? A major problem arises as to the process by which the evidence regarding psychiatric treatments is to be evaluated. I believe there are serious deficiencies in our current professional and governmental arrangements for evaluating psychiatric treatments. In the case of drugs, we have the Food and Drug Administration, which makes such judgments according to established legal statutes and regulatory processes. There is no comparable statutory mandate for assessing the efficacy and safety of non-pharmacological treatments such as radiation, surgery, and psychotherapy.

In this situation, I believe the public has the right to expect that the medical profession will provide appropriate judgments as to the state of the evidence for treatments and establish criteria for standards of care. I maintain that the psychiatric profession has been lax in this responsibility and that the absence of professional consensus statements in our field leaves it open for the courts to be used by individuals, such as Dr. Osheroff, who feel they have been poorly treated and who believe they are entitled to redress of their grievances.

The fact that evidence changes is to my mind irrelevant to any policy or clinical discussion. The judgment on treatment of individual patients should be made according to the state of knowledge and professional practice at the time the individual patient is treated. In the case of *Osheroff*, this was 1979.

My strong preference would be for the profession to be more vigorous and more responsible in accepting this responsibility. I have stated these views on numerous occasions.

Alan A. Stone, "Law, Science, and Psychiatric Malpractice: A Response to Klerman's Indictment of Psychoanalytic Psychiatry"

Malcolm's book* reports that Dr. Osheroff was married three times before his hospitalization. His first marital relationship began while he was in college and ended in divorce after 21 months because his wife had been unfaithful. He thought of leaving medical school but saw a psychiatrist who convinced him to return. During his internship he met and married a nurse. The second marriage lasted much longer but deteriorated after the birth of two children. Dr. Osheroff saw a psychiatrist again during these years while he was establishing his practice. According to Malcolm, he wrote about this period of time in his autobiography, which he entitled *A Symbolic Death*:

> All during the early years of my [second] marriage, I had been rather immature and insensitive and my energies seemed to be devoted to and

---

*Editor's note: The author refers here to John Malcolm, *Treatment Choices and Informed Consent* (Springfield, IL: Charles C. Thomas, 1988).

focused on my career, that I perhaps was not listening and if I was listening, perhaps I wasn't hearing. I was seemingly oblivious to the stresses that were developing in my marriage at the time.

Psychotherapy for Dr. Osheroff and marital therapy for the couple did not save the marriage. His second wife left the children with him and went off with another man. Dr. Osheroff lost 40 pounds during this time, living "a life that was almost devoid of the usual types of satisfaction." His nephrology practice, nonetheless, grew and prospered as he opened his own dialysis center. He then met his third wife, a medical student on her clinical clerkship, and married her after a "whirlwind romance." This was at first a happy and successful marriage, and symptoms of depression apparently disappeared. He and his wife were, in his words, "one of the most celebrated and sought after medical couples in the . . . area."

There were continuing conflicts, however, with his second wife, who now wanted custody of their two children. Conflicts also began with his third wife. They were precipitated, according to her, by his seemingly inconsiderate behavior during the birth of their first child (his third) and his lack of attention to the baby and her.

Dr. Osheroff also began to have serious disagreements with his professional associates in practice. With these conflicts and the deterioration of his third marriage, he saw at least three different psychiatrists, two of whom prescribed antidepressive medication, which was not successful—perhaps because of lack of compliance. It is well recognized that "drug manipulation and drug compliance are anticipated problems" in patients whose affective symptoms are complicated by personality disorders.* No doubt, such problems can be even greater when the patient is himself a physician and may have his own opinions about treatment.

I do not mean to suggest that Klerman intentionally selected from the history only those features which support his diagnosis and the basic thesis of his paper. Perhaps the kinds of subjective experiences revealed in Dr. Osheroff's autobiographical account and the interpersonal difficulties he experienced with the important people in his life, which suggest problems

---

*Author's note: J. O. Cole and P. S. Sunderland III, "The Drug Treatment of Borderline Patients," in Psychiatry 1982: The American Psychiatric Association Annual Review ed. L. Grinspoon (Washington, DC: American Psychiatric Association, 1982).

in the sphere of object relations and character, have become less relevant to psychiatrists who tend to overemphasize *DSM-III's* axis I in comparison with axis II. Perhaps these two quite different histories indicate that there is an incorrigible diagnostic and conceptual difference between Klerman's school and traditional psychiatrists. The "scientific" psychiatrist now looks for the symptoms. The traditional psychiatrist still looks for the person. Each school can criticize the blindness of the other on the basis of its own criteria.

In any event, when Dr. Osheroff entered Chestnut Lodge he was not a neophyte as to psychiatry or its various therapeutic approaches, nor was he professionally or personally ignorant about depression. He was a physician who, I have no doubt, had already several times in his life been diagnosed, fully informed about his diagnosis, and treated exactly in the manner recommended by Klerman in his paper. Those treatment methods had failed. All of this seems relevant to any judgment about Chestnut Lodge's alleged negligence and the lessons Klerman claims are to be learned from this litigation.

THE TREATMENT

The breakdown of Dr. Osheroff's third marriage and his professional conflicts, which precipitated his hospitalization, could reasonably have been understood at the time as classic examples of the kind of psychosocial crises that destroy the precarious balance of the narcissistic personality. Even if Klerman believes that this kind of psychodynamic formulation and approach to treatment is no longer "scientifically" acceptable, there can be little doubt that it was well within the collective sense of the profession in 1979. Thus, I suggest that the initial treatment program for Dr. Osheroff was acceptable, particularly in light of a history of previous unsuccessful drug treatment provided by a leading psychopharmacologist and implemented by his traditional psychotherapist.

With only this psychodynamically oriented psychotherapy, however, the patient's condition obviously deteriorated. Whatever the original diagnosis and treatment plan were, reevaluation and consultation are required at some point when a treatment regimen has such obviously negative consequences. I have no doubt that during the 1950s, 1960s, and 1970s at Chestnut Lodge and other similarly oriented hospitals, traditional therapists did persist in exclusive psychoanalytic psychotherapy, despite similar situations of obvious symptomatic deterioration. My own clinical experience at McLean Hospital during these years certainly confirms this impression.

If Klerman had stayed with this narrow fact of the situation and stated that exclusively psychoanalytic treatment of a hospitalized patient in the face of obvious psychotic deterioration is no longer clinically acceptable, I believe he could have claimed to speak for the collective sense of the profession, including the vast majority of traditional psychotherapists.

It is important to recognize that this marks an important historical moment of transition in modern psychiatry. Many new considerations as well as efficacy studies have led to this change. The biological dimensions of serious mental disorders and their treatment have been better understood, and this understanding has been more widely accepted. The consequences of longer periods of psychotic decompensation have been more fully recognized. The distinction between social recovery with improvement of symptoms and the cure of serious mental illness has been better appreciated, and psychiatric hospitalization has increasingly focused on the former. The negative implications of long-term hospitalization of patients with psychotic disorders have been well documented. Psychiatrists have recognized the importance of improvement in symptoms for the therapeutic alliance and, therefore, as a necessary part of treatment with seriously disturbed patients. The limitations of traditional therapy with psychotic patients are widely accepted, and successful treatment is more often attributed to the unique qualities of the therapist or the relationship rather than to the method of the psychotherapy. All of these factors and not just the available efficacy studies have led to the changes in the collective sense of the profession.

At Chestnut Lodge, Dr. Osheroff apparently developed a negative therapeutic reaction and a negative transference to both the therapist and the hospital. The person suffering from these serious symptoms of depression was in revolt against his treatment. The recommendation to change hospitals seems to me eminently sound on psychodynamic grounds. Klerman suggests that Dr. Osheroff's remarkable cure at the Silver Hill Foundation was a function of his finally being provided the efficacious combination of tricyclics and phenothiazines. If all patients like Dr. Osheroff had such remarkable cures with these drugs, psychiatry would be a different profession. But Dr. Osheroff's psychological response to Silver Hill Foundation, as described in his autobiography, suggests that other, equally important, psychodynamic factors were involved. He had escaped, if not narcissistically triumphed over, Chestnut Lodge and his therapist. His negative transference had been vindicated. Such psychodynamic conceptions still seem as relevant to our clinical understanding of such remarkable cures as does psychopharmacology.

BIOLOGICAL VERSUS PSYCHODYNAMIC PSYCHIATRY

Klerman and Klein have both objected to my characterization of the *Osheroff* dispute as one between biological and psychodynamic psychiatry. Klerman here states that it is, rather, a matter of opinion versus evidence. Klein* has made the same point in stronger and more colorful language. Both of them contend that they are speaking as scientists and that the issue is one of scientific evidence versus dogmatic opinion. Klerman makes this a thesis of his current paper, applying it as a standard to all psychiatric treatments. I believe both men ignore the very real problem of differing opinions about scientific evidence and the canons of science within the psychiatric profession. Klerman and Klein surely recognize that the quality of evidence, even in their own impressive research, leaves room for other scientists to make interpretations and raise questions. The basic assumption on which clinical research on depression and panic states proceeds are subject to fundamental questions by serious scientists. Klerman is no doubt correct that at a meeting of scientists, the person with evidence should take precedence over the person without evidence. Even a small amount of evidence is better than opinion when the question is what can science say about a subject. But that does not mean the science is good enough to create a uniform policy or to dictate to clinicians the clinical standards of care. . . .

EFFICACY RESEARCH AND PUBLIC POLICY CONCERNS

There is an apocryphal story told about male lawyers. One asks the other, "How is your spouse?" The other replies, "Compared to what?" "Compared to what" is the appropriate perspective to bring to Klerman's discussion of efficacy research and policy. He compares psychotherapy and drugs. In that comparison he criticizes the failure of various government agencies

---

*Author's note: D. F. Klein, "The *Osheroff* Case: A Rebuttal," *Psychiatric News* 7 April 1989: 26.

at the federal and state levels. He also criticizes his colleagues in research and in professional associations. When compared to Food and Drug Administration safety and efficacy standards for drugs, the regulation of psychotherapy seems to stand out as a public policy disaster. But virtually everything Klerman says about psychotherapy applies with equal force to surgery and almost everything that physicians do which does not come under the Food and Drug Administration's authority. Much of what all physicians do has no demonstrated effectiveness—even the prescription of supposedly efficacious medication. Thus, if psychotherapy is compared to surgery, for example, one might get a totally different impression about the nature and significance of the public policy problem posed by traditional psychotherapy. It turns out that the Food and Drug Administration is quite unique, holding the massive pharmaceutical industry hostage and able to require it to invest vast resources in research into efficacy and safety. Thus, Klerman's use of the Food and Drug Administration as a model is less relevant and less meaningful than it seems.

All health policy experts are concerned about efficacy. Indeed, efficacy research has become the central requirement of what Relman* called the third revolution in medical care, requiring increased attention to assessment and accountability. In order to meet the pressing objectives of quality and cost control, however, Relman wrote, "We will also need to know much more about the relative costs, safety, and effectiveness of all the things physicians do or employ in the diagnosis, treatment and prevention of disease." Relman was commenting on an article by Roper et al. of the Health Care Financing Administration, who described new "effectiveness initiatives." These will increasingly involve the federal government in the collection and distribution of efficacy and outcome data concerning many branches of medicine. Roper et al.,[†] along with Relman, stated that more comprehensive assessment of medical effectiveness will eventually improve the quality of care and eventually help curtail costs. Unlike Klerman, they suggested that the science of efficacy research currently available in the rest

---

*Author's note: A. S. Relman, "Assessment and Accountability: The Third Revolution in Medical Care (Editorial)," *New England Journal of Medicine* 319 (1988): 1220–1222.

†Author's note: W. L. Roper, W. Winkenwerder, G. M. Hackbarth, et al., "Effectiveness in Health Care: An Initiative to Evaluate and Improve Medical Practice," *New England Journal of Medicine* 319 (1988): 1197–1202.

of medicine is inadequate to the task. The focus of the Health Care Financing Administration was on surgery. For example, they cited carotid endarterectomy and the implantation of cardiac pacemakers as examples of surgical practices often used inappropriately because of the lack of adequate efficacy studies. More money is certainly spent on these procedures than on all of the traditional psychotherapy provided in the United States—and the immediate risks of their use or misuse are much greater. Roper et al. clearly recognized what Klerman has not: that the "science of health care evaluation, still in its formative stages, requires certain resources: money, data, and people trained in the evaluative sciences" and that "methods of gathering and synthesizing data on health outcomes and effectiveness are correspondingly underdeveloped."

Roper et al. made it clear that a whole new infrastructure for gathering data is necessary before sensible public policy can be developed to control clinical practice. They did not blame the medical profession for this gap in our scientific knowledge. Klerman's paper, in contrast, seems to be a rush to judgment, with the first stop at the courthouse. Klerman does not even acknowledge that there is any legitimate opposition to his views. He is prepared to argue that "the absence of professional consensus statements in our field leaves it open for the courts to be used by individuals, such as Dr. Osheroff, who feel they have been poorly treated and who believe they are entitled to redress of their grievances." This is to suggest that the psychiatric profession is now being punished for its own sins of laxity, which opened the door to the courtroom. This is simply nonsense. Every legal scholar writing on the subject of psychiatric malpractice has pointed to the lack of professional consensus in psychiatry as a major cause for the remarkable dearth of such litigation compared to other specialties over the past century. In fact, any experienced lawyer would say that Dr. Osheroff was able to litigate because he was able to obtain expert witnesses like Klerman and his distinguished colleagues, who were willing to testify that there is a consensus about efficacious treatment. Indeed, Klerman's paper is an attempt to assert and establish this thesis.

The use of the courtroom and malpractice litigation to enforce a consensus policy on efficacy would have serious consequences for biological psychiatry as well as for the field as a whole. The history of neuroleptic medication for psychiatric disorders presents a striking example. Psychiatry's understanding of efficacious doses and deleterious side effects has changed dramatically over the past two decades. We have gone from smaller doses to megadoses back to smaller doses. We have gone from routine maintenance to selective intramuscular "neurolepticization" for acute psychotic disorders and abandoned it. All of these changing standards of care were based on clinical experience, available scientific evidence, and a genuine concern for providing effective treatment. If, at any early point in this history, biological psychiatrists had gone to court or to any other official authority to impose efficacious dose standards on all their colleagues, it would have been a disaster for our patients and for biological psychiatry. If it is Klerman's idea that psychiatry should be ruled by the courts applying the prevailing scientific evidence of the day, he has a recipe for disaster.*

From G. L. Klerman, "The Psychiatric Patient's Right to Effective Treatment: Implications of Osheroff v. Chestnut Lodge," *American Journal of Psychiatry* 147 (1990): 409–418 and A. A. Stone, "Law, Science, and Psychiatric Malpractice: A Response to Klerman's Indictment of Psychoanalytic Psychiatry," *American Journal of Psychiatry* 147 (1990): 419–427. Reprinted with permission from the *American Journal of Psychiatry*, American Psychiatric Association. Copyright 1990.

---

*Editor's note: Only those notes have been included in which the authors name a specific citation in the main text.

Appendix

Bibliography of First-Person Narratives of Madness in English

(Fourth Edition)

Gail A. Hornstein

This bibliography is in four sections: (1) personal accounts of madness written by survivors themselves; (2) narratives written by family members; (3) anthologies and critical analyses of the madness narrative genre; and (4) Web sites featuring oral histories and other first-person madness accounts.

Last revised in November 2008 with assistance from Cheryl McGraw, Catherine Riffin, and Moriah Silver.

Please send corrections, additions, comments or inquiries to

Gail A. Hornstein
Professor of Psychology
Mount Holyoke College
South Hadley, MA 01075
USA
ghornste@mtholyoke.edu

Personal Accounts of Madness by Survivors Themselves

Abrams, Albert. 1895. *Transactions of the Antiseptic Club*. New York: E. B. Treat.

Adams, Brian. 2003. *The Pits and the Pendulum: A Life with Bipolar Disorder*. London: Jessica Kingsley.

Adams, Joe Kennedy. 1971. *Secrets of the Trade: Notes on Madness, Creativity, and Ideology*. New York: Viking.

Adler, George J. 1854. *Letters of a Lunatic: A Brief Exposition of My University Life during the Years 1853–1854*. New York: The Author.

Agnew, Anna. 1886. *From under a Cloud; or, Personal Reminiscences of Insanity*. Cincinnati: Robert Clarke.

Aldrin, Edwin E. "Buzz," Jr. With Wayne Warga. 1973. *Back to Earth*. New York: Random House.

Alexander, Rosie. 1995. *Folie à Deux: An Experience of One-to-One Therapy*. London: Free Association Books.

Alexandra [Messenger]. 1984. *I Speak for the Silent*. Enfield, UK: Alexandra Press.

Alexson, Jacob. 1941. *The Triumph of Personal Thought and How I Became a Mason*. Washington: Ransdell.

Allan, Clare. 2006. *Poppy Shakespeare*. London: Bloomsbury.

Allen, Rosealine. 2005. *It's Happening to Me*. London: Chipmunka.

Alper, T. G. 1948. "An Electric Shock Patient Tells His Story." *Journal of Abnormal and Social Psychology* 43:201–210.

Altenberg, P. 1960. *Evocations of Love*. Translated by Alexander King. New York: Simon & Schuster.

Anderson, Anna Eisenhart. 1979. *Pain: The Essence of a Mental Illness*. Fort Lauderdale, FL: Exposition-Phoenix.

Anderson, Dwight. With Page Cooper. 1950. *The Other Side of the Bottle*. New York: A. A. Wyn.

Anne. "Coping with Schizophrenia." 1979. *Mind Out*.

Anonymous. 1620. *The Petition of the Poor Distracted People in the House of Bedlam*. London.

———. 1842. "Letter by 'a Friend of the Insane.'" *Asylum Journal* 1 (5): 2.

———. 1842. "Scenes in a Private Madhouse." *Asylum Journal* 1 (1): 1.

———. 1844. "Case VIII." *American Journal of Insanity* 1:52–71.

———. 1846. *Bedlamiana; or, Selections from the "Asylum Journal."* Lowell, for the Compiler. [MA?]

———. 1846. "Illustrations of Insanity." *American Journal of Insanity* 3:212–226, 333–348.

———. 1848. "Illustrations of Insanity Furnished by the Letters and Writings of the Insane." *American Journal of Insanity* 4:290–303.

———. 1849. *Five Months in the New York State Lunatic Asylum, by an Inmate*. Buffalo, NY: L. Danforth.

———. 1850. "The Ohio Lunatic Asylum." *Journal of Psychological Medicine and Mental Pathology* 3:456–490.

———. 1852. "A Letter from a Patient." *Opal: A Monthly Periodical of the New York State Lunatic Asylum, Devoted to Usefulness* 2:245–246.

———. 1854. "A Chapter from Real Life: By a Recovered Patient." *Opal: A Monthly Periodical of the New York State Lunatic Asylum at Utica* 4:48–50.

———. 1855. "Life in the Asylum." *Opal: A Monthly Periodical of the New York State Lunatic Asylum, Edited by Patients* 5:4–6.

———. 1855. *Scenes from the Life of a Sufferer: Being the Narrative of a Residence in Morningside Asylum.* Edinburgh: Royal Asylum Press.

———. 1867. *Life in a Lunatic Asylum: An Autobiographical Sketch.* London: Houlston & Wright.

———. 1884. *A Palace Prison; or, The Past and the Present.* New York: Fords, Howard & Hulbert.

———. 1896. "The Confessions of a Nervous Woman." *Post Graduate Monthly: Journal of Medicine and Surgery* 11:364–368.

———. 1898. *A Madman's Musings: Being a Collection of Essays Written by a Patient during His Detention in a Private Madhouse.* London: A. E. Harvey.

———. 1901. *Five Months in a Mad-House: An Actual Experience, by an Inmate.* New York: Press Exchange.

———. 1930. "Wondering: The Impressions of an Inmate." *Atlantic Monthly* 145:669.

———. 1932. *I Lost My Memory: The Case as the Patient Saw It.* London: Faber.

———. 1934. *Autobiography of a Suicide.* Lawrence, L. I: Golden Galleon.

———. 1935. *Crook Frightfulness: By a Victim.* London: Moody Bros.

———. 1938. "They Said I Was Mad." *Forum and Century* 100:231–237.

———. 1940. "Insulin and I." *American Journal of Orthopsychiatry* 10:810–814.

———. 1945. *I Question.* Nashville, TN: n.p.

———. 1951. *Autobiography of a Schizophrenic.* Bristol: J. Baker & Son.

———. 1952. [Mrs. F. H.]. "Recovery from a Long Neurosis." *Psychiatry* 15:161–177.

———. 1971. "Life on a Psychiatric Ward." *Mind.*

———. 1974. "Ordeal in a Mental Hospital." *Radical Therapist.*

———. 1974. "What It's Like—from the Receiving End." Special issue, *Mind Out.*

———. 2005. *Out of It: An Autobiography of the Experience of Schizophrenia.* Lincoln, NE: iUniverse.

Ansite, Pat. 1977. *No Longer Lonely.* Van Nuys, CA: Bible Voice.

Antonieta, Susanne. 2005. *A Mind Apart: Travels in a Neurodiverse World.* New York: Jeremy P. Tarcher.

Arisoy, Suzan. 2008. *Bi-polar Recovery: Twenty Years of Manic Depression and Medication.* London: Chipmunka.

Artaud, Antonin. 1965. *Antonin Artaud Anthology.* San Francisco: City Lights Books.

Balt, John. 1967. *By Reason of Insanity.* New York: New American Library.

Balter, M., and R. Katz. 1991. *Nobody's Child.* Reading, MA: Addison-Wesley.

Barlow, Brigit. 1975. "How I Conquered Claustrophobia." *Mind Out.*

Barnes, Mary, and Joseph Berke. 1971. *Mary Barnes: Two Accounts of a Journey through Madness.* New York: Harcourt, Brace, Jovanovich. Reprint, New York: Other Press, 2002.

———. With Ann Scott. 1989. *Something Sacred: Conversations, Writings, Paintings.* London: Free Association Books.

Barnett, Francis. 1823. *The Hero of No Fiction; or, Memoirs of Francis Barnett.* Boston: C. Ewer and T. Bedlington.

Barry, Anne. 1971. *Bellevue Is a State of Mind*. New York: Harcourt, Brace, Jovanovich.

Barrymore, Diana. 1957. *Too Much, Too Soon*. New York: Holt.

Bassman, Ronald. 2001. "Overcoming the Impossible: My Journey through Schizophrenia." *Psychology Today*, February, 34–40.

———. 2007. *A Fight to Be: A Psychologist's Experience from Both Sides of the Locked Door*. New York: Tantamount Press.

Bauer, Hanna. 1973. *I Came to My Island: A Journey through the Experience of Change*. Seattle: Straub.

B.C.A. 1909. *My Life as a Dissociated Personality*. With an introduction by Morton Prince, MD. Boston: Badger.

Beecher, Catherine. 1855. *Letters to the People on Health and Happiness*. New York: Harper & Brothers.

Beers, Clifford. 1908. *A Mind That Found Itself*. Pittsburgh: University of Pittsburgh Press.

Behrman, Andy. 2003. *Electroboy: A Memoir of Mania*. New York: Random House.

Belcher, William. 1796. *Address to Humanity, Containing a Letter to Dr. Thomas Monro; a Receipt to Make a Lunatic, and Seize his Estate and a Sketch of a True Smiling Hyena*. London: The Author.

Benjamin, Bianca. 2005. *Madness at Midnight*. London: Chipmunka.

Benson, Arthur Christopher. 1907. *The House of Quiet*. New York: Dutton.

———. 1912. *Thy Rod and Thy Staff*. London: Smith, Elder.

Benson, Frederic. 2005. *Bi-polar Dreams*. London: Chipmunka.

Benziger, Barbara Field. 1969. *The Prison of My Mind*. New York: Walker.

Bergen, Marja. 1999. *Riding the Roller Coaster: Living with Mood Disorders*. Kelowna, BC: Northstone.

Berger, Marie. 2007. *From the Prison of My Mind: A Collection of Works*. London: Chipmunka.

Berlow, Joshua. 2000. *Insanity Factory*. Lincoln, NE: iUniverse.

Bernard, Susan. 2008. *Bi-polar Depression Unplugged: A Survivor Speaks Out*. London: Chipmunka.

Berryman, John. 1973. *Recovery*. New York: Dell.

Berzon, Betty. 2002. *Surviving Madness: A Therapist's Own Story*. Madison: University of Wisconsin Press.

Black, Michael. 2008. *Angels, Cleopatra, and Psychosis*. London: Chipmunka.

Blackbridge, Persimmon. 1996. *Sunnybrook: A True Story with Lies*. Vancouver, BC: Press Gang.

———. 1997. *Prozac Highway*. Vancouver, BC: Press Gang.

Blackburn, Lorraine. 2007. *Alive with Bipolar*. London: Chipmunka.

Blackwell, Sean. 2008. *A Quiet Mind*. London: Chipmunka.

Bly, Nellie [Elizabeth Cochrane]. 1887. *Ten Days in a Madhouse; or, Nellie Bly's Experience on Blackwell's Island: Feigning Insanity in Order to Reveal Asylum Horrors*. New York: Norman L. Munro.

Boisen, Anton T. 1936. *The Exploration of the Inner World*. New York: Harper & Row, 1936.

———. 1960. *Out of the Depths*. New York: Harper & Row.

Bojko, Annemarie. 2007. *While Shepherds Watched Their Flocks*. London: Chipmunka.

Bowers, M. B. 1974. *Retreat from Sanity*. New York: Human Sciences.

Brando, A. K. 1978. *Brando for Breakfast*. New York: Crown.

Brandon, David. 1980. "Three Meetings with Madness." *Mind Out*.

Brandt, Anthony. 1975. *Reality Police: The Experience of Insanity in America*. New York: Morrow.

Brea, Alton. 1968. *Half a Lifetime*. New York: Vantage.

Brinkle, Andriana P. 1887. "Life among the Insane." *North American Review* 144:190–199.

Brinson, Jean Small. 1994. *Murderous Memories: One Woman's Hellish Battle to Save Herself*. Far Hills, NJ: New Horizon.

Brocklesby, Anne. 2005. *Move Over Manic Depression, Here I Am!* London: Chipmunka.

Brokenshire, Norman. 1954. *This Is Norman Brokenshire: An Unvarnished Self-Portrait*. New York: David McKay.

Broughton, Stephen. 2006. *Big Dick, Little Dick*. London: Chipmunka.

Brown, Carlton. 1944. *Brainstorm*. New York: Farrar & Rinehart.

Brown, Henry Collins. 1937. *A Mind Mislaid*. New York: E. P. Dutton.

Bruckshaw, Samuel. 1774. *The Case, Petition, and Address of Samuel Bruckshaw, who Suffered a Most Severe Imprisonment, for Very Near the Whole Year, Loaded with Irons, without Being Heard in his Defense, Nay Even without Being Accused, and at Last Denied an Appeal to a Jury. Humbly Offered to the Perusal and Consideration of the Public*. London: The Author.

———. 1774. *One More Proof of the Iniquitous Abuse of Private Madhouses*. London: The Author.

Buck, Peggy. 1978. *I'm Depressed—Are You Listening Lord?* Valley Forge, PA: Judson.

Bukovskii, V. 1978. *To Build a Castle: My Life as a Dissenter*. London: Andre Deutsch.

Bullitt-Jonas, Margaret. 1999. *Holy Hunger: A Memoir of Desire*. New York: Knopf.

Burke, Ross David. 1995. *When the Music's Over: My Journey into Schizophrenia*. Edited by Richard Gates and Robin Hammond. New York: Basic Books.

Caine, Linda, and Robin Royston. 2003. *Out of the Dark*. London: Bantam Press.

Camp, Joseph. 1882. *An Insight into an Insane Asylum*. Louisville, KY: The Author.

Campbell, E.J. Moran. 1988. *Not Always on a Level*. Cambridge: Cambridge University Press.

Cantor, Carla. With Brian Fallon. 1996. *Phantom Illness: Shattering the Myth of Hypochondria*. Boston: Houghton Mifflin.

Capponi, Pat. 1992. *Upstairs in the Crazy House: The Life of a Psychiatric Survivor*. Toronto: Penguin Books.

———. 2003. *Beyond the Crazy House*. New York: Penguin.

Cardinal, Marie. 1983. *The Words to Say It*. Cambridge, MA: VanVactor & Goodheart.

———. 1995. *In Other Words*. Bloomington: Indiana University Press.

Casey, Joan F., and Lynn Wilson. 1991. *Flock: The Autobiography of a Multiple Personality*. New York: Ballantine Books.

Castle, Kit, and S. Bechtel. 1989. *Katherine, It's Time: An Incredible Journey into the World of a Multiple Personality*. New York: Harper & Row.

Chadwick, Peter K. 1993. "The Stepladder to the Impossible: A First Hand Phenomenological Account of a Schizoaffective Psychotic Crisis." *Journal of Mental Health* 2:239–250.

Chaloner, John Armstrong. 1906. *The Lunacy Law of the World: Being That of Each of the Forty-eight States and Territories of the United States, with an Examination Thereof and Leading Cases Thereon; Together with That of the Six Great Powers of Europe—Great Britain, France, Italy, Germany, Austria-Hungary, and Russia.* Roanoke Rapids, NC: Palmetto Press.

————. 1914. *Who's Looney Now?* Roanoke Rapids, NC.: Palmetto.

Chamberlin, Judi. 1978. *On Our Own: Patient-Controlled Alternatives to the Mental Health System.* New York: Hawthorn Books.

Chambers, Julius. 1876. *A Mad World and Its Inhabitants.* New York: Appleton.

Chaning-Pearce, Melville [Nicodemus]. 1942. *Midnight Hour.* London: Faber & Faber.

Chase, Trudi. 1987. *When Rabbit Howls: The Troops for Trudi Chase.* With an introduction and epilogue by Robert A. Phillips. New York: Dutton.

Cheney, Terri. 2008. *Manic: A Memoir.* New York: HarperCollins.

Chisholm, Kate. 2002. *Hungry Hell.* London: Short Books.

Cienin, Pawel. 1972. *Fragments from the Diary of a Madman.* London: Gryf.

Clare, John. 1931. *Sketches in the Life of John Clare.* First published with an introduction, notes, and additions, by Edmund Blunden. London: Cobden-Sanderson.

Clark, Nick. 2008. *Love in the Prison of Psychosis.* London: Chipmunka.

Cleaves, Margaret A. 1910. *The Autobiography of a Neurasthenic.* Boston: Badger.

Clemens, Louisa Perina Courtauld. 1870. *Narrative of a Pilgrim and Sojourner on Earth, from 1791 to the Present Year, 1870.* Edinburgh.

Clements, Philip. 2005. *Sweet and Bitter Fool: A Priest's Journey through Manic Depression.* London: Chipmunka.

Clements, Richard M. 2006. *Defender.* London: Chipmunka.

Cline, Jean Darby. 1997. *Silencing the Voices: One Woman's Experience with Multiple Personality Disorder.* New York: Berkley Books.

Clover. 1999. *Escape from Psychiatry: The Autobiography of Clover.* 2nd ed. Ignacio, CO: Rainbow.

Coate, Morag. 1964. *Beyond All Reason.* London: Constable.

Colas, Emily. 1998. *Just Checking: Scenes from the Life of an Obsessive-Compulsive.* New York: Simon & Schuster.

Cole, Joshua. 2008. *No One Knows.* London: Chipmunka.

Coleman, Emily Holmes. 1930. *The Shutter of Snow.* New York: Viking.

Coleman, Ron. 1999. *Recovery: An Alien Concept.* Gloucester, UK: Handsell.

Collins, William J. 1971. *Out of the Depths.* New York: Doubleday.

Colme, Mairi. 2006. *A Divine Dance of Madness.* London: Chipmunka.

Connolly, Justin. 2008. *Is a Durham Degree a Passport to Madness?* London: Chipmunka.

Cooper, Janet. 2008. *The Huddle.* London: Chipmunka.

Cooper, Lisa. 2008. *The Most Outrageous Rollercoaster: Bipolar—a True Life Story.* London: Chipmunka.

Cottier, Lizzie D. 1885. *The Right Spirit.* Buffalo, NY: Courier.

Cowper, William. 1816. *Memoir of the Early Life of William Cowper.* New York: Taylor & Gould.

Coyle, Charles. 1983. "Life in an Insane Asylum." *Overland Monthly.* 13:161–171.

Coyne, Margaret. 2001. *Breakingdown, Breakingthrough: My Thorn-Paved Road to Healing via Altered States and Near Madness.* Dublin: Oxwood Print Solutions.

Crawford, Paul. 2002. *Nothing Purple, Nothing Black*. Lewes, UK: Book Guild.

Cresswell, Janet. 2005. *Ox-Bow*. London: Chipmunka.

Crowe, Anne Mary. 1811. *A Letter to Dr. R. D. Willis: to Which are Added, Copies of Three Other Letters: Published in the Hope of Rousing a Humane Nation to the Consideration of the Miseries Arising from Private Madhouses: with a Preliminary Address to Lord Erskine*. London: The Author.

Crowley, Kathleen. 1995. *The Day Room: A Memoir of Madness and Mending*. Kennedy Carlisle.

Cruden, Alexander. 1739. *The London-Citizen Exceedingly Injured; or, a British Inquisition Display'd, in an Account of the Unparallel'd Case of a Citizen of London, Bookseller to the Late Queen, Who Was in a Most Unjust and Arbitrary Manner Sent on the 23rd of March Last, 1738, by One Robert Wightman, a Mere Stranger, to a Private Madhouse*. London: T. Cooper.

———. 1740. *Mr. Cruden Greatly Injured: An Account of a Trial between Mr. Alexander Cruden, Bookseller to the Late Queen, Plaintif, and Dr. Monro, Matthew Wright, John Oswald, and John Davis, Defendants; in the Court of the Common-Pleas in Westminster Hall July 17, 1739, on an Action of Trespass, Assault and Imprisonment: the Said Mr. Cruden, Tho' in His Right Senses, Having Been Unjustly Confined and Barbarously Used in the Said Matthew Wright's Private Madhouse at Bethnal-Green for Nine Weeks and Six Days, till He Made His Wonderful Escape May 31, 1738. To Which is Added a Surprising Account of Several Other Persons, Who Have Been Mostly Unjustly Confined in Private Madhouses*. London: A. Injured.

———. 1754. *The Adventures of Alexander the Corrector, Wherein Is Given an Account of His Being Unjustly Sent to Chelsea, and of His Bad Usage during the Time of his Chelsea Campaign . . . with an Account of the Chelsea-Academies, or the Private Places for the Confinement of such as Are Supposed to Be Deprived of the Exercise of Their Reason*. London: The Author.

Custance, John [pseud.]. 1952. *Wisdom, Madness, and Folly: The Philosophy of a Lunatic*. New York: Pelligrini & Cudahy.

———. 1954. *Adventure into the Unconscious*. London: Christopher Johnson.

Cutting, Linda Katherine. 1997. *Memory Slips: A Memoir of Music and Healing*. New York: HarperCollins.

Dahl, Robert G. 1959. *Breakdown*. Indianapolis: Bobbs-Merrill.

Dailey, Abram H. 1984. *Mollie Fancher: The Brooklyn Enigma; an Authentic Statement of Facts in the Life of Mary J. Fancher; the Psychological Marvel of the Nineteenth Century*. Brooklyn, NY: New Library Press.

Dallett, Janet O. 1988. *When the Spirits Come Back*. Toronto: Inner City Books.

Dangarembga, Tsitsi. 1988. *Nervous Conditions*. London: Women's Press. Reprint, Seattle: Seal Press, 1996.

Danquah, Meri Nana-Ama. 1998. *Willow Weep for Me: A Black Woman's Journey through Depression*. New York: Ballantine.

Davenport, Eloise. 1960. *I Can't Forget*. New York: Carlton.

David [pseud.]. 1946. *The Autobiography of David*. Edited by Ernest Raymond. London: Victor Gollancz.

Davidson, D. 1912. *Remembrances of a Religio-Maniac*. Stratford-on-Avon, UK: Shakespeare.

Davis, Phebe E. 1855. *Two Years and Three Months in the New York State Lunatic Asylum at Utica, Together with the Outline of Twenty Years' Peregrinations in Syracuse*. Syracuse: The Author.

Davys, Sarah. 1971. *A Time and a Time*. London: Calder and Bozars.

Dawson, Jennifer. 1961. *The Ha-Ha*. Boston: Little, Brown.

Day, Beth. 1957. *No Hiding Place*. New York: Henry Holt.

Deane, Ruth. 2005. *Washing My Life Away: Surviving Obsessive-Compulsive Disorder*. London: Jessica Kingsley.

Delilez, Francis. 1888. *The True Cause of Insanity Explained; or, The Terrible Experience of an Insane, Related by Himself*. Minneapolis: Kimball.

Denny, Lydia B. 1862. *Statement of Mrs. Lydia B. Denny, Wife of Reuben S. Denny, of Boston, in Regard to Her Alleged Insanity*. N.p.

Denzer, Peter W. 1954. *Episode: A Record of Five Hundred Lost Days*. New York: Dutton.

Derby, John Barton. 1838. *Scenes in a Mad House*. Boston: Samuel N. Dickinson.

Dietrick, Frances I. 1992. *I'm Not Crazy: The True Story of Frances Dietrick's Flight from a Psychiatric Snake Pit to Freedom*. Far Hills, NJ: New Horizon Press.

Diski, Jenny. 1997. *Skating to Antarctica*. London: Granta.

Doe, Jane [pseud.]. 1966. *Crazy*. New York: Hawthorne.

Donaldson, Kenneth. 1976. *Insanity Inside Out*. New York: Crown.

Drake, John H. 1847. *Thirty-two Years of the Life of an Adventurer*. New York: The Author.

Drory, Irene. 1978. *Another World*. New York: Vantage.

Duffy, James. 1939. *The Capital's Siberia*. Middletown, ID: Boise Valley Herald.

Dukakis, Kitty. With J. Srovell. 1990. *Now You Know*. New York: Simon & Schuster.

Dukakis, Kitty, and Larry Tye. 2006. *Shock: The Healing Power of Electroconvulsive Therapy*. New York: Avery.

Duke, Patty. With K. Turan. 1987. *Call Me Anna: The Autobiography of Patty Duke*. New York: Bantam.

Duke, Patty. With Gloria Hochman. 1992. *A Brilliant Madness: Living with Manic-Depressive Illness*. New York: Bantam.

Dully, Howard, and Charles Fleming. 2007. *My Lobotomy*. New York: Crown.

Durmush, Fatma. 2006. *Nothing Sacred*. London: Chipmunka.

―――. 2008. *Hot Flowers*. London: Chipmunka.

Dyzantae, Adnandus. 2008. *The Ill Literate*. London: Chipmunka.

Edmonds, Helen Woods [Anna Kavan]. 1940. *Asylum Piece*. Garden City, NJ: Doubleday.

Edwards, Kenneth. 2006. *Psychosis from the Horse's Mouth*. London: Chipmunka.

Eliot, Jane. 1946. "My Way Back to Sanity." *Ladies Home Journal* 63 (10): 54–55, 242–250.

Ellis, William B. 1928. *Sanity for Sale: The Story of the Rise and Fall of William B. Ellis, by Himself*. Advance, NC: Advance.

―――. 1929. *Sanity for Sale: The Story of American Life since the Civil War*. Advance, NC: Advance.

Endler, Norman S. 1982. *Holiday of Darkness*. New York: Wiley. Rev. ed., Toronto: Wall & Thompson, 1990.

Etchell, Mabel. 1865. *Two Years in a Lunatic Asylum*. London: Simpkin, Marshall.

Etten, Howard J. 1972. *Memoirs of a Mental Case*. New York: Vantage.

Evans, Kim. 2008. *Memories of Mania*. London: Chipmunka.

Evans, Margiad. 1943. *Autobiography*. Oxford: Basil Blackwell.

―――. n.d. *A Ray of Darkness*. New York: Roy.

Farmer, Frances. 1972. *Will There Really Be a Morning?* New York: Putnam.

Farmer, John Harrison. 1975. *Road to Love: An Autobiography.* New York: Exposition.

Feldman, Harry. 1960. *In a Forest Dark.* New York: Thomas Nelson & Sons.

Ferguson, Sarah. 1973. *A Guard Within.* London: Chatto & Windus.

Ferland, Carol. 1980. *The Long Journey Home.* New York: Knopf.

Feugilly, Mary Heustis. 1885. *Diary Written in the Provincial Lunatic Asylum.* [St. John, N.B.?]: The Author.

Field, E. 1964. *The White Shirts.* Los Angeles: E. Field.

Fink, Harold Kenneth. 1954. *Long Journey: A Verbatim Report of a Case of Severe Psychosexual Infantilism.* New York: Julian.

Firestone, Shulamith. 1998. *Airless Spaces.* New York: Semiotext(e).

Fischer, Augusta Catherine. 1937. *Searchlight: An Autobiography.* Seattle.

Fleming, E. G. 1893. *Three Years in a Mad House.* Chicago: Donohue, Henneberry.

Fleming, Mark. 2008. *BrainBomb.* London: Chipmunka.

Foley, Nancy. 2002. "A Room with a View." *Valley Advocate* (Northampton, MA), March 7.

Folkland, Lynne. 1992. *The Rock Pillow: A Personal Account of Schizophrenia.* Freemantle, Western Australia: Freemantle Arts Centre.

Fox, George. 1919. *George Fox: An Autobiography.* Philadelphia: Friends' Book Store.

Frame, Janet. 1961. *Faces in the Water.* New York: George Braziller.

————. 1984. *An Angel at My Table: An Autobiography.* New York: George Braziller.Francis, Joseph H. 1915. *My Last Drink.* Chicago: Empire Books.

Fraser, Sarah. 1975. *Living with Depression—and Winning.* Wheaton, IL: Tyndale House.

Freeman, C.P.L., et al. 1980. "Three Essays on Patients' Experiences of ECT." *British Journal of Psychiatry* 137:8–16, 17–25, 26–37.

Freeman, Lucy. 1951. *Fight against Fears.* New York: Crown.

Frolick, Vernon. 2004. *Descent into Madness: The Diary of a Killer.* Blaine, WA: Hancock House.

Fry, Jane. 1974. *Being Different: The Autobiography of Jane Fry.* New York: John Wiley & Sons.

Fuller, Robert. 1833. *An Account of the Imprisonment and Sufferings of Robert Fuller, of Cambridge.* Boston: The Author.

Fullerton, James. 1912. *Autobiography of Roosevelt's Adversary.* Boston: Roxbaugh.

Funk, Wendy. 1998. *What Difference Does It Make? (The Journey of a Soul Survivor).* Cranbrook, BC: Wildflower.

Garfield, Johanna. 1986. *The Life of a Real Girl.* New York: St. Martin's Press.

Garner, Edward Dixon. 1974. *Sketchbook from Hell.* Durham, NC: Moore.

Gary, Looney Lee [pseud.]. 1940. *The Bridge of Eternity.* New York: Fortuny's.

George. 1981. "I Can't Imagine Life Without Mental Illness." *Mind Out.*

Geraghty, Deirdre. 2007. *Cracking Up: My Experiences of Schizophrenia.* London: Chipmunka.

Gibson, M. 1976. *The Butterfly Ward.* Toronto: HarperCollins.

Gifford, Patsy. 2008. *Fighting the Corners.* London: Chipmunka.

Gilbert, William. 1864. *The Monomaniac, or Shirley Hall Asylum.* New York: James G. Gregory.

Gilman, Charlotte Perkins. 1892. "The Yellow Wallpaper." *New England Magazine* 5 (5): 647–656.

————. 1935. *The Living of Charlotte Perkins Gilman*. New York: Appleton-Century.

Gilmour, Jimmy. 2008. *I Thought I Was the King of Scotland*. London: Chipmunka.

Gluck, Jeremy. 2008. *Victim of Dreams: Civil War in the Soul*. London: Chipmunka.

Gorbanevskaya, N. 1972. *Red Square at Noon*. London: Andre Deutsch.

Gordon, Barbara. 1979. *I'm Dancing as Fast as I Can*. New York: Harper & Row.

Gordon, Emily Fox. 2000. *Mockingbird Years: A Life in and out of Therapy*. New York: Basic Books.

Gotkin, Janet, and Paul Gotkin. 1975. *Too Much Anger, Too Many Tears: A Personal Triumph over Psychiatry*. New York: Quadrangle.

Goulet, Robert. 1973. *Madhouse*. Chicago: J. P. O'Hara.

Grandin, Temple. 1985. *Thinking in Pictures, and Other Reports from My Life with Autism*. New York: Doubleday.

Grant, Linda. 1998. *Remind Me Who I Am Again*. London: Granta.

Grant-Smith, Rachel. 1922. *The Experiences of an Asylum Patient*. London: Allen & Unwin.

Graves, Alonzo. 1942. *The Eclipse of a Mind*. New York: Medical Journal Press.

Gray, Jerry. 1949. *The Third Strike*. New York: Abingdon-Cokesbury.

Greally, Hanna. 1971. *Bird's Nest Soup*. Dublin: Attic Press.

Green, Rosemary. 1995. *Diary of a Fat Housewife: A True Story of Humor, Heartbreak, and Hope*. New York: Warner.

Greenberg, Joanne [Hannah Green]. 1964. *I Never Promised You a Rose Garden*. New York: Holt, Rinehart & Winston.

Greene, Julie. 2002. *Breakdown Lane, Traveled*. Bloomington, IN: Author House.

Greene-McCreight, Kathryn. 2006. *Darkness Is My Only Companion: A Christian Response to Mental Illness*. Ada, MI: Brazos Press.

Greiner, S. 1943. *Prelude to Sanity*. Fort Lauderdale: Master.

Griffin, Sarah. 2007. *Sarah's Diary*. London: Virgin Books.

Grigorenko, P. G. 1976. *The Grigorenko Papers*. Boulder, CO: Westview.

Grimes, Green. 1846. *The Lily of the West: On Human Nature, Education, the Mind, Insanity, with Ten Letters as a Sequel to the Alphabet; the Conquest of Man, Early Days; a Farewell to My Native Home, the Song of the Chieftain's Daughter, Tree of Liberty, and the Beauties of Nature and Art, by G. Grimes, an Inmate of the Lunatic Asylum of Tennessee*. Nashville.

————. 1846. *A Secret Worth Knowing: A Treatise on the Most Important Secret in the World: Simply to Say, Insanity, by G. Grimes, an Inmate of the Lunatic Asylum of Tennessee*. Nashville: Nashville Union.

————. 1847. *A Secret Worth Knowing: A Treatise on Insanity, the Only Work of the Kind in the United States or, Perhaps in the Known World: Founded on General Observation and Truth, by G. Grimes, an Inmate of the Lunatic Asylum of Tennessee*. New York: W. H. Graham.

Hackett, Paul. 1952. *The Cardboard Giants*. New York: Putnam.

Haizmann, Christoph. 1956. *Schizophrenia, 1677: A Psychiatric Study of an Illustrated Autobiographical Record of Demoniacal Possession*. Edited by Ida Macalpine and Richard Hunter. London: William Dawson & Sons.

Halban, Emily. 2008. *Perfect: Anorexia and Me*. London: Vermilion.

Hales, Ella [pseud.]. 1958. *Like a Lamb*. London: Christopher Johnson.

Hall, Roger. 1977. *Clouds of Fear*. London: Coronet.

Hamilcar, Marcia. 1910. *Legally Dead: Experiences during Seventeen Weeks' Detention in a Private Asylum*. London: John Ouseley.

Hamill, Pete. 1994. *A Drinking Life: A Memoir*. Boston: Little, Brown.

Hampton, Russell K. 1975. *The Far Side of Despair: A Personal Account of Depression*. Chicago: Nelson-Hall.

Handler, Lowell. 1999. *Twitch and Shout: A Touretter's Tale*. New York: Penguin.

Hannon, Bill. 1997. *Agents in My Brain: How I Survived Manic Depression*. Chicago: Open Court.

Harding, Len. 1985. *Born a Number*. London: Mind.

Hardwick, William J. 1993. *The Mind of a Madman: An Autobiographical Account*. [England?]: The Author.

Harlan, Olivia. 1941. "Minds in the Mending." *Atlantic Monthly* 168:330–334.

Harris, E. Lynn. 2003. *What Becomes of the Brokenhearted?* New York: Anchor Books.

Harris, Tracy L. 2001. *The Music of Madness*. Lincoln, NE: iUniverse.

Harrison, Maude. 1941. *Spinner's Lake*. London: John Lane, The Bodley Head.

Harrison, P. G.. 1974. "Visions of a Madman." In *Madness Network News Reader*, edited by S. Hirsh, J. K. Adams, and I. R. Frank. San Francisco: Glide.

Hart, Linda. 1995. *Phone at Nine Just to Say You're Alive*. London: D. Elliot.

Harvey, Sheila. 2003. *Sheila's Book: A Shared Journey Through "Madness."* Taunton, UK: Somerset Virtual College NHS.

Harvin, Emily [pseud.]. 1948. *The Stubborn Wood*. Chicago: Ziff-Davis.

Haselton, Anthony. 2006. *A Modern Medical Miracle*. London: Chipmunka.

Haskell, Ebenezer. 1869. *The Trial of Ebenezer Haskell, in Lunacy, and His Acquittal Before Judge Brewster, in November, 1868, Together with a Brief Sketch of the Mode of Treatment of Lunatics in Different Asylums in this Country and in England, with Illustrations, Including a Copy of Hogarth's Celebrated Painting of a Scene of Old Bedlam, in London, 1635*. Philadelphia: E. Haskell.

Haslam, John, ed. 1810. *Illustrations of Madness: Exhibiting a Singular Case of Insanity, and a No Less Remarkable Difference in Medical Opinion: Developing the Nature of Assailment, and the Manner of Working Events; with a Description of the Torture Experienced by Bomb-Bursting, Lobster-Cracking, and Lengthening the Brain*. London: G. Haydon.

Havecamp, Katharina. 1978. *Love Comes in Buckets*. London: Boyars.

Hayes, Billy. With W. Hoffer. 1977. *Midnight Express*. New York: Dutton.

Heaslip, Barbara. 1972. *Saints and Strait Jackets: An Intimate View of Life in an Australian Psychiatric Hospital, by an Ex-Patient*. The Author.

Heater, Sandra Harvey. 1983. *Am I Still Visible? A Woman's Triumph over Anorexia Nervosa*. White Hall, VA: White Hall Books.

Hebald, Carol. 2001. *The Heart Too Long Suppressed: A Chronicle of Mental Illness*. Boston: Northeastern University Press.

Hellmuth, Charles F. 1977. *Maniac: Anatomy of a Mental Illness*. Philadelphia: Dorrance.

Helmbold, Henry T. 1877. *Am I a Lunatic? Or, Dr. Henry T. Helmbold's Exposure of his Personal Experience in the Lunatic Asylums of Europe and America*. New York.

Hennell, Thomas Barcley. 1938. *The Witnesses*. London: Davies.

Hewitt, Harald. 1923. *From Harrow School to Herrison House Asylum*. London: C. W. Daniel.

Hill, Clare. 2005. *Living without Marbles*. London: Chipmunka.

Hill, Philip. 2008. *Living "out" of the Book: The Journey from a Diagnosis of Learning Difficulties through Periods of Mental Illness to a Career as a Professional Social Worker*. London: Chipmunka.

Hillyer, Jane. 1926. *Reluctantly Told*. New York: Macmillan.

Hodgins, Eric. 1964. *Episode: Report on the Accident inside My Skull*. New York: Atheneum.

Hoffman, R. 1995. *Half the House: A Memoir*. New York: Harcourt Brace.

Hornbacher, Marya. 1999. *Wasted: A Memoir of Anorexia and Bulimia*. New York: HarperCollins.

———. 2008. *Madness: A Bipolar Life*. New York: Houghton Mifflin.

Howland, Bette. 1974. *W-3*. New York: Viking.

Hughes, John S., ed. 1993. *The Letters of a Victorian Madwoman [Andrew M. Sheffield]*. Columbia: University of South Carolina Press.

Hummel, James E. [James H. Ellis]. 1953. *To Hell and Back: The Story of an Alcoholic*. New York: Vantage.

Hunt, Isaac H. 1851. *Astounding Disclosures! Three Years in a Mad House, by a Victim. A True Account of the Barbarous, Inhuman and Cruel Treatment of Isaac H. Hunt, in the Maine Insane Hospital, in the Years 1844, '45, '46 and '47, by Drs. Isaac Ray, James Bates, and Their Assistants and Attendants*. Skowhegan: The Author.

———. 1852. *Astounding Disclosures! Three Years in a Mad House, by a Victim. Contains Also: A Short Account of Miss Elizabeth T. Stone in the McLean Asylum at Somerville, Mass. and a Short Account of the Burning of the Maine Asylum, Dec. 4th, 1850*. Skowhegan, [ME?]: The Author.

Hunt, Morton M. 1962. *Mental Hospital*. New York: Pyramid.

Hurley, Tony. 2004. *Why Me?* London: Chipmunka.

Hurry, A. 1977. "My Ambition Is to Be Dead." *Journal of Child Psychotherapy* 4 (3): 66–83.

Inmate Ward Eight [Marion Woodson]. 1932. *Behind the Door of Delusion*. New York: Macmillan.

Jackson, C. 1944. *The Lost Weekend*. New York: Farrar, Strauss & Cudahy.

James, William. 2003. *A Journey through Madness: Bonds Unshackled*. N.p.: Writers Club Press.

Jamieson, Patrick E. 2006. *Mind Race: A Firsthand Account of One Teenager's Experience with Bipolar Disorder*. New York: Oxford University Press.

Jamison, Kay Redfield. 1995. *An Unquiet Mind: A Memoir of Moods and Madness*. New York: Random House.

Jayson, Lawrence M. 1937. *Mania*. New York: Funk & Wagnalls.

Jefferson, Lara [pseud.]. 1947. *These Are My Sisters: An "Insandectomy."* Tulsa, OK: Vickers. Reprint, Garden City, NJ: Doubleday, 1974.

Jensen, Jan Lars. 2004. *Nervous System: The Story of a Novelist Who Lost His Mind*. Vancouver: Raincoast Books.

John, Otto. 1972. *Twice through the Lines: The Autobiography of Otto John*. New York: Harper.

Johnson, Donald McIntosh. 1949. *A Doctor Regrets, Being the First Part of "A Publisher Presents Himself."* London: Johnson.

———. 1952. *Bars and Barricades, Being the Second Part of "A Publisher Presents Himself."* London: Johnson.

———. 1956. *A Doctor Returns, Being the Third Part of "A Publisher Presents Himself."* London: Johnson.

Johnston, Jill. 1973. *Lesbian Nation.* New York: Simon & Schuster.

Johnstone, Nick. 2003. *A Head Full of Blue.* London: Bloomsbury.

Joyce, John A. 1883. *A Checkered Life.* Chicago: S. P. Rounds.

Karr, Mary. 1995. *The Liar's Club: A Memoir.* New York: Viking.

Kaysen, Susanna. 1993. *Girl, Interrupted.* New York: Random House.

Kempe, Margery. 1940. *The Book of Margery Kempe.* Edited and introduced by Sanford Brown Meech and Hope Emily Allen. Oxford: Oxford University Press. (Orig. manuscript 1436.)

———. 1944. *The Book of Margery Kempe.* Rendered into modern English by W. Butler-Bowdon. New York: DevinAdair.

Kent, Patricia. 1967. *An American Woman and Alcohol.* New York: Holt, Rinehart & Winston.

Kerkoff, Jack. 1952. *How Thin the Veil: A Newspaperman's Story of His Own Mental Crackup and Recovery.* New York: Greenberg.

Kesey, Ken. 1975. *One Flew over the Cuckoo's Nest.* New York: Picador.

Kettlewell, Caroline. 1999. *Skin Game.* New York: St. Martin's Press.

Kinder, Elaine F. 1940. "Postscript on a Benign Psychosis." *Psychiatry* 3:527–534.

King, Alexander. 1958. *Mine Enemy Grows Older.* New York: Simon & Schuster.

King, L. Percy [pseud.]. ca. 1940. *Criminal Complaints with Probable Causes (a True Account).* Bound, circular letter.

King, Marian. 1931. *The Recovery of Myself.* New Haven: Yale University Press.

King, Philippa. 2008. *A Mind Taut with Pain.* London: Chipmunka.

Kirk, Anne. 1937. *Chronicles of Interdict No. 7807.* Boston: Meador.

Knapp, Caroline. 1996. *Drinking: A Love Story.* New York: Dial.

Knauth, Percy. 1956. *A Season in Hell.* New York: Harper.

Knight, Paul Slade. 1827. *Observations on the Causes, Symptoms, and Treatment of Derangement. Founded on an Extensive Moral and Medical Practice in the Treatment of Lunatics. Together With the Particulars of the Sensations and Ideas of a Gentleman During Mental Alternation, Written by Himself during His Confinement.* London: Longman.

Knight, Suzannah. 2007. *Black Magic.* London: Chipmunka.

Knipfel, Jim. 2000. *Quitting the Nairobi Trio.* New York: Putnam.

Knox, Sandy. 2008. *Bi-polar on Benefits (I Can't Be the Only One).* London: Chipmunka.

Kops, Bernard. 1962. *The World Is a Wedding.* New York: Coward-McCann.

———. 1978. *On Margate Sands.* London: Secker & Warburg.

Krauch, Elsa. 1937. *A Mind Restored: The Story of Jim Curran.* New York: G. P. Putnam's Sons.

Krim, Seymour. 1948. *Views of a Nearsighted Cannoneer.* New York: E. P. Dutton.

Kruger, Judith. 1959. *My Fight for Sanity.* London: Hammond.

Kumin, Philip A. 1998. *Ex-inmate in Exile: The Autobiography of Philip A. Kumin.* Victoria, BC: Trafford.

Kurelek, William. 1973. *Someone with Me: The Autobiography of William Kurelek.* Edited by J. Maas. Ithaca: Cornell University Center for the Improvement of Undergraduate Education.

Kwok, Caroline Fei-Yeng. 2006. *Free to Fly: A Story of Manic-Depression.* Toronto: Inclusion Press.

La Marr, Dressler [Jinxy R Howell]. 1965. *All the Hairs on My Head Hurt.* New York: Exposition.

Labrunie, Gerard [Gerard De Nerval]. 1923. *Daughters of Fire: Sylvia—Emilie—Octavie.* Translated from the 1862 French edition. London: Heineman.

———. 1933. *Dreams and Life.* Translated from the 1855 French edition. London: First Edition Club and Boar's Head Press of Manaton, Devon.

Lane, Edward X. 1963. *I Was a Mental Statistic.* New York: Carlton.

Larkin, Joy. 1979. *Strangers No More: Diary of a Schizo.* New York: Vantage.

A Late Inmate of the Glasgow Royal Asylum for Lunatics at Gartnavel (James Frame). 1947. *The Philosophy of Insanity.* London: Fireside Press. (Orig. pub. 1860.)

Lathrop, Clarissa Caldwell. 1890. *A Secret Institution.* New York: Bryant.

Lazell, David. 1973. *I Couldn't Catch the Bus Today: The True Story of a Nervous Breakdown That Became a Pilgrimage.* Guildford, UK: Lutterworth Press.

Leach, John E. 1969. *Fear No Evil.* New York: Vantage.

Leah, Shane. 2008. *Dead City Streets.* London: Chipmunka.

Lee, Judy. 1980. *Save Me! A Young Woman's Journey through Schizophrenia to Health.* New York: Doubleday.

Lee, Kate [pseud.]. 1902. *A Year at Elgin Insane Asylum.* New York: Irving.

Lee-Houghton, Melissa. 2008. *Patterns of Mourning.* London: Chipmunka.

Lelchuk, Alan. 1978. *Shrinking.* New York: Little, Brown.

Leonard, William Ellery. 1927. *The Locomotive God.* New York: Appleton-Century.

———. 1933. *Two Lives.* New York: Viking.

———. 1945. *A Man Against Time: An Heroic Dream.* New York: Appleton-Century.

Levant, Oscar. 1965. *Memoirs of an Amnesiac.* Hollywood, CA: Samuel French (republished 1989).

———. 1968. *The Unimportance of Being Oscar.* New York: Putnam's Sons.

Lewis, Gwyneth. 2002. *Sunbathing in the Rain.* London: Flamingo.

Lewis, Mindy. 2002. *Life Inside: A Memoir.* New York: Atria Books.

Lloyd, Ronald. 1968. *Born to Trouble: Portrait of a Psychopath.* London: Cassirer.

Logan, Joshua. 1976. *Josh: My up and down, in and out Life.* New York: Delacorte, 1976.

Lorenz, Sarah E. 1963. *And Always Tomorrow.* New York: Holt, Rinehart & Winston.

Lott, Tim. 1996. *The Scent of Dried Roses.* London: Viking.

Lovelace, David. 2008. *Scattershot: My Bipolar Family.* New York: Dutton.

Lowe, Louisa. 1883. *The Bastilles of England; or, The Lunacy Laws at Work.* London: Crookenden, 1883.

———. 1872. *Gagging in Madhouses as Practised by Government Servants in a Letter to the People, by One of the Gagged.* London: Burns.

———. 1872. *How an Old Woman Obtained Passive Writing and the Outcome Thereof.* London: Burns.

———. 1872. *The Lunacy Laws and Trade in Lunacy in a Correspondence with the Earl of Shaftesbury.* London: Burns.

———. 1872. *My Outlawry: A Tale of Madhouse Life.* London: Burns.

———. 1872. *A Nineteenth Century Adaptation of Old Inventions to the Repression of New Thoughts and Personal Liberty.* London: Burns.

———. 1872. *Report of a Case Heard in Queen's Bench, November 22nd, 1872, Charging the Commissioners in Lunacy with Concurring in the Improper Detention of a Falsely-Alleged Lunatic and Wrongfully Tampering with her Correspondence.* London: Burns.

Lundgren, Jodi. 1999. *Touched*. Vancouver, BC: Anvil.

Lunt, Adeline. 1871. *Behind Bars*. New York: Lee, Shepard, & Dillingham.

Lytton, Rosina Bulwer. 1996. *A Blighted Life: A True Story*. Bristol: Thoemmes Press. (Orig. pub. 1880.)

Mabey, Richard. 2005. *Nature Cure*. London: Chatto & Windus.

Macard, Lotti. 2006. *To Live with Myself*. London: Chipmunka.

MacLane, Mary. 1902. *The Story of Mary MacLane by Herself*. Chicago: Herbert S. Stone. Reprint, n.p.: Riverbend, 2002.

———. 1917. *I, Mary MacLane: A Diary of Human Days*. New York: Frederick A. Stokes.

Maine, H. 1947. *If a Man Be Mad*. New York: Doubleday.

Mairs, Nancy. 1986. *Plaintext: Essays*. Tucson: University of Arizona Press.

Manna, Marci M. 2008. *Into the Darkness*. London: Chipmunka.

Manning, Martha. 1994. *Undercurrents: A Therapist's Reckoning with Her Own Depression*. New York: HarperCollins.

Marchenko, Anatoly. 1969. *My Testimony*. New York: Dutton.

Marks, Jan. 1959. *Doctor Purgatory*. New York: Citadel.

Marshall, Des. 2002. *Journal of an Urban Robinson Crusoe: London and Brighton*. Sussex, UK: Saxon Books.

Martel, S. 1961. *In the Forests of the Night*. London: George Randid.

Martens, David. 1946. *The Abrupt Self*. New York: Harper & Brothers.

Martin, Wanda. 1966. *Woman in Two Worlds: A Personal Story of Psychological Experience*. Norwalk, CT: Silvermine.

Mays, John Bentley. 1996. *In the Jaws of the Black Dogs: A Memoir of Depression*. Toronto: Penguin.

McCall, Lenore. 1947. *Between Us and the Dark*. Philadelphia: Lippincott.

McCormick, Patricia. 2000. *Cut*. New York: Push.

McDonald, Norma. 1960. "Living with Schizophrenia." *Canadian Medical Association Journal* 82:218–222.

McFadden, Benjamin. 2008. *Withdrawals from a Legal Drug*. London: Chipmunka.

McGarr, Margaret Atkins. 1953. *And Lo, the Star*. New York: Pageant.

McHarg, Alistair. 2007. *Invisible Driving*. Charleston, SC: BookSurge.

McIntyre, Alistair. 2007. *A Journey into Madness: A Story of Schizophrenia*. London: Chipmunka.

McKean, Thomas A. 1994. *Soon Will Come the Light: A View from inside the Autism Puzzle*. Arlington, TX: Future Horizons.

McLean, Richard. 2003. *Recovered, Not Cured: A Journey through Schizophrenia*. Crows Nest, NSW, Australia: Allen and Unwin.

McMeekin, Michelle. 2008. *Poles Apart*. London: Chipmunka.

McNeight, Tom. 2008. *Beyond Psychosis*. London: Chipmunka.

McNeill, Elizabeth. 1978. *Nine and a Half Weeks*. New York: Dutton.

McPherson, Bess Howard. 2006. *A Smoker's and Dog's Guide to the Gal-Alexy*. London: Chipmunka.

Medvedev, Zhores A. 1971. *A Question of Madness*. Translated from the 1971 Russian edition. New York: Knopf.

Merivale, Herman Charles. 1879. *My Experience in a Lunatic Asylum, by a Sane Patient*. London: Chatto and Windus.

Merritt, Stephanie. 2008. *The Devil Within*. London: Vermilion.

Metcalf, Ada. 1876. *Lunatic Asylums: And How I Became an Inmate of One.* Chicago: Ottaway & Colbert.

Metcalf, Urbane. 1818. *The Interior of Bethlehem Hospital.* London: The Author.

Middle-Aged Man [pseud.]. 1853. *Passages from the History of a Wasted Life.* Boston: Benj. B. Mussey.

Millett, Kate. 1990. *The Loony-Bin Trip.* New York: Simon & Schuster.

Mingus, Charles. 1971. *Beneath the Underdog, His World as Composed by Mingus.* Edited by N. King. New York: Knopf.

Mitford, John. 1825. *A Description of the Crimes and Horrors in the Interior of Warburton's Private Mad-House at Hoxton, Commonly Called Whibmore House.* London: Benbow.

————. 1825. *Part Second of the Crimes and Horrors of the Interior of Warburton's Private Mad-Houses at Hoxton and Bethnal Green and of These Establishments in General with Reasons for Their Total Abolition.* London: Benbow.

Modrow, John. 1992. *How to Become a Schizophrenic.* Lincoln, NE: iUniverse. 3rd ed., 2003.

Moeller, Helen. 1968. *Tornado: My Experience with Mental Illness.* Westwood, NJ: F. H. Revell.

Molony, William O'Sullivan. 1935. *New Armor for Old.* New York: Holt.

Money, John, Gordon Wainwright, and David Hingsburger. 1991. *The Breathless Orgasm.* Buffalo, NY: Promethean.

Moody, Rick. 2002. *The Black Veil: A Memoir with Digressions.* New York: Little, Brown.

Moon, Annie. 2008. *To Schizophrenia and Back.* London: Chipmunka.

Mooney, Jonathan. 2007. *The Short Bus: A Journey beyond Normal.* New York: Holt.

Moore, Teresa. 2005. *For Endings to End, Beginnings Have to Begin.* London: Chipmunka.

Moore, William L. 1955. *The Mind in Chains (Autobiography of a Schizophrenic).* New York: Exposition.

Morrison, Isabella Millar. 1956. *A Tale Told by a Lunatic.* Dumfries: Robert Dinwiddle.

Mowrer, Orval Hobart. 1983. *Leaves from Many Seasons: Selected Papers.* New York: Praeger.

Mumford, Edwin. 1965. *Diary of a Paranoiac.* New York: Exposition.

Mundfrom, G. F. 1990. *My Experiences With Clinical Depression.* Osceola, WI: Mercy & Truth.

Nakhla, Fayek, and Grace Jackson. 1993. *Picking Up the Pieces: Two Accounts of a Psychoanalytic Journey.* New Haven: Yale University Press.

Neary, John. 1975. *Whom the Gods Destroy.* New York: Atheneum.

Nekipelov, Viktor. 1980. *Institute of Fools.* New York: Farrar, Straus & Giroux

Nelson, Dianne. 2008. *Unveiling Schizophrenia.* Frederick, MD: PublishAmerica.

Nelson, Robert Quentin. 1970. *Mental.* Chichester, UK: Quentin Nelson.

Nerval, Gérard de. 1957. *Selected Writings.* Translated by Geoffrey Wagner. New York: Grove Press.

Newman, Katherine A. 1998. *Sorority of Survival.* Commack, NY: Kroshka Books.

Newport, Jerry, Mary Newport, and Johnny Dodd. 2007. *Mozart and the Whale: An Asperger's Love Story.* New York: Touchstone Books.

Neyer, Dix. 1977. *Wander, Wander: A Woman's Journey into Herself.* Englewood Cliffs, NJ: Prentice-Hall.

Nijinsky, Vaslav. 1999. *Diary of Vaslav Nijinsky*. Edited by Joan Accocella. New York: Farrar, Straus & Giroux. (Orig. pub. 1936.)

Noël, Barbara. With Kathryn Watterson. 1992. *You Must Be Dreaming*. New York: Poseidon Press.

Nolan, M. J. 1928. *Exposure of the Asylum System*. N.p.

Noone, Mary [pseud.]. 1961. *Sweetheart, I Have Been to School*. New York: Harcourt, Brace & World.

North, Carol S. 1987. *Welcome Silence: My Triumph over Schizophrenia*. New York: Simon & Schuster.

O'Brien, Barbara [pseud.]. 1958. *Operators and Things: The Inner Life of a Schizophrenic*. London: Ace.

Ogdon, John Andrew Howard. 1947. *The Kingdom of the Lost*. London: Bodley Head.

O'Hagan, Mary. 1993. *Stopovers on My Way Home from Mars*. London: Survivors Speak Out.

Oliver, Maureen. 2006. *Breaking Down: The Diary of a Survivor*. London: Chipmunka.

———. 2008. *Being Icarus*. London: Chipmunka.

Olson, Sarah E. 1997. *Becoming One: A Story of Triumph over Multiple Personality Disorder*. Pasadena, CA: Trilogy Books.

O'Neill, Cherry Boone. 1982. *Starving for Attention*. New York: Continuum.

Osborne, Luther. 1939. *The Insanity Racket: A Story of One of the Worst Hell Holes in This Country*. Oakland, CA.

Owens, Emerson D. [North 3–1]. 1929. *Pick Up the Pieces*. New York: Doubleday, Doran.

Packard, Elizabeth Parsons Ware. 1866. *Marital Power Exemplified in Mrs. Packard's Trial and Self-defense from the Charge of Insanity; or, Three Years Imprisonment for Religious Belief, by the Arbitrary Will of a Husband, with an Appeal to the Government to So Change the Laws as to Afford Legal Protection to Married Women*. Hartford, CT: Case, Lockwood.

———. 1868. *Mrs. Olsen's Narrative of Her One Year Imprisonment, at Jacksonville Insane Asylum; with the Testimony of Mrs. Minard, Mrs. Shedd, Mrs. Yates, and Mrs. Lake, All Corroborated by the Investigating Committee of the Legislature of Illinois*. Chicago: A.B. Case.

———. 1868. *The Prisoners' Hidden Life; or, Insane Asylums Unveiled: As Demonstrated by the Report of the Investigating Committee of the Legislature of Illinois. Together with Mrs. Packard's Coadjutors' Testimony*. Chicago: The Author.

———. 1874. *A Bill to Remedy the Evils of Insane Asylums, and Mrs. Packard's Argument in Support of the Same*. Presented to the Massachusetts Legislature, April 28, 1874. Boston: n.p.

———. 1874. *Modern Persecutions; or, Insane Asylums Unveiled, as Demonstrated by the Report of the Investigating Committee of the Legislature of Illinois, Volumes I & II. Vol. 2, Modern Persecutions; or, Married Woman's Liabilities, as Demonstrated by the Action of the Illinois Legislature*. Hartford, CT: Case, Lockwood, & Brainard.

———. 1886. *The Mystic Key; or, The Asylum Secret Unlocked*. Hartford: Case, Lockwood & Brainard.

———. 1973. *Modern Persecution; or, Insane Asylums Unveiled*. New York: Arno Press (Orig. pub. 1873.)

————. 1974. *Great Disclosures of Spiritual Wickedness!! In High Places: with an Appeal to the Government to Protect the Inalienable Rights of Married Women.* New York: Arno Press (Orig. pub. 1865.)

Pagett, Nicola. 1997. *Diamonds behind My Eyes.* London: Gollancz.

Pahlson-Moller, Lovisa. 2005. *Little Girl Lost.* London: Chipmunka.

Painter, Charlotte. 1971. *Confessions from the Malaga Madhouse: A Christmas Diary.* New York: Dial Press.

Parker, Beulah. 1972. *A Mingled Yarn.* New Haven: Yale University Press.

Partyka, Joseph J. 1968. *Never Come Early.* Mountain View, CA: The Author.

Paternoster, Richard. 1841. *The Madhouse System.* London: The Author.

Paul, Brenda Dean. 1935. *My First Life: A Biography, by Brenda Dean Paul, Written By Herself.* London: J. Long.

Pauley, Jane. 2004. *Skywriting: A Life out of the Blue.* New York: Random House.

Pegler, Jason. 2002. *A Can of Madness: An Autobiography on Manic Depression.* Brentwood, UK: Chipmunka.

Penn, Arthur. 1941. *California Justice: Is This Supposed to Be a Democracy?* San Francisco.

Pennell, Lemira Clarissa. 1883. *The Memorial Scrapbook. A Combination of Precedents.* Boston: n.p.

————. 1884. *Another Section of the "M.S.B." by L.C.P. A Boomerang for a Swarm of B.B.B.'s.* Boston: n.p.

————. 1885. *Prospectus of Hospital Revelations. How Opinions Vary.* N.p.

————. 1886. *This Red Book Is Partly a Reprint of What Was Published in 1883, and Later. And Earlier Letters from Prominent Men. Instructions to Dr. Harlow, from Springfield, His Letters from the Hospitals, and Much Else.* Boston: n.p.

————. 1888. *Hospital Revelations.* N.p.

————. 188[?]. *An Explanation to the Public as to Why Mrs. Lemira Clarissa Pennell Was Confined in the Insane Hospital and the Portland Poor House.* Augusta, ME: n.p.

————. 1890. *New Horrors.* N.p.

————. n.d. *Leave to Withdraw.* Boston: n.p.

Perceval, John. 1830, 1840. *A Narrative of the Treatment Experienced by a Gentleman, during a State of Mental Derangement; Designed to Explain the Causes and the Nature of Insanity, and to Expose the Injudicious Conduct Pursued towards Many Unfortunate Sufferers Under That Calamity.* 2 vols. London: Effingham Wilson. Republished, with an introduction by Gregory Bateson, Stanford, CA: Stanford University Press, 1961.

Perkins, Robert. 1996. *Talking to Angels: A Life Spent at High Latitudes.* Boston: Beacon Press.

Peters, Fritz. 1949. *The World Next Door.* New York: Farrar Strauss.

Pettican, Phil. 2003. *Don't Look Back in Anger.* London: Chipmunka.

Pfau, Father Ralph. 1959. *Prodigal Shepherd.* New York: Popular Library.

Phillips, J. 1995. *The Magic Daughter: A Memoir of Living with Multiple Personality Disorder.* New York: Viking.

Pierce, S. W., and J. T. [pseud.]. 1929. *The Layman Looks at Doctors.* New York: Harcourt, Brace.

Piersall, James, and Albert Hirshberg. 1955. *Fear Strikes Out: The Jim Piersall Story.* Boston: Little, Brown.

Plath, Sylvia. 1963. *The Bell Jar.* New York: Bantam.

Plyushch, Leonid. 1976. *The Case of Leonid Plyushch*. Translated by Marie Sapiets. Boulder, CO: Westview.

———. 1979. *History's Carnival*. New York: Harcourt Brace Jovanovich.

Pole, John L. 1929. *When: A Record of Transition*. London: Chapman & Hall.

Pollard, Marc. 2003. *In Small Doses: A Memoir about Accepting and Living with Bipolar Disorder*. Mill Valley, CA: Vision Books International.

Pollitt, Basil Hubbard. 1954. *Justice and Justices*. Daytona Beach, FL: College.

———. 1958. *A Lawyer's Story in and out of the World of Insanity*. Miami: B. H. Pollitt.

Powers, Barbara W., and W. Diehl. 1965. *Spy Wife*. New York: Pyramid.

Pratt, Ann. 1860. *Seven Months in the Kingston Lunatic Asylum, and What I Saw There*. Kingston: G. Henderson Savage.

Previn, Dory. 1976. *Midnight Baby: Autobiography*. New York: Macmillan.

———. 1980. *Bog-Trotter*. New York: Doubleday.

Prince-Hughes, Dawn. 2004. *Songs of the Gorilla Nation: My Journey through Autism*. New York: Harmony Books.

Prouty, Olive Higgins. 1961. *Pencil Shavings: Memoirs*. Cambridge: Riverside.

Putnam, Daniel. 1885. *Twenty-five Years with the Insane*. Detroit: John MacFarlane.

Quivers, Robin. 1995. *Quivers*. New York: Regan Books.

Raphael, Maryanne. 2002. *Along Came a Spider: A Personal Look at Madness*. Lincoln, NE: iUniverse.

Read, Sue. 1990. *Only for a Fortnight: My Life in a Locked Ward*. London: Bloomsbury.

Reason, Brendan. 2006. *An Introvert in a State of Angst*. London: Chipmunka.

Rebeta-Burditt, Joyce. 1977. *The Cracker Factory*. New York: Macmillan.

Redfield, Mary Ellen [Ellen Field]. 1964. *The White Shirts*. Los Angeles: The Author.

Reed, David. 1976. *Anna*. London: Secker & Warburg.

Reid, Eva Charlotte. 1910. "Autopsychology of the Manic-Depressive." *Journal of Nervous and Mental Diseases* 37:606–620.

Reilly, Patrick. 1984. *A Private Practice*. New York: Macmillan.

Remington, Michele G., and Carl S. Burak. 1995. *The Cradle Will Fall*. New York: Leisure Books.

Rhodes, Laura, and Lucy Freeman. 1964. *Chastise Me with Scorpions*. New York: GP Putnam's Sons.

Riggall, Mary. 1929. *Reminiscences of a Stay in a Mental Hospital*. London: A. H. Stockwell.

Rittmaye, Jane. 1979. *Life-Time*. New York: Exposition.

Riviere, Pierre. 1975. *I Pierre Riviere, Having Slaughtered My Mother, My Sister, and My Brother . . . : A Case of Parricide in the 19th Century*. Edited by Michel Foucault. Translated from 1973 French edition. New York: Random House.

Roane, Wilbur E., Jr. 1982. *First Day*. The Author.

Roberts, Marty. 1970. *Sojourn in a Palace for Peculiars*. New York: Carlton.

Robertson, N. 1988. *Getting Better: Inside Alcoholics Anonymous*. New York: William Morrow.

Robinson, Martha. 1979. *Schizophrenia: The Hell Within*. Community Care.

Robison, John Elder. 2007. *Look Me in the Eye: My Life with Asperger's*. New York: Crown.

Rogers, Annie. 1995. *A Shining Affliction: A Story of Harm and Healing in Psychotherapy*. New York: Viking.

Rogers, Hope. 1975. *Time and the Human Robot*. Vinton, IA: Ink Spot Press.

Roman, Charles. 1909. *A Man Remade; Or, Out of Delirium's Wonderland*. Chicago: Reilly & Britton.

Ronen, Tammie. 2001. *In and out of Anorexia: The Story, the Client, the Therapist, and Recovery*. London: Jessica Kingsley.

Ross, Barney. 1963. *No Man Stands Alone: The True Story of Barney Ross*. New York: Simon & Schuster.

Ross, James. 1964. *Truth Forever on the Scaffold: I Tried to Help My Country*. New York: Pageant Press.

Rossiter, Anthony. 1969. *The Pendulum*. New York: Helix.

———. 1970. *The Golden Chain*. London: Hutchinson.

Roth, Lillian. With Mike Connolly and Gerald Frank. 1954. *I'll Cry Tomorrow*. New York: F. Fell.

Runyon, Brent. 2004. *The Burn Journals*. New York: Knopf.

Russell, A. B. 1998. *A Plea from the Insane by Friends of the Living Dead*. Minneapolis: Roberts.

Russell, James William. 1968. *The Stranger in the Mirror*. New York: Harper.

Rutherford, Mark. 1885. *The Autobiography of Mark Rutherford*. New York: Dodd, Mead.

Rutz-Rees, Janet E. 1888. "Hospitals for the Insane: Viewed from the Standpoint of Personal Experience, by a Recovered Patient." *Alienist and Neurologist* 9:51–57.

Ryan, Michael. 1995. *Secret Life: An Autobiography*. New York: Pantheon.

Rzecki, Catherine. 1996. *Surfing the Blues*. Sydney: HarperCollins.

Saks, Elyn. 2007. *The Center Cannot Hold: My Journey through Madness*. New York: Hyperion.

Sanger, William Cary. 1937. *1935–1936*. Newark: Newark Press.

Saunders, Q. T. 2006. *Heart of Hurts*. London: Chipmunka.

Savage, Mary. 1975. *Addicted to Suicide: A Woman Struggling to Live*. Santa Barbara, CA: Capra.

Sawyer, Vanessa Y. 2005. *Journey from Madness to Serenity*. Lincoln, NE: iUniverse.

Scally, Anthony. 2007. *Eyebrows and Other Fish*. London: Chipmunka.

Schaffer, Evan. 2008. *For Madmen Only*. London: Chipmunka.

Schiller, Lori, and Amanda Bennett. 1994. *The Quiet Room: A Journey out of the Torment of Madness*. New York: Warner Books.

Schneilin, Laura Hargrove. 2007. *Broken Syntax*. London: Chipmunka.

Scholinski, Daphne. 1997. *The Last Time I Wore a Dress: A Memoir*. New York: Riverhead.

Schreber, Daniel Paul. 1955. *Memoirs of My Nervous Illness*. Edited by Ida Macalpine and Richard Hunter. Translated from the 1903 German edition. London: William Dawson & Sons. Reprint, New York Review of Books, 2000.

Schumacher, John L. 1959. *Cynicism and Realism of a Psychotic*. New York: Vantage.

Scot, B. J. 1995. *Prairie Reunion*. New York: Farrar, Straus & Giroux.

Scott, James. 1931. *Sane in Asylum Walls*. London: Fowler Wright.

Seabrook, William. 1935. *Asylum*. New York: Harcourt Brace.

———. 1942. *No Hiding Place: An Autobiography*. Philadelphia: Lippincott.

Sechehaye, Marguerite, ed. 1951. *Autobiography of a Schizophrenic Girl*. Translated from the 1950 French edition. New York: New American Library.

Sen, Dolly. 2005. *The World is Full of Laughter*. London: Chipmunka.

⸻. 2006. *Am I Still Laughing?* London: Chipmunka.

⸻. 2007. *Eloquent*. London: Chipmunka.

Seng, Quek Lai. 1977. *A Case between Mentally Sound and Mentally Unsound*. New York: Vantage.

Sexton, Anne. 1960. *To Bedlam and Part Way Back*. New York: Houghton Mifflin.

Shaw, Fiona. 1998. *Composing Myself: A Journey through Postpartum Depression*. South Royalton, VT: Steerforth Press.

Siebert, Al. 1995. *Peaking Out: How My Mind Broke Free from the Delusions in Psychiatry*. Portland, OR: Practical Psychology Press.

Simon, Lizzie. 2002. *Detour: My Bipolar Road Trip in 4-D*. New York: Simon & Schuster.

Simpson, Doris G. 1957. *The Plague of Psychiatry*. New York: Greenwich Books.

Simpson, Jane. 1958. *The Lost Days of My Life*. London: Allen & Unwin.

Simpson, William. 1925. *Cruelties in an Edinburgh Asylum*. Edinburgh: The Author.

Singer, Mickie R. 2008. *The Mystery that Binds Me Still*. London: Chipmunka.

Sizemore, Chris Costner, and Elen Sain Pittillo. 1977. *I'm Eve*. New York: Doubleday.

⸻. 1989. *A Mind of My Own*. New York: William Morrow.

Skram, Bertha Amalia. 1899. *Professor Hieronymous*. Translated from the 1895 Norwegian edition. London: John Lane.

Slater, Lauren. 1996. *Welcome to My Country: A Therapist's Memoir of Madness*. New York: Random House.

⸻. 1998. *Prozac Diary*. New York: Random House.

Smith, Cherry. 1985. *Snowblind*. London: Jonathan Cape.

Smith, Coralyn. 2006. *Cutting It Out: A Journey through Psychotherapy and Self-Harm*. London: Jessica Kingsley.

Smith, Jeffery. 1999. *Where the Roots Reach for Water*. New York: North Point Press.

Smith, Lydia Adeline Jackson Button. 1879. *Behind the Scenes; or, Life in an Insane Asylum*. Chicago: Culver.

Smith, Nancy Covert. 1973. *Journey out of Nowhere*. Waco, TX: Word Books.

Snider, Benjamin S. 1869. *The Life and Travels of Benjamin S. Snider: His Persecution, Fifteen Times a Prisoner*. Washington: The Author.

Snyder, Kurt, Raquel E. Gur, and Linda Wasmer Andrews. 2007. *Me, Myself, and Them: A Firsthand Account of One Young Person's Experience with Schizophrenia*. New York: Oxford University Press.

Solomon, Andrew. 2001. *The Noonday Demon: An Atlas of Depression*. New York: Scribner.

Solomon, C. 1989. *Emergency Messages: An Autobiographical Miscellany*. Edited by J. Tytell. New York: Paragon House.

Solomon, C. 1966. *Mishaps, Perhaps*. San Francisco: City Lights Books.

⸻. 1968. *More Mishaps*. San Francisco: City Lights Books.

Sombre, Dyce. 1849. *Mr. Dyce Sombre's Refutation of the Charge of Lunacy Brought against Him in the Court of Chancer*. Paris: Sombre.

Somers, S. 1988. *Keeping Secrets*. New York: Warner.

Southcott, Joanna. 1801. *The Strange Effects of Faith with Remarkable Prophecies.* Exeter, UK: Brill.

―――. 1813. *The Second Book of Wonders.* London: Marchant & Galubin.

Spencer, Walter Steward [W. S. Stewart]. 1964. *The Divided Self: The Healing of a Nervous Disorder.* London: Allen & Unwin.

Splain, Susan. 2008. *Darkened Light.* London: Chipmunka.

Stafford, Chad. 2004. *The Sublime Detour: My Experience with Madness; the True Story of Chad Stafford's Hallucinations.* Frederick, MD: Publish America.

Starr, Margaret. 1904. *Sane or Insane? Or How I Regained Liberty.* Baltimore: Fosnot.

Stebel, S. L. 1980. *The Shoe Leather Treatment: The Inspiring Story of Bill Thomas' Triumphant Nine-Year Fight for Survival in a State Hospital for the Criminally Insane as Told to S. L. Stebel.* Los Angeles: J. P. Tarcher.

Steele, Ken. With Claire Berman. 2001. *The Day the Voices Stopped: A Memoir of Madness.* New York: Perseus.

Stefan, Gregory. 1965. *In Search of Sanity: The Journal of a Schizophrenic.* New York: University Books.

Stein, Judith Beck. 1973. *The Journal of Judith Beck Stein.* Washington, DC: Columbia Journal.

Stern, Bill, and Oscar Fraley. 1959. *The Taste of Ashes: An Autobiography.* New York: Holt.

Stone, Elizabeth. 1842. *A Sketch of the Life of Elizabeth T. Stone, and of Her Persecution, with an Appendix of Her Treatment and Sufferings while in the Charleston McLean Asylum Where She was Confined under the Pretence of Insanity.* Boston: The Author.

―――. 1843. *Remarks by Elizabeth T. Stone, upon the Statements Made by H. B. Skinner, in the Pulpit of the Hamilton Chapel, on Sunday Afternoon, 18th of June 1843, in Reference to What She Had Stated Concerning His Being Chaplain in the Charlestown McLean Asylum: and Also a Further Relation on Her Suffering while Confined in That Place for 16 Months and 20 Days.* Boston: The Author.

―――. 1859. *Elizabeth T. Stone, Exposing the Modern Secret Way of Persecuting Christians in Order to Hush the Voice of Truth. Insane Hospitals Are Inquisition Houses. All Heaven Is Interested in This Crime.* Boston: The Author.

―――. 1861. *The American Godhead: or, the Constitution of the United States Cast down by Northern Slavery, or by the Power of Insane Hospitals.* Boston: The Author.

Stoneman, Linda. 2008. *From Heights to Depths and Somewhere in Between.* London: Chipmunka.

Stowell, Peter. 2006. *The Quest for Peter's Truth: An Analysis of Schizophrenia from a Sufferer's Perspective.* London: Christmas Press.

Strindberg, August. 1902. *Inferno.* Translated by M. Sandbach. London: Hutchinson.

―――. 1925. *The Confession of a Fool.* Translated by Ellie Scheussner. New York: Viking Press.

Styron, William. 1990. *Darkness Visible: A Memoir of Madness.* New York: Random House.

Sugar, Frank Emery. 1978. *Mindrape: A Diary of Endogenous Depression.* New York: Exposition.

Supeene, Shelagh Lynne. 1990. *As for the Sky, Falling: A Critical Look at Psychiatry and Suffering.* Toronto: Second Story.

Sutherland, Stuart. 1976. *Breakdown*. New York: New American Library.

Sutton, Tiffany. 2007. *Schizophrenia: One Woman's Story*. London: Chipmunka.

Swan, Moses. 1874. *Ten Years and Ten Months in Lunatic Asylums in Different States*. Hoosick Falls, NY: The Author.

Swart, Jonathan R. 2007. *Sewer*. London: Chipmunka.

Symonds, John. 1951. *The Great Beast: The Life of Aleister Crowley*. London: Rider.

Symons, Arthur. 1905. *Spiritual Adventures*. London: Constable.

———. 1930. *Confessions: A Study in Pathology*. New York: Fountain Press.

Tarsis, Valeriy. 1965. *Ward Seven: An Autobiographical Novel*. Translated from the 1965 Russian edition. New York: Dutton.

Telso, A. 1899. *Experience of a Criminal*. New York.

Tempest, John. 1830. *Narrative of the Treatment Experienced by John Tempest, Esq., of Lincoln's Inn, Barrister at Law during Fourteen Months Solitary Confinement under a False Imputation of Lunacy*. London: The Author.

Tew, Raya Eksola. 1978. *How Not to Kill a Cockroach*. New York: Vantage.

Thach, Harell G. 1964. *God Gets in the Way of a Sailor*. Smithtown, NY: Exposition.

Thaw, Harry K. 1926. *The Traitor: Being the Untampered with, Unrevised Account of the Trial and All that Led to It*. Philadelphia: Dorrance.

Thelmar, E. 1909. *The Maniac: A Realistic Study of Madness from the Maniac's Point of View*. New York: Books for the Few.

Thomas, M. 1984. *Home from Seven North*. San Diego: Libra,.

Thompson, Florence S., and George W. Galvin. 1920. *A Thousand Faces*. Boston: Four Seas.

Thompson, Peter. 1972. *Bound for Broadmoor*. London: Hodder & Stoughton.

———. 1974. *Back from Broadmoor*. London: Hodder & Stoughton.

Thompson, Tracy. 1995. *The Beast: A Reckoning with Depression*. New York: Putnam.

Titus, Mrs. Ann H. 1870. *Lunatic Asylums: Their Use and Abuse*. New York.

Tocher, Suzanne. 2001. *Well Connected: Journey to Mental Health*. Wellington, NZ: Philip Garside.

Traig, Jennifer. 2004. *Devil in the Details: Scenes from an Obsessive Girlhood*. New York: Little, Brown.

Trosse, George. 1714. *The Life of the Reverend Mr. George Trosse, Late Minister of the Gospel in the City of Exon, Who Died January 11th, 1712/13. In the Eighty Second Year of His Age, Written by Himself and Published According to His Order*. Exon, UK: Printed by Joseph Bliss for Richard White.

———. 1974. *The Life of the Reverend Mr. George Trosse: Written by Himself, and Published Post-humously According to His Order in 1714*. Edited by A. W. Brink. Montreal: McGill Queen's University Press.

Turner, Cyrus S. 1912. *Eight and One-Half Years in Hell*. Des Moines: Turner.

Turner, Mary. 1981. "Thoughts of Suicide." *Mind Out*.

Unzicker, Rae. 1989. "On My Own: A Personal Journey through Madness and Re-emergence." *Psychosocial Rehabilitation Journal* 13:71–77.

Vakin, Sam. 1999. *Malignant Self Love: Narcissism Revisited*. Prague: Narcissus.

———. 2002. *Diary of a Narcissist*. Prague: Narcissus.

Valentine, Christina M. 1957. *The God Within*. Pasadena: Avante.

Van Atta, Winfred. 1961. *Shock Treatment*. New York: Doubleday.

Van Gogh, Vincent. 1937. *Dear Theo: The Autobiography of Vincent Van Gogh*. Edited by Irving Stone. Cambridge, MA: Riverside Press.

Victor, Sarah M. 1887. *The Life Story of Sarah Victor*. Cleveland: Williams.

Vidal, Lois. 1934. *Magpie: The Autobiography of a Nymph Errant*. Boston: Little, Brown.

Vilar, Irene. 1996. *A Message from God in the Atomic Age*. Translated by Gregory Rabassa. New York: Pantheon.

Vincent. 1919. "Confessions of an Agoraphobic Victim." *American Journal of Psychology* 30:295–299.

Vincent, John. 1948. *Inside the Asylum*. London: Allen & Unwin.

Vincent, Roy. 2008. *Listening to the Silences in a World of Hearing Voices*. London: Chipmunka.

Vonnegut, Mark. 1975. *The Eden Express*. New York: Praeger. Reprint, New York: Seven Stories Press, 2002.

Voyce, Andrew. 2008. *The Durham Light and Other Stories: A Personal History of Homelessness and Schizophrenia*. London: Chipmunka.

Wagner, Pamela Spiro, and Carolyn Spiro. 2005. *Divided Minds: Twin Sisters and Their Journey through Schizophrenia*. New York: St. Martin's Press.

Wagner, Petti. 1992. *Murdered Heiress, Living Witness*. Shippensburg, PA: Destiny Image.

Walford, William. 1851. *Autobiography of the Rev. William Walford*. London: Jackson & Walford.

Wallace, Clare Marc. 1962. *Nothing to Lose*. London: Hurst & Blackett.

———. 1965. *Portrait of a Schizophrenic Nurse*. London: Hammond, Hammond & Co.

Walsh, Sheila. 1996. *Honestly*. Grand Rapids, MI: Zondervan.

Walter, Steve. 2006. *Fast Train Approaching: Breaking away from Breaking Down*. London: Chipmunka.

Walton, Neil. 2006. *Bi-polar Expedition*. London: Chipmunka.

Wannack [pseud.]. 1931. *Guilty but Insane: A Broadmoor Autobiography*. London: Chapman & Hall.

Ward, Mary Jane. 1946. "Out of the Dark Ages." *Woman's Home Companion*, August, 34–35, 91–92.

———. 1946. *The Snake Pit*. New York: New American Library.

———. 1969. *Counter-clockwise*. New York: Avon.

———. 1970. *The Other Caroline*. New York: Avon.

Warde, James Cook. 1902. *Jimmy Warde's Experiences as a Lunatic. A True Story. A Full Account of What I Thought, Saw, Heard, Did, and Experienced Just before and during My Confinement of One Hundred and Eighty-one Days as a Lunatic in the Arkansas Lunatic Asylum*. Little Rock: Tunnah Pittard.

Watson, Lesley. 2007. *Through the Eyes of a Manic*. London: Chipmunka.

Wegefarth, G. C. 1937. *A Patient's Memoirs*. Baltimore: "The Rocket Buster."

Weisskopf-Joelson, E., ed. 1988. *Father Have I Kept My Promise? Madness as Seen from Within*. West Lafayette: Purdue University Press.

Weldon, Georgina. 1878. *The History of My Orphanage; or, the Outpourings of an Alleged Lunatic*. London: The Author.

———. 1882. *How I Escaped the Mad Doctors*. London: The Author.

Wellon, Arthur. 1967. *Five Years in Mental Hospitals: An Autobiographical Essay*. New York: Exposition.

West, Cameron. 1999. *First Person Plural: My Life as a Multiple*. New York: Hyperion.

West, Robert Frederick. 1959. *Light beyond Shadows: A Minister and Mental Health*. New York: Macmillan.

Weston, Joss Smith. 2006. *Aargh!* London: Chipmunka.

Wharton, William. 1979. *Birdy*. New York: Penguin.

White, John. 1955. *Ward N-1*. New York: A. A. Wyn.

Wilcox, Gerald Erasmus [Thomas G. E. Wilkes]. 1953. *Hell's Cauldron*. Atlanta: Stratton-Wilcox.

Wiley, Lisa. 1955. *Voices Calling*. Cedar Rapids, IA: Torch Press.

Williams, Donna. 1992. *Nobody Nowhere: The Extraordinary Autobiography of an Autistic*. New York: Times Books.

———. 1994. *Somebody Somewhere: Breaking Free from the World of Autism*. New York: Times Books.

Williamson, Wendell. 2001. *Nightmare: A Schizophrenic Narrative*. Durham, NC: Mental Health Communication Network.

Wilson, Bertrand. 1974. *A Quest for Justice: My Confinement in Two Institutions*. Hicksville, NY: Exposition Press.

Wilson, Margaret Isabel. 1940. *Borderland Minds*. Boston: Meador.

Wilson, Wilma. 1940. *They Call Them Camisoles*. Los Angeles: Lymanhouse.

Wingfield, A. 1958. *The Inside of the Cup*. London: Angus & Robertson.

Wolfe, Ellen. 1969. *Aftershock*. New York: GP Putnam's Sons.

Woods, Daryl M. 1984. *Afraid of Everything: A Personal History of Agoraphobia*. Saratoga, CA: R & E.

Wurtzel, Elizabeth. 1994. *Prozac Nation: Young and Depressed in America*. Boston: Houghton Mifflin.

———. 2002. *More, Now, Again: A Memoir of Addiction*. New York: Simon & Schuster.

Yalom, Irvin, and Ginny Elkin. 1974. *Every Day Gets a Little Closer: A Twice-Told Therapy*. New York: Basic Books.

Yesenin-Volpin, A. 1971. *A Leaf of Spring*. New York: Praeger.

Zuendel, Friedrich. 2000. *The Awakening: One Man's Battle with Darkness*. Farmington, PA: Plough.

Zurn, John. 2008. *The Bi-polar Challenge*. London: Chipmunka.

Zwiren, Scott. 1996. *God Head*. Dalkey Archive Press.

Narratives by Family Members

Anstadt, Sera. 2007. *All My Friends Are Crazy*. Translated from 1983 Dutch edition. London: Chipmunka.

Arthur, Jonathan. 2002. *The Angel and the Dragon: A Father's Search for Answers to His Son's Mental Illness and Suicide*. Deerfield Beach, FL: Health Communications.

Bass, Elaine. 2006. *A Secret Madness: The Story of a Marriage*. London: Profile Books.

Berger, Diane, and Lisa Berger. 1991. *We Heard the Angels of Madness: One Family's Struggle with Manic Depression*. New York: William Morrow.

Bottoms, Greg. 2001. *Angelhead: My Brother's Descent into Madness*. London: Headline.

Brown, Josephine. 2007. *Betrayal of Minds*. London: Chipmunka.

Carrigan, John. 2008. *The Other Side of Harry*. London: Chipmunka.

Copeland, James. 1976. *For the Love of Ann: The True Story of an Autistic Child.* London: Severn House.

Craig, Eleanor. 1994. *The Moon Is Broken: A Mother's True Story.* New York: Signet.

Davis, Hope Hale. 1994. *Great Day Coming: A Memoir of the 1930s.* South Royalton, VT: Steerforth Press.

Day, G.W.L. 1939. *Rivers of Damascus.* London: Rider.

Early, Pete. 2006. *Crazy: A Father's Search through America's Mental Health Madness.* New York: Putnam.

Evans, Stan A. 2003. *Box of Mustaches: The Darkly Funny True Story of How Twin Brothers Survived Their Mother's Madness.* Lincoln, NE: iUniverse.

Ford, Joy. 2007. *One in Four.* London: Chipmunka.

Greenberg, Michael. 2008. *Hurry Down Sunshine.* New York: Other Press.

Gregory, Julie. 2003. *Sickened: The Memoir of a Munchausen by Proxy Childhood.* New York: Random House.

Hackett, Marie. 1954. *The Cliff's Edge.* New York: McGraw-Hill, 1954.

Helfgott, Gillian, with Alissa Tanskaya. 1997. *Love You to Bits and Pieces: Life with David Helfgott.* New York: Penguin.

Hillman Paterson, Judith. 1997. *Sweet Mysteries: A Southern Memoir of Family Alcoholism, Mental Illness, and Recovery.* New York: Farrar, Straus & Giroux.

Hinshaw, Stephen P. 2002. *The Years of Silence Are Past: My Father's Life with Bipolar Disorder.* Cambridge: Cambridge University Press.

Johnston, Jean. 2005. *To Walk on Eggshells (Is to Care for a Mental Illness).* Helensburgh, UK: Cairn.

Kaufman, Barry Neil. 1976. *Son Rise.* New York: Harper & Row.

Kingsley, Jo, and Alice Kingsley. 2005. *Alice in the Looking Glass: A Mother and Daughter's Experience of Anorexia.* London: Piatkus Books.

Lachenmeyer, Nathaniel. 2000. *The Outsider: A Journey into My Father's Struggle with Madness.* New York: Broadway Books.

Loudon, Mary. 2006. *Relative Stranger: A Sister's Life after Death.* London: Canongate.

Lyden, Jacki. 1997. *Daughter of the Queen of Sheba: A Memoir.* New York: Houghton Mifflin.

Moorman, Margaret. 1992. *My Sister's Keeper: Learning to Cope with a Sibling's Mental Illness.* New York: Norton.

Naylor, Phyllis. 1977. *Crazy Love.* New York: William Morrow.

Neale, R. M. 1998. *To Challenge or Not to Challenge: A Family's Response to a Son's Illness.* Kelso, Scotland: Curlew.

Neugeboren, Jay. 1997. *Imagining Robert: Brothers, Madness, and Survival; A Memoir.* New York: William Morrow.

Pines, Paul. 2007. *My Brother's Madness.* Willimantic, CT: Curbstone Press.

Raeburn, Paul. 2005. *Acquainted with the Night: A Parent's Quest to Understand Depression and Bipolar Disorder in His Children.* New York: Broadway Books.

Shields, Mary Lou. 1981. *Sea Run: Surviving My Mother's Madness.* New York: Seaview.

Simon, Clea. 1998. *Mad House: Growing Up in the Shadow of Mentally Ill Siblings.* New York: Penguin.

Spungen, Deborah. 1984. *And I Don't Want to Live This Life.* London: Corgi Books.

Steel, Danielle. 2000. *His Bright Light: The Story of Nick Traina*. New York: Dell.

Steinem, Gloria. 1983. "Ruth's Song (Because She Could Not Sing It)." In *Outrageous Acts and Everyday Rebellions*. New York: Holt, Rinehart & Winston.

Swados, Elizabeth. 1991. *The Four of Us: A Family Memoir*. New York: Farrar, Straus & Giroux.

Tebb, Barry, ed. 2004. *Kith and Kin: Experiences in Mental Health Caring*. Leeds, UK: Sixties Press.

Townsend, Martin. 2008. *The Father I Had*. London: Transworld.

Tracey, Patrick. 2008. *Stalking Irish Madness: Searching for the Roots of My Family's Schizophrenia*. New York: Bantam.

Van Amber, James Anthony. 2000. *Regina's Record*. Marlow, UK: AnSer House.

Wilson, Louise. 1968. *This Stranger, My Son*. New York: Putnam.

Woolson, Arthur. 1962. *Good-Bye, My Son*. London: Frederick Muller.

Wyden, P. 1998. *Conquering Schizophrenia: A Father, His Son, and a Medical Breakthrough*. New York: Knopf.

Anthologies, Narrative Analyses, and Criticism

Alvarez, Walter C. 1961. *Minds That Came Back*. Philadelphia: J. B. Lippincott.

Aswell, Mary Louise. 1947. *The World Within, Fiction Illuminating Neuroses of Our Time; with an Introduction and Analyses by Frederic Wertham*. New York: Whittlesey House.

Barker, Phil, Peter Campbell, and Ben Davidson, eds. 1999. *From the Ashes of Experience: Reflections on Madness, Survival, and Growth*. London: Whurr.

Beard, Jean J., and Peggy Gillespie, eds. 2002. *Nothing to Hide: Mental Illness in the Family*. New York: New Press.

Berlin, Richard M., ed. 2008. *Poets on Prozac: Mental Illness, Treatment, and the Creative Process*. Baltimore: Johns Hopkins University Press.

Berman, Jeffrey, and Patricia Hatch Wallace. 2007. *Cutting and the Pedagogy of Self-Disclosure*. Amherst: University of Massachusetts Press.

Bird, Ann, ed. n.d. *Living with Mental Illness*. Peterborough, UK: Foundery Press.

Boyd, Julia. 1999. *Can I Get a Witness? Black Women and Depression*. New York: Plume.

Brandon, David. 1981. *Voices of Experience: Consumer Perspectives on Psychiatric Treatment*. London: Mind.

———, ed. 1980. *Voices from the Institution*. London: Mind.

Brandon, David, et al. 1980. *The Survivors*. London: Routledge & Kegan Paul.

Bridges Creative Writing Group. 1999. *I Am God's Goldfish and Other Writings*. UK: Breckland Print Solutions.

Burstow, Bonnie, and Don Weitz, eds. 1988. *Shrink Resistant: The Struggle Against Psychiatry in Canada*. Vancouver, BC: New Star.

Caminero-Santangelo, Marta. 1998. *The Madwoman Can't Speak: Or Why Insanity Is Not Subversive*. Ithaca: Cornell University Press.

Casey, Nell, ed. 2001. *Unholy Ghost: Writers on Depression*. New York: William Morrow.

Clark, Mary. 1994. *Altered Lives: Personal Experiences of Schizophrenia*. Victoria, Australia: Schizophrenia Fellowship, 1994.

Clay, Sally (ed.) 2005. *On Our Own, Together: Peer Programs for People with Mental Illness*. Nashville: Vanderbilt University Press.

Clift, Elayne, ed. 2002. *Women's Encounters with the Mental Health Establishment: Escaping the Yellow Wallpaper*. New York: Routledge.

Cohen, Bruce M. Z. 2008. *Mental Health User Narratives: New Perspectives on Illness and Recovery*. Basingstoke, UK: Palgrave Macmillan.

Copeland, Mary Ellen, ed. 2008. *The WRAP Story: First Person Accounts of Personal and System Recovery and Transformation*. West Dummerston, VT: Mental Health Recovery.

Crisp, Arthur H., ed. 2004. *Every Family in the Land*. Rev ed. London: Royal Society of Medicine Press.

Cullen, Rosie, ed. 1991. *Looking Back: An Anthology of Writing from the Pastures Hospital*. Leicester, UK: East Midlands Shape.

Curtis, Ted, Robert Dellar, Esther Leslie, and Ben Watson, eds. 2000. *Mad Pride: A Celebration of Mad Culture*. London: Spare Change Books.

Davies, Kerry. 2002. "Narratives beyond the Walls: Patients' Experiences of Mental Health and Illness in Oxfordshire Since 1948." PhD diss., Oxford Brookes University.

Donley, Carol, and Sheryl Buckley, eds. 2000. *What's Normal? Narratives of Mental Illness and Emotional Disorders*. Kent: Kent State University Press.

Dyer, Lindsey. 1985. *Wrong End of the Telescope*. London: Mind.

Elfenbein, Debra, ed. 1995. *Living with Prozac and Other Selective Serotonin Reuptake Inhibitors (SSRIs): Personal Accounts of Life on Anti-Depressants*. New York: HarperCollins.

———. 1996. *Living with Tricyclic Antidepressants (TCAs): Personal Accounts of Life on Imipramine, Nortiptyline, Amitriptyline, and Others*. New York: HarperCollins.

Fadiman, James, and Donald Kewman. 1973. *Exploring Madness: Experience, Theory, and Research*. Monterey, CA: Brooks/Cole.

Farber, Seth. 1993. *Madness, Heresy, and the Rumor of Angels: The Revolt against the Mental Health System*. Chicago: Open Court.

Fenton, Steve, and Azra Sadiq. 1993. *The Sorrow in My Heart: Sixteen Asian Women Speak about Depression*. London: Commission for Racial Equality.

Furst, Lilian R. 1999. *Just Talk: Narratives of Psychotherapy*. Lexington: University Press of Kentucky.

Geller, Jesse, and Maxine Harris, eds. 1994. *Women of the Asylum: Voices from Behind the Walls, 1840–1945*. New York: Anchor.

Gittins, Diana. 1998. *Madness in Its Place: Narrative of Severalls Hospital, 1913–1997*. London: Routledge.

Glenn, Michael, ed. 1974. *Voices from the Asylum*. New York: Harper & Row.

Glickman, Mark, and Mary Flannery. 1996. *Fountain House: Portraits of Lives Reclaimed from Mental Illness*. Center City, MN: Hazeldon.

Gray, Penny, ed. 2006. *The Madness of Our Lives: Experiences of Mental Breakdown and Recovery*. London: Jessica Kingsley.

Grobe, Jeanine, ed. 1995. *Beyond Bedlam: Contemporary Women Psychiatric Survivors Speak Out*. Chicago: Third Side Press.

Hinshaw, Stephen P. 2008. *Breaking the Silence: Mental Health Professionals Disclose Their Personal and Family Experiences of Mental Illness*. New York: Oxford University Press.

Hirsch, Sherry, et al., eds. 1974. *Madness Network News Reader*. San Francisco: Glide.

Hodgkin, Katharine. 2007. *Madness in Seventeenth-Century Autobiography*. Basingstoke, UK: Palgrave Macmillan.

Hornstein, Gail A. 2002. "Narratives of Madness, as Told from Within." *Chronicle Review*, 25 January.

————. 2003. "Witnessing Courageously." *OpenMind*, September/October.

————. 2009. *Agnes's Jacket: A Psychologist's Search for the Meanings of Madness*. New York: Rodale Books.

Hubert, Susan J. 2002. *Questions of Power: The Politics of Women's Madness Narratives*. Newark: University of Delaware Press.

Hughes, John S., ed. 1993. *The Letters of a Victorian Madwoman [Andrew M. Sheffield]*. Columbia: University of South Carolina Press.

Ingram, Allan, ed. 1997. *Voices of Madness*. Gloucestershire, UK: Sutton.

Inside, Outside: Women's Experiences of Mental Distress. 1995. Exeter, UK: Outsider.

Jackson, Vanessa. *In Our Own Voice: African-American Stories of Oppression, Survival, and Recovery in Mental Health Systems*. Available from PO Box 10796, Atlanta, GA 30310.

Jacobson, N. 2001. "Experiencing Recovery: A Dimensional Analysis of Recovery Narratives." *Psychiatric Rehabilitation Journal* 24:248–257.

Johnson, Donald McIntosh, and Norman Dodds, eds. 1957. *The Plea for the Silent*. London: Christopher Johnson.

Kaplan, Bert. 1964. *The Inner World of Mental Illness: A Series of First Person Accounts of What It Was Like*. New York: Harper & Row.

Keitel, Evelyne. 1989. *Reading Psychosis*. Oxford, UK: Blackwell.

Landis, Carney, and Fred Mettler. 1964. *Varieties of Psychopathological Experience*. New York: Holt, Rinehart & Winston.

Lehman, Peter, ed. 2002. *Coming off Psychiatric Drugs*. Berlin: Peter Lehman.

McCagby, Charles, and James K. Skipper. 1968. *In Their Own Behalf: Voices from the Margin*. New York: Appleton.

McDonnell, Flora, ed. 2003. *Threads of Hope: Learning to Live with Depression*. London: Short Books.

Mead, Shery, and Mary Ellen Copeland. 2000. "What Recovery Means to Us: Consumers' Perspectives." *Community Mental Health Journal* 36:315–328.

Mental Patients Association. 1973. *Madness Unmasked: Mental Patients Association Creative Writing Book*. Vancouver, BC: Mental Patient Publishing Project.

Mental Patients Liberation Front. 1977. *Our Journal*. Somerville, MA: n.p.

Miller, Chel, and Susan Mason. 2002. *Diagnosis Schizophrenia*. New York: Columbia University Press.

National Council on Disability. 2000. *From Privileges to Rights: People Labeled with Psychiatric Disabilities Speak for Themselves*. Washington, DC: Government Printing Office.

Newnes, Craig, Guy Holmes, and Cailzie Dunn, eds. 1999. *This Is Madness*. Ross-on-Wye, UK: PCCS Books.

————. 2001. *This Is Madness, Too*. Ross-on-Wye, UK: PCCS Books.

Norwich Mind Resource Centre Members and Staff. 2004. "Escape to Reality: Five Life Stories from Individuals Who Share Experience of Mental Illness and Real Recovery." [Norwich, UK?]: Norwich Mind.

Nunes, Julia, and Scott Simmie. 2004. *Beyond Crazy: Journeys through Mental Illness*. Toronto: McClelland and Stewart.

Oakes, J. G., and D. Kennison, eds. 1991. *In the Realms of the Unreal: "Insane" Writings*. New York: Four Walls Eight Windows.

Oettli-van Delden, Simone. 2003. *Surfaces of Strangeness: Janet Frame and the Rhetoric of Madness*. Wellington, NZ: Victoria University Press.

Pedler, Margret. 2001. *Shock Treatment: A Survey of People's Experiences of ECT*. London: MIND.

Peterson, Dale, ed. 1982. *A Mad People's History of Madness*. Pittsburgh: University of Pittsburgh Press.

Pinn, Paul. 1997. *Scattered Remains: A Celebration of 750 Years of Bedlam*. Leicester, UK: Tanjen.

Porter, Roy. 1988. *A Social History of Madmen: The World through the Eyes of the Insane*. New York: Weidenfeld & Nicolson.

Porter, Roy, Helen Nicholson, and Bridget Bennet, eds. 2003. *Women, Madness, and Spiritualism*. London: Routledge.

Pow, Tom. 2008. *Dear Alice: Narratives of Madness*. Cambridge, UK: Salt.

Prince-Hughes, Dawn, ed. 2002. *Aquamarine Blue 5: Personal Stories of College Students with Autism*. Athens, OH: Swallow Press.

Ramsay, Rosalind, Anne Page, Tricia Goodman, and Deborah Hart, eds. 2002. *Changing Minds: Our Lives and Mental Illness*. London: Royal College of Psychiatrists.

Raphael, Winifred. 1977. *Psychiatric Hospitals Viewed by Their Patients*. London: King Edward's Hospital Fund.

Read, Jim, and Jill Reynolds, eds. 1996. *Speaking Our Minds: An Anthology of Personal Experiences of Mental Distress and Its Consequences*. Milton Keynes, UK: Open University Press.

Reaume, Geoffrey. 2000. *Remembrance of Patients Past: Patient Life at the Toronto Hospital for the Insane, 1870–1940*. New York: Oxford University Press.

Ridgeway, Priscilla. 2001. "Restorying Psychiatric Disability: Learning from First Person Recovery Narratives." *Psychiatric Rehabilitation Journal* 24:335–344.

Rippere, Vicky, and Ruth Williams, eds. 1985. *Wounded Healers: Mental Health Workers' Experiences of Depression*. Chichester, UK: Wiley.

Rodgers, John, Martin Came, Karl Romilly Pitts, and John Furness. n.d. *Outside, inside: A Collection of Writings by People Who Have Been Mentally Distressed*. Exeter, UK: Outsider.

Romme, Marius, and Sandra Escher. 1993. *Accepting Voices*. London: MIND.

Shannonhouse, Rebecca, ed. 2000. *Out of Her Mind: Women Writing on Madness*. New York: Modern Library.

Shavelson, Lonny. 1986. *I'm Not Crazy, I Just Lost My Glasses: Portraits and Oral Histories of People Who Have Been in and out of Mental Institutions*. Berkeley, CA: DeNovo Press.

Shimrat, Irit. 1997. *Call Me Crazy: Stories from the Mad Movement*. Vancouver, BC: Press Gang.

Smith, Barbara Holler. 2000. "Skirting Bedlam: Women's Autobiographies of Mental Illness." PhD diss., Rutgers University.

Smith, Dorothy E., and Sara J. David, eds. 1975. *Women Look at Psychiatry*. Vancouver, BC: Press Gang.

Sommer, Robert, and Humphrey Osmond. 1983. "A Bibliography of Mental Patients' Autobiographies, 1960–1982." *American Journal of Psychiatry* 140:1051–1054.

Stanford, Gene. 1973. *Strangers to Themselves: Readings on Mental Illness.* New York: Bantam.

Steir, Charles. 1978. *Blue Jolts: True Stories from the Cuckoo's Nest.* Washington, DC: New Republic Books.

Susko, Michael A., ed. 1991. *Cry of the Invisible: Writings of the Homeless and Survivors of Psychiatric Hospitals.* Baltimore: Conservatory Press.

Taylor, Kate, ed. 2008. *Going Hungry: Writers on Desire, Self-denial, and Overcoming Anorexia.* New York: Anchor Books.

Ten Ex-patients. n.d. *Breakthru—Dear Society, Open Your Mind: Ten Ex-patients of Hillcrest Psychiatric Hospital Tell Their Stories.* [Adelaide?], Australia: Liberation.

Thornton, Joan, ed. 1996. *Out of Mind, out of Sight: Experiences of Mental Illness.* Castleford, UK: Yorkshire Art Circus.

Wilentz, Gay. 2000. *Healing Narratives: Women Writers Curing Cultural Dis-Ease.* New Brunswick: Rutgers University Press.

Winslow, L. Forbes. 1898. *Mad Humanity.* New York: Mansfield.

Wood, Mary Elene. 1994. *The Writing on the Wall: Women's Autobiography and the Asylum.* Urbana: University of Illinois Press.

Web Sites Featuring First-Person Madness Narratives

Alaska Mental Health Consumers Website: http://www.akmhcweb.org
Antipsychiatry Coalition: http://www.antipsychiatry.org
Asylum Magazine: http://www.asylumonline.net
ECT: http://www.ect.org
Freedom Center: http://www.freedom-center.org
Hearing Voices Network: http://www.hearing-voices.org
Icarus Project: http://www.theicarusproject.net
Institute for the Study of Human Resilience: http://www.bu.edu/resilience
International Community for Hearing Voices: http://www.intervoiceonline.org
International Guide to the World of Alternative Mental Health:
    http://www.alternativementalhealth.com
Law Project for Psychiatric Rights: http://psychrights.org
M-Power: http://www.m-power.org
Mad Not Bad: http://www.madnotbad.co.uk
Mad Pride: http://www.ctono.freeserve.co.uk
Mental Health Client Action Network of Santa Cruz County:
    http://www.mhcan.org
Mental Health in the UK: http://www.zoo.pwp.blueyonder.co.uk
Mental Health Media: http://www.mhmedia.com
Mind: http://www.mind.org.uk
Mind Freedom International: http://www.mindfreedom.org
National Association for Rights Protection and Advocacy: http://www.narpa.org
National Empowerment Center: http://www.power2u.org
Pennsylvania Mental Health Consumers Association: http://www.pmhca.org
People Who: http://www.peoplewho.org
Prinzhorn Collection: http://prinzhorn.uni-hd.de/index_eng.shtml
Psychiatric Survivor Archives: http://psychiatricsurvivorarchives.com
Successful Schizophrenia: http://www.successfulschizophrenia.org
Survivors Art Foundation: http://www.survivorsartfoundation.org

Index

About the Editor

Greg Eghigian is Director of the Science, Technology, and Society Program and Associate Professor of Modern History at Penn State University. A historian of psychiatry and the human sciences as well as of modern Germany, he has written on the history of such topics as disability, criminal deviance, pain and suffering, and the politics of science. His is the author and coeditor of numerous books, including *Making Security Social: Disability, Insurance, and the Birth of the Social Entitlement State in Germany*; *Pain and Prosperity: Reconsidering Twentieth-Century German History*; and *The Self as Project: Politics and the Human Sciences in the Twentieth Century*.